ESSENTIALS OF NUTRITION AND DIET THERAPY

ESSENTIALS OF NUTRITION AND DIET THERAPY

Y. H. HUI

Humboldt State University

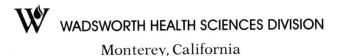
WADSWORTH HEALTH SCIENCES DIVISION

Monterey, California

The selection and dosage of drugs presented in this book are in accord with standards accepted at the time of publication. The author and publisher have made every effort to provide accurate information. However, research, clinical practice, and government regulations often change the accepted standard in this field. Before administering any drug, the reader is advised to check the manufacturer's product information sheet for the most up-to-date recommendations on dosage, precautions, and contraindications. This is especially important in the case of drugs that are new or seldom used.

Wadsworth Health Sciences Division
A Division of Wadsworth, Inc.

Printed in the United States of America

10 9 8 7 6 5 4 3 2 1

Library of Congress Cataloging in Publication Data

Hui, Y. H. (Yiu H.)
    Essentials of nutrition and diet therapy.

    Condensed version of: Human nutrition and diet therapy. 1983.
    Includes bibliographies and index.
    1. Nutrition. 2. Diet therapy. I. Hui, Y. H.
(Yiu H.) Human nutrition and diet therapy. II. Title.
[DNLM: 1. Diet Therapy. 2. Nutrition. QU 145 H899h]
QP141.H772   1985   612.3   84-25753
ISBN 0-534-04380-1

Sponsoring Editor   Thomas J. Keating
Editorial Assistants   Mary Beth McDavid and Corinne Kibbe
Production Editor   Constance D. Brown
Manuscript Editor   Lillian Rodberg
Permissions Editor   Mary Kay Hancharick
Interior and Cover Design   Lois Stanfield
Cover and Part Opening Illustrations   Lois Stanfield
Art Coordinator   Judith Macdonald
Typesetting   G & S Typesetters, Inc., Austin, Texas
Printing and Binding   Maple-Vail Book Manufacturing Group

PREFACE

This book is a condensed version of *Human Nutrition and Diet Therapy* (Hui, Wadsworth Health Sciences, 1983). It contains about 25 to 30% of the most relevant materials presented in the larger volume.

At present there are many instructional and clinical programs accredited to train registered nurses. They differ, among other criteria, in content of curriculum and length of training period. Accordingly, nursing instruction in basic nutrition and diet therapy varies with specific programs. Many current college textbooks, similar to *Human Nutrition and Diet Therapy*, are used as a standard text in many of these educational programs. However, most of these books are unsuitable for some nursing programs for various reasons. Some programs require shorter and more intensive training periods, integrated curriculums, extensive class-distributed instructional materials, use of multiple specialty books on subject matter, etc. This small volume on nutrition and diet therapy is written specifically to satisfy these needs.

Nutritional and dietary services for patient care are currently contributed by other professionals apart from physicians, nurses, and dietitians. They include dietetic aides/assistants/technicians, nursing aides and assistants, practical and licensed vocational nurses, medical and dental assistants, dental hygienists, and other allied health personnel. At present, few books are available to prepare these health workers in the basics of nutritional and dietary services in patient care. The new text will introduce them to the elements of normal and therapeutic nutrition.

The main objective of this book is to provide students in nursing and allied health fields with some basic information related to normal and therapeutic nutrition. With this background knowledge, these health professionals should be able to educate the general public about sound nutritional practices and to provide proper nutritional and dietary care to patients with specific diseases.

In reference to sophistication, coverage, and writing style, a background in biology and chemistry will enable the student to gain a more in-depth understanding of the chemical and biological bases of the information presented in the book. The lack of this knowledge will not be a handicap in following most of the basic facts and principles discussed in Parts One to Three. However, some elementary training in biology, human physiology, and chemistry is necessary to follow the contents of Part Four. Information coverage in this book is comprehensive at the level of expected student competency.

This book is divided into three parts: nutrients and body physiology, nutrition during the life cycle, and basics of diet therapy and patient care. Part One discusses nutrients according to definitions and occurrences in foods, terminology, essentiality, daily requirements, deficiency and toxicity symptoms (if any), relationship to health, and ingestion, digestion, absorption, and metabolism. Part Two deals with undernutrition in the United States and throughout the world and describes ways being undertaken to alleviate this problem.

Part Two also traces nutrition through the cycles of life. We will investigate the special nutritional needs of pregnant women, the variations between infant nutrition and child nutrition, adolescent nutrition as a bridge to adult nutrition, and the special nutritional needs of the elderly. Thus, Part Three analyzes the life cycle by discussing the nutritional needs and requirements, nutritional status, and nutrition-related health problems and controversial issues of each stage.

Part Three is devoted entirely to the nutrition and dietary care of patients with clinical disorders such as diseases of the gastrointestinal tract, liver, kidney, and cardiovascular system. Surgical, cancer, burn, diabetic, and obese patients are also studied. These diseases will be discussed according to causes, symptoms, diagnoses, medical management, and nutritional and dietary care.

The information presented in this book has been derived mainly from the latest books, journal articles, conferences, and symposia on the subject matter. These references are provided at the end of each chapter.

The major problem in a health science textbook of this size is the difficulty of including as much relevant information as possible. Every attempt has been made to achieve this. However, it is hoped that the instructor will provide supplementary information for any area that may need improvement due to the brevity of discussion.

Special clinical case studies are provided in the instructor's manual to supplement the information in Part Four. This manual also contains a variety of materials designed to familiarize the instructor with the objectives of the book. Other features include activities, discussions and projects, a test bank of matching quizzes and multiple-choice questions, and a list of audiovisual and journal resources keyed to each chapter. The instructor's manual is intended to supplement the knowledge and experience each teacher brings to the subject of nutrition and diet therapy.

The glossary at the end of the book includes many terms not covered in the text. This is an attempt to provide the students with a wider frame of reference.

The appendices present tables of major reference data, including food composition tables, growth curves, blood and urine analyses, and Recommended Daily Dietary Allowances. These tables serve two important purposes: They assist a student in completing classroom assignments and, together with the text materials, they serve as a useful reference source for health professionals who may be directly or indirectly responsible for the nutritional and dietary care of a patient.

ACKNOWLEDGMENTS

Ms. Jackie Glenn of *ABC Words* (Eureka, California) deserves the most credit for the completion of this book. She assisted me in editing *Human Nutrition and Diet Therapy* (Hui, Wadsworth Health Sciences Division, 1983) and reducing it to the size and level of this book. The reader is the best judge of her expertise and professionalism. However, I assume full responsibility for the final result, since the rewritten material was subject to my final approval and further modification.

Mrs. Mary Farr, Miss Dorothy Bissell and Dr. Darlena Blucher are three friends who have stood by me year after year. They have complete faith in my endeavors and help me in all aspects of my research and writing whenever they can. I will always be grateful to them. The entire staff of reference librarians at Humboldt State University is always there to provide assistance whenever I need it. They have my sincere appreciation.

I thank all authors who have permitted me to reproduce their work. However, one person deserves special appreciation. Professor Samuel Dreizen, M.D., D.D.S., of the University of Texas Dental Branch, has been most generous and helpful with his wonderful collection of slides on nutritional deficiency symptoms. Not only has he permitted the use of his work in three of my books, he has sent me the original color slide of every picture I need. It is appropriate to state that without his contribution, the educational value of this book would be reduced.

No matter how many times I have expressed my thanks to Mr. James

Keating, the sponsoring editor for this book, I feel that my appreciation is inadequate. Mr. Keating has played an important part in my professional life. We will always be good friends.

This book has been produced under the management of Wadsworth Health Sciences of Monterey, California. The excellent quality and professionalism of its work is self-evident. Miss Diane Brown is one of those persons in a working team in book production that does most of the headache work. Somehow, I always have difficulty forgetting individuals such as Miss Diane who took care of the plethora of details that go with the tedious process of producing a book.

Finally, I am deeply grateful to my family for their indispensable and long-enduring patience and support.

To all who have assisted in the preparation of this textbook, I express gratitude and recognize that factual errors, which may appear in the text, are solely my responsibility.

Y. H. Hui

CONTENTS

PART TWO NUTRITION DURING THE LIFE CYCLE 151

PART THREE   BASICS OF DIET THERAPY AND PATIENT CARE   225

Part One

NUTRIENTS AND BODY PHYSIOLOGY

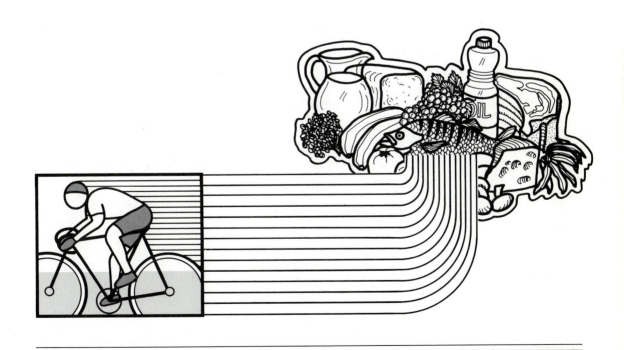

1

DIET, NUTRITION, AND HEALTH

Today, the health professions and the general public are becoming increasingly aware that food intake is closely related to health and a sense of well-being. Claims that every factor in the diet is linked to some disease are exaggerated, of course. But knowing how overall nutrition as well as specific nutrients influences our well-being can help us make important decisions about how long and how well we live.

The controversial nutritional issues reviewed in this chapter concern you as a health professional as well as the public. Among them are the relationship between health and diet, health foods, food safety, adding nutrients to foods, the role of exercise, and world hunger. We also discuss briefly how health professionals with a background in foods, nutrition, diet therapy, and related fields fit into the health care system. First, however, let us look at what *nutrition* means.

WHAT NUTRITION MEANS

According to *Webster's Third International Dictionary*, **nutrition** is the "sum of the processes by which an animal or plant takes in and utilizes food substances . . . typically involving ingestion, digestion, absorption, and assimilation." The Council on Foods and Nutrition of the American Medical Association (AMA) defines nutrition as the "science of food, the nutrients and other substances therein, their action, interaction, and balance in relation to health and disease and the processes by which the organism ingests, absorbs, transports, utilizes and excretes food substances." These definitions outline the areas covered in this text.

During the last 100 years, the science of nutrition has made a great deal of progress. For example, most of the essential nutrients have by now been identified. Nutritional deficiency diseases such as scurvy, rickets, and goiter have been either eliminated or greatly reduced. The average American can now anticipate a life expectancy of more than 70 years, as compared with 40 at the turn of this century, at least partially because of improvements in nutritional knowledge. But even though the many nutritional advances have enhanced our quality of life, researchers continue to seek—and find—additional knowledge.

EAT RIGHT AND BE HEALTHY

Much of the research now in progress concerns the relationship between food choices and health. Although many scientists believe that the average modern diet contributes to certain chronic diseases, evidence remains inconclusive.

When experts disagree, how can the average food shopper help being confused? First of all, consider the tremendous variety of foods available to us—more than 10,000 food products, in fact—and their conflicting claims. Then consider the additional complications of staying within a food budget; planning meals around different work, school, and play schedules; and coping with special diets.

On the other hand, the bewildering variety at the supermarket offers us many benefits, for research indicates that our nutrient and energy needs are best met if we eat a variety of foods. Foods can be purchased fresh, frozen, canned, or dried; partially or completely prepared; or fortified with nutrients. The price range, too, is flexible.

While the food choices we make are influenced by our individual tastes, budgets, and cultural beliefs, learning to select a diet that is both enjoyable and healthful has advantages for all of us. As shown in Chapter 11, nutritionists have simplified selection of desirable foods by providing guides. These guides suggest the kinds and amounts of foods needed for a good nutritional foundation. Good nutrition adds to the enjoyment of living by affecting how we look, how we feel, and how well we work and play.

HEALTH FOODS

The advantages claimed for health foods over conventionally grown and marketed products are now being hotly debated. We are bombarded with claims that health, organic, and natural foods are safer and more nutritious than others. The implication is that our food supply is unsafe or inadequate in meeting our nutritional needs. Since we know that modern farming involves the use of chemical fertilizers, for example, it is hard to separate fact from fiction.

Claims that organic foods are more nutritious than conventional foods have no scientific basis. The fact is, plant roots absorb nutrients in an inorganic form, regardless of the source. Differences in the nutrient content of food from plants of the same species depend on their genetic nature, the climate, the nutrients available for growth, the stage of maturity at which they were harvested, and the conditions under which they are stored.

Most chemically and organically grown foods do not differ in looks, taste, or chemical analysis. The best thing to do is to use care and common sense by eating a balanced diet from a wide variety of foods.

FOOD SAFETY

Consumers have expressed increasing concern about the safety of our food supply since the late 1960s. Such issues as the effects of drinking coffee, the use of hormones to raise cattle, and the possible dangers of food additives have been raised.

In the United States, two major regulatory agencies have been charged by the federal government with safeguarding the public from potentially dangerous foods. The Department of Agriculture (USDA) is concerned mainly with meat and poultry products, while the Food and Drug Administration (FDA) is responsible for practically all other edible items. However, such factors as public pressure, vague laws, and inconclusive scientific research have hampered the work of the FDA.

Controversies over the strictness of government controls and the legislation of food safety further complicate the process of policing the food supply.

ADDING NUTRIENTS TO FOODS

The enrichment and fortification of foods, begun in an effort to prevent deficiencies, has helped eliminate certain major nutritional deficiency conditions. Once-common deficiency disorders such as beriberi, pellagra, goiter, and rickets have almost disappeared in the United States.

Some nutritionists now want to increase the use of nutrient addition to further improve public health. They point out that we are eating less, possibly short-changing ourselves on nutrients. These professionals are skeptical about people's willingness to change their poor food habits. Why not try to make the foods people do eat—including "junk foods"—more nutrient dense?

Although the use of additives has improved the nutritional quality of foods, some observers question the safety of this practice. One problem is that nutritional needs and eating patterns vary from one individual to another. Persons whose requirement of a specific nutrient is low may ingest more than their bodies can handle safely.

A second problem is that few people have sufficient information concerning the nutrients in foods and their own need of those nutrients. For example, many experts believe most Americans consume adequate daily protein. Fortifying "junk" foods with protein, therefore, would be pointless and perhaps even dangerous.

The possibility of creating chemical imbalances in our bodies is a third concern surrounding the indiscriminate use of additives. Many nutrients must apparently interact at appropriate levels to create optimal health.

Finally, nutrients added to foods must be in a form that the body can use and that will not detract from the taste, appearance, or freshness of the food. Determining appropriate combinations of foods and additives is a complex process that requires specialized knowledge.

Government agencies have established some guidelines governing the use of food additives. In general, the government encourages food manufacturers to: (1) correct nutritional deficiencies; (2) restore foods to nutrient levels present before processing, storage, and handling; (3) balance the nutrient content of a food in proportion to its total caloric content.

EXERCISE AND DIET

Good health is difficult to legislate. Overeating and underexercising, for example, have made obesity a national problem. Leisure activities for half of our population involve sitting around or going to bars, restaurants, or movies. But how could laws address this situation without seriously curtailing people's freedom?

On the other hand, half of all Americans exercise regularly to keep in shape. According to the President's Council on Physical Fitness and Sports, running and jogging, bicycling, and swimming are of particular benefit to weight loss.

In addition to weight loss benefits, regular exercise makes people feel better, have more energy, and require less sleep. As muscle strength and flexibility improve, people begin to feel better about themselves. Certain preventive benefits to body systems also may result from exercise. A notable example is prevention of cardiovascular disease, which is two and a half times less likely to develop in people who exercise regularly.

WORLD HUNGER*

Many of the world's people are hungry. Especially in developing countries, undernutrition and even severe malnutrition are common problems. By comparison, the extent of undernourishment in Western nations is definitely not as serious.

Some people use the term *world hunger* to refer to famine—a local lack of food caused by war or crop failure that can lead to starvation if no outside force intervenes. Thanks to the increasing concern and aid from individuals and countries with greater resources, death tolls from famines are going down.

A second interpretation of the term world hunger is the less visible crisis of *chronic undernutrition*. It is estimated that one quarter of the people in the world are chronically undernourished. That is, they habitually or seasonally eat less protein and calories than they need to be active and healthy. Among undernourished people, energy intake is low, infant mortality rates are high, and resistance to infectious diseases is decreased. The capacity for concentration, motivation, and learning is impaired. Victims of malnourishment have little power to effect change. Over half of these victims are children under 5, and far more women are malnourished than men.

Alleviating World Hunger

Many industrialized Western countries are attempting to solve the problems of world hunger. Chronic undernutrition has been identified as the major world hunger problem today. It is estimated that by the year 2000 the world is likely to face a major food supply crisis unless steps are taken now to significantly increase food production in developing nations.

Increasing the food supply is not the only answer to the problem of hunger, however. Political issues, problems of distribution, and indiscriminate population growth also must be considered. The central cause of hunger is poverty, a condition deeply rooted in political, economic, and social realities.

As the largest producer, consumer, and trader of food in the world, the United States has a major role in alleviating world hunger. However, the hungry people of the world can best be helped by a cooperative effort among the Western nations aimed at helping developing nations

* The information in this section has been adapted from: *Overcoming world hunger: The challenge ahead*, Presidential Commission on World Hunger, 1980.

help themselves. This aid will require long-term economic and political support and the development of public awareness if hunger is to be conquered at home and in other nations.

NUTRITION EDUCATION

In addition to educating the public about the problem of hunger, we need to educate individuals about the importance of nutrition to their own health. Health professionals as well as people in the helping professions—social workers, physical and recreational therapists, counselors, and psychologists—are in a unique position to emphasize the important role of proper nutrition, but often they themselves have inadequate backgrounds in nutrition. These people should be encouraged to learn more about food and how it affects health.

Improper diet and sedentary life styles are currently thought to be two major risk factors leading to disease and early death. Proper eating patterns and frequent exercise are certainly important, but health professionals must also be aware of other major public health concerns such as dental care, blood pressure control, alcohol consumption, smoking, drug abuse, and maternal and child care. The health profession's role in nutrition-related preventive medicine—nutrition education and public-health and community nutrition—is undergoing important changes.

NUTRITION IN HEALTH CARE

Nutrition is one of the youngest branches of medical science. Its role in achieving and maintaining good health is both preventive and therapeutic. Advances in nutritional science have increased the role of diet therapy in patient care in the last decade. Part III of this book discusses in detail the principles and application of diet therapy.

Dietary care and patient management are becoming increasingly specialized. A team approach to inpatient, outpatient, and community health care is being used more and more often. The team approach not only provides better diagnosis, treatment, and overall patient care, but the patient is more likely to be treated as a whole person rather than as a disease or a collection of symptoms.

Those who work closely with patients every day have especially good opportunities to tailor meals to a wide range of individual tastes and needs. Whether the nutritional focus is on prevention or therapy, health care professionals must learn to view their clients as individuals with unique feelings about eating, rather than as insensitive food-ingesting machines.

The issues raised in this chapter are explored throughout this book. To begin with, we need a good background in the basic principles of nutrition, to be discussed in the next eight chapters.

REFERENCES

Berg, A. 1981. *Malnourished people, a policy view*. Washington, D. C.: World Bank.

Blaxter, K., ed. 1980. *Food chains and human nutrition*. Barking, Great Britain: Applied Science Publications.

Connor, W. E. 1979. Too little or too much: the case for preventive nutrition. *Amer. J. Clin. Nutr.* 32:1975.

Ducanis, A. J., and Golin, A. K. 1979. *The interdisciplinary health care team: a handbook*. Rockville, MD.: Aspen Systems.

Goodhart, R. S., and Shils, M. E., eds. 1980. *Modern nutrition in health and disease*, 6th ed. Philadelphia: Lea & Febiger.

Graham, H. D. 1980. *The safety of foods*. 2nd ed. Westport, CT.: AVI Publishing.

Guggenheim, K. Y. 1981. *Nutrition and nutritional diseases: the evolution of concepts*. Lexington, Mass.: Callamore Press.

Hui, Y. H. 1983. *Human nutrition and diet therapy*. Monterey, CA.: Wadsworth Health Sciences Division.

Lowenberg, M. E., et al. 1979. *Food and people*. 3rd ed. New York: Wiley.

U. S. Department of Health, Education and Welfare. 1979. *Healthy people: the Surgeon General's report on health promotion and disease prevention*. PHS publ. no. 79-55071.

U. S. Senate. 1977. *Dietary goals for the United States*. 2nd ed. Select Committee on Nutrition and Human Needs.

2 CARBOHYDRATES

Carbohydrates are a major source of food energy for most people. For example, Americans obtain approximately half their energy requirement from carbohydrates. Because carbohydrates are generally an inexpensive source of food energy, they are consumed in greater quantities by the poor. In developing countries, 80 to 90 percent of people's food energy may come from carbohydrates.

In this chapter, we will first look at what carbohydrates are, how they are classified, and how our bodies use them. The final sections of the chapter will discuss how much carbohydrate our bodies need to survive, if any, and how the amounts and types of carbohydrates we consume affect our health. A more detailed discussion of the absorption, digestion, and metabolism of carbohydrates may be found in Chapter 8.

FORMS OF CARBOHYDRATES

Plant carbohydrates are the most abundant organic substances on earth. They supply the major portion of the human body's energy needs. In the process of photosynthesis, all green plants convert carbon dioxide and water, with the assistance of sunlight, into carbohydrates and oxygen. Plant carbohydrates exist in two forms: wood structure or cellulose and sugar and starch storages. Two factors determine the relative amounts of sugar and starch stored in plant foods: (1) the plant's maturity (ripeness) and (2) environmental conditions such as temperature, humidity, acidity, moisture, fertility, contamination, and storage conditions.

Some carbohydrates are available in milk and dairy products (see

Percentage	Food sources
10%	Milk and other dairy products
30%	Regular table sugar including that used in pastries, desserts, candies, and beverages. Items such as syrup are included.
60%	Starchy foods such as grains, cereal products, starchy vegetables, and fruits.

FIGURE 2-1. Relative contribution of digestible carbohydrates by different food sources in the American diet.

Figure 2-1), but we get most of our carbohydrates from eating sugar, starch, grains, vegetables, and fruits. Whatever its source, a carbohydrate is always made up of carbon, hydrogen, and oxygen in the ratio $1:2:1$—that is, one molecule of carbon, two molecules of hydrogen, and one molecule of oxygen. Because there are two molecules of hydrogen to one of oxygen, as in water, the term **carbohydrate** literally means "hydrated carbon" (or water attached to carbon).

The many different kinds of carbohydrates are broken down into four major categories: monosaccharides, oligosaccharides, polysaccharides and organic acids. Table 2-1 classifies carbohydrates and gives some common examples.

Monosaccharides, because they cannot be split (hydrolyzed) into simpler forms, are considered to be the simplest carbohydrate molecules (*mono-* means one, or single). When a carbohydrate contains many units and each unit is made up of two to ten monosaccharides chemically joined, it is called an **oligosaccharide** (*oligo-* means few). In **polysaccharides,** the repeating units contain hundreds to thousands of monosaccharides (*poly-* means many). Oligosaccharides can be hydrolyzed so that all the monosaccharides are released and exist in their free forms.

Organic acids are also carbohydrates. Citric acid, tartaric acid, and others are common organic acids occurring in many foods we eat. You can find more detailed information about organic acids in a standard textbook on food science.

How the four major types of carbohydrates are metabolized by the body is discussed in Chapter 8. The unique properties of many common carbohydrates are presented below.

TABLE 2-1. Classification and Common Examples of Carbohydrates

---

A. Monosaccharides
1. 6-carbon sugars: glucose, fructose, galactose, mannose
2. 5-carbon sugars: D-ribose, D-2-deoxyribose, L-arabinose, D-xylose
3. 6-carbon sugar alcohols: sorbitol, mannitol, dulcitol, inositol
4. 5-carbon sugar alcohols: xylitol

B. Oligosaccharides
1. Disaccharides: sucrose, lactose, maltose, trehalose
2. Trisaccharides: raffinose
3. Tetrasaccharides: stachyose

C. Polysaccharides
1. Homopolysaccharides: starch, cellulose, dextrans, glycogen, dextrins, inulin
2. Heteropolysaccharides: mucopolysaccharides, glycolipids, glycoprotein

D. Organic acids
Acetic acid, citric acid, tartaric acid, and others

Monosaccharides

Six-carbon sugars (hexoses) are the most common monosaccharides. These include glucose, fructose, galactose, and mannose. Five-carbon sugars (pentoses), six-carbon sugar alcohols, and five-carbon sugar alcohols are among the other monosaccharides. All these monosaccharides can be absorbed in the intestine of a healthy person, though the extent and rate of absorption vary. Monosaccharides also vary in known importance to human health.

Glucose

The only known six-carbon monosaccharide existing in significant amounts in the human body is **glucose.** Found mainly in the blood, glucose is an important and readily available energy fuel. When needed, the glucose in a cell is oxidized to form water, carbon dioxide, and energy. A normal person has from 70 to 100 mg of glucose per 100 mL of blood. **Hyperglycemia** refers to a higher than normal level of blood glucose, whereas **hypoglycemia** refers to a lower than normal level. If glucose is found in the urine, diabetes is suspected, since the disease is associated with hyperglycemia.

TABLE 2-2. Approximate Contents of Glucose, Fructose, and Sucrose in Selected Fruits and Vegetables*

Food Item	% of Fresh Weight		
	Glucose	Fructose	Sucrose
Asparagus	1	1.4	0.3
Celery	0.5	0.5	0.4
Onion	2	1.2	0.9
Tomato	1.1	1.4	0.01
Swiss corn	0.35	0.35	2.9
Apple	1.2	6.2	4
Grape	6	6	2
Pear	1	6.5	1.5
Plum	3.2	1.5	4.5
Strawberry	2	2.2	1.5
Lima bean	0.03	0.1	2.5
Cowpea	0.1	0.05	1.6

*These data are the average values obtained from the results of different investigators. The contents of these monosaccharides vary widely in different plant products. This table is intended to serve as a guide only.

Glucose—also called D-glucose, fruit sugar, corn sugar, and, commercially, dextrose—is about 70 percent as sweet as table sugar. Free glucose is found in very few foods other than those mentioned above.

Commercially, glucose is made from starch or corn by the action of heat, acid, or enzymes, all of which can hydrolyze (break down) a polysaccharide into its component monosaccharides. Commercial glucose exists in two forms. Anhydrous dextrose contains less than 0.5% water, and dextrose hydrate contains about 9% water. Dextrose hydrate is used frequently in food processing.

Glucose occurs as a chemical component in combination with other monosaccharides in table sugar, milk sugar, and starch. The glucose contents of selected foods are shown in Table 2-2. A comprehensive review of the physiological properties of glucose may be found in Chapter 8.

Fructose

Fructose is commonly found in many fruits, in honey, and in plant saps, and is sometimes called fruit sugar or levulose. Although their chemical structure is different, fructose and glucose are alike in that both are fruit sugars containing six carbons. The body uses fructose in much the same way as glucose: When consumed with other foods, fructose will eventually be changed to glucose in the liver or broken down into carbon dioxide, water, and energy.

Fructose is one of the two monosaccharides in table sugar. Commercial fructose is extremely sweet. It is used in the pharmaceutical industry and in food processing.

Fructose has recognized clinical potential. Among its advantages is its ability to speed up alcohol metabolism. Because fructose does not induce drastic changes in blood glucose level, it may be useful for diabetics. Fructose may also be used as an intravenous nutrient. It is not as likely as sucrose to cause dental cavities. A possible drawback to the use of fructose is that it may increase the level of fatty chemicals in the blood, thus enhancing the risk of heart disease.

Table 2-2 lists the fructose contents of a number of common food items.

Galactose and Mannose

Galactose, a six-carbon monosaccharide, does not exist as a free sugar. It is usually found in milk. The body can convert galactose to glucose and vice versa. Abnormal metabolism of this chemical may lead to cataract formation.

The six-carbon monosaccharide **mannose** exists in small amounts as a free sugar in peaches, apples, oranges, and the food manna as well as in baker's yeast and plant saps. Like galactose, mannose can be converted in the liver to glucose and vice versa.

Five-Carbon Sugars (Pentoses)

Although the five-carbon sugars, also known as **pentoses,** are of little or no importance as a source of energy for the human body, they are synthesized by humans and are present in small amounts in all cells. Although they are not an energy source in themselves, pentoses nevertheless play an important role in releasing and forming energy in the body.

Most pentoses ingested in the free form are not utilized but instead are eliminated in the urine and feces. This characteristic has led to the use of certain pentoses as "markers" to determine the absorptive function of the human intestine.

Six-Carbon Sugar Alcohols

Fruits such as apples, cherries, pears, and plums are good sources of **sorbitol,** the most common six-carbon sugar alcohol. Less sweet than table sugar, sorbitol is a major ingredient in many dietetic foods, such as jams, canned fruit, and soft drinks. Its absorption and utilization in the human body have little effect on blood glucose level. Diarrhea may result from ingesting more than 50 g of sorbitol, since the body does not absorb the substance well.

When mannose and galactose are hydrogenated, they form the six-carbon sugar alcohols *mannitol* and *dulcitol*, respectively. Both occur naturally; for example, mannitol is found in a certain seaweed. Both substances also can be prepared commercially and are used as food additives in food processing (mannitol, for instance, is used in sugarless gum). They are also used occasionally in testing for the normality of kidney clearance.

Inositol occurs naturally in different foods, especially cereal brans. **Phytic acid,** found in whole wheat flour, is a form of inositol that is suspected of interfering with the absorption of calcium, iron, and zinc.

Though inositol is claimed to be a vitamin, its need by humans has not been substantiated. More information about phytic acid is available in Chapter 7.

Five-Carbon Sugar Alcohols

Many berries contain **xylitol,** a naturally occurring five-carbon sugar alcohol. Xylitol may also be extracted from wood and farm crop residues such as unused hulls, straw, and stalks. The human body synthesizes xylitol, and commercial production is also possible. The substance is sweeter than table sugar.

Because xylitol does not affect blood glucose levels, it is suitable as a sugar substitute for patients with diabetes and liver disease. It may also protect teeth from developing cavities. In some countries it is used in intravenous feeding.

Oligosaccharides

As indicated earlier, oligosaccharides are carbohydrates containing many individual units, each of which is made up of two to ten monosaccharides. The best known of the oligosaccharides are the **disaccharides,** made up of many units, each of which contains two monosaccharides that are chemically joined. This section will describe three common disaccharides: sucrose, lactose, and maltose.

Sucrose

Probably the best known disaccharide is **sucrose** or common table sugar. It is usually obtained from sugar cane or sugar beets.

Many repeating units, each a chemical combination of glucose and fructose, make up sucrose. Under laboratory conditions, heat, enzymes, or acid can split each unit into its constituents, glucose and fructose. In the human intestine, sucrose must be broken down to its components by the intestinal enzyme *sucrase* before absorption.

Cooking and commercial food processing make extensive use of sucrose. Because of its sweetness and digestibility, sucrose is also used in the production of drug tablets.

Lactose

The monosaccharides glucose and galactose make up the disaccharide **lactose.** Sometimes called milk sugar because of its almost universal presence in the milk of mammals, lactose is very insoluble in water and not very sweet.

Lactose facilitates the absorption of calcium in the human intestine. A breast-fed infant is likely to receive more calcium than a formula-fed baby, because breast milk contains greater amounts of lactose. To compensate for this difference, lactose is now added to many commercial infant formulas. Lactose is also used in food processing and in pharmaceutical preparations.

An enzyme called *lactase* can digest lactose in the intestine. Under certain conditions, the enzyme may disappear, taking with it the individual's ability to digest and absorb lactose. Symptoms include cramps, bloating, and gas.

Maltose

The disaccharide **maltose,** also known as "malt sugar," is not very sweet, as indicated in Table 2-3, a comparison of the sweetness of certain carbohydrates. Maltose may be obtained by the malting of barley, among other methods. Each unit within maltose is made up of two molecules of glucose. A mixture of maltose and dextrose is used commercially in "instant" foods and in bakery products.

Polysaccharides

The **polysaccharides** are carbohydrates made up of more than ten monosaccharides. *Homopolysaccharides* contain carbohydrates only; they include starch, glycogen, cellulose, dextrins, dextrans, and inulin. Polysaccharides that contain both carbohydrates and noncarbohydrates are called *heteropolysaccharides*; some examples are seaweed extracts, heparin, and pectin.

TABLE 2-3. The Relative Sweetening Power of Selected Carbohydrates and Carbohydrate-Rich Foods

Carbohydrate or Food	Relative Sweetening Power
Sucrose (table sugar)	100
Fructose	140–170
Honey	120–170
Molasses	110
Glucose	75
Corn syrup	60
Sorbitol	60
Mannitol	50
Galactose	30
Maltose	30
Lactose	15

Starch

A polysaccharide of many units, **starch** contains hundreds or thousands of glucose molecules that are chemically joined. Starch is stored in granules within plant seeds and roots such as grains, cereals, beans, and rice. As the major energy storage of a plant, starch is made up of two types of polysaccharides: amylose and amylopectin.

About 15 to 20 percent of starch is made up of **amylose,** which is composed of many glucose units joined together in a straight line. The remaining 75 to 80 percent of starch is made up of **amylopectin,** which also is composed of many units of glucose joined together, but in branched patterns. Because of its insolubility in water, amylopectin causes gravy to thicken when heated.

When first obtained from plants (i.e., when raw) starch granules barely dissolve in water. Cooking increases the digestibility of a starch food and can make it taste sweeter by releasing its glucose molecules.

Glycogen (Animal Starch)

Glycogen, or *animal starch,* is the form in which energy is stored in an animal. Only small amounts of glycogen occur in land animals, but a more significant amount is found in shellfish, especially oysters and scallops.

Glycogen resembles amylopectin, except that glycogen's 30 to 60 thousand glucose molecules are more branched. Another difference is that glycogen is fairly soluble in water. Although land animals do not contribute a significant amount of dietary glycogen, the human body is able to manufacture this compound from other carbohydrates. Glucose and other monosaccharides are converted to glycogen in the liver and muscles. This stored glycogen is an important and readily available source of glucose. When needed, the glycogen releases glucose, which can be metabolized to form energy and eventually carbon dioxide and water.

People undergoing strenuous activity particularly need glycogen. About 5 to 6 oz of glycogen are contained in human muscle; the liver contains another 2 to 3 oz. The digestive system makes more glucose available for absorption by splitting glycogen into individual glucose molecules.

Heat, as in cooking, also allows glycogen to release glucose. The glycogen content of certain cooked shellfish, such as oysters, scallops, and lobster, is responsible for the delicate sweet flavor of these foods.

Cellulose

Cellulose is a polysaccharide made up of many molecules that are chemically joined. (Formerly, the term referred to dietary fiber, or roughage.) Cellulose is one of a number of indigestible substances including hemicellulose A, hemicellulose B, pectin, lignin, mucilages, and gums. There is no accurate method for determining available versus unavailable carbohydrate in food.

Dietary fiber serves several different purposes in the body. It provides bulk in the diet, thus satisfying hunger. It also maintains good intestinal motility, establishes regular bowel movements, and prevents constipation. Some researchers speculate that among Western populations, where daily consumption of roughage has decreased, the risk of developing certain diseases and clinical problems may have increased. These conditions include: hiatus hernia, appendicitis, diverticular diseases, irritable bowel syndrome, constipation, hemorrhoids, cancer of the colon, gallstones, varicose veins, obesity, dental cavities, diabetes, and cardiovascular diseases.

Dextrins

Dextrins are small polysaccharides with five to six glucose units. Dextrins occur naturally in the leaves of starch-forming plants. The human alimentary tract also produces dextrins through the digestion of starch. In this process, the long chains of glucose (as in starch) are broken down to a smaller number of glucose units (as in dextrins) per molecule. Another fair source of dextrins is the crust and toast of bread, produced when starch is broken down by moist heat.

Commercially, dextrins are very important. They are moderately sweet—sweeter than starch but not as sweet as glucose. Dextrins are present in corn syrup and in beer. "Liquid glucose" is actually a mixture of dextrins, maltose, glucose, and water, and is given to hospitalized patients who are unable to digest regular carbohydrate food.

Dextrans

Like starch, glycogen, cellulose, and dextrins, **dextrans** are another polysaccharide made up of many glucose molecules that are chemically joined. Found naturally in yeast and bacteria, dextrans when mixed with sugar make up the slime we normally associate with surfaces coated with bacterial or other molds.

Dextrans can be easily manufactured in the laboratory and are of potential use as a blood plasma substitute. Because dextrans can increase blood volume and prevent shock, they have been recommended for patients with blood loss. The value of dextrans for human use has not, however, been established.

Dextrans may contribute to the formation of dental cavities. Bacteria present in the mouth can change certain carbohydrate molecules such as sucrose, glucose, and fructose into dextrans, which are the slimy substances on or near teeth edges and surfaces. These surfaces create a medium in which other carbohydrates are readily fermented to form lactic acid, which can produce cavities.

Basic

CARBOHYDRATE REQUIREMENTS

Although current evidence does not indicate that carbohydrate is an essential nutrient for the human body—that is, the body seems able to survive without carbohydrate—many nutritionists recommend the daily consumption of a minimal quantity of this nutrient. Carbohydrate is the main source of energy fuel for the body, chiefly in the form of glucose. If little or no carbohydrate is consumed, the body derives its energy mainly from protein and fat in the diet or from the body tissues (as in starvation). When protein is used for energy, it is no longer available to build muscles and bones. Carbohydrates could be said, then, to "spare" protein.

The extensive breakdown of fat and protein for energy results in the formation and accumulation of acids, thus upsetting the body's acid balance. A second result of the excessive use of protein for energy is that there is an accompanying loss of water and electrolytes, such as sodium, calcium, potassium, magnesium, and phosphorus. A minimum daily intake of 100 g of carbohydrate will prevent acid imbalance and undue loss of water and electrolytes.

Eating meat protein and animal fat in lieu of carbohydrate will raise blood cholesterol and triglyceride levels, possibly increasing the individual's tendency toward heart disease. In addition, the person may be predisposed to gout and kidney stones.

Carbohydrates may have some functions that other nutrients cannot perform. For example, brain cells and cells of the eye lens and nervous tissues depend specifically on glucose as a main source of energy. Carbohydrates also play an important role in body metabolic processes and the structural formation of cells, tissues, and organs. Even the indigestible parts of dietary carbohydrates such as roughage or fiber serve special purposes in the body.

Eating carbohydrates often supplies us with other essential nutrients as well, since few foods apart from table sugar, honey, and syrup are made up of carbohydrates alone. Foods such as potatoes, rice, corn, and bread are high-carbohydrate foods, but they also contain additional nutrients, such as vitamins, minerals, and small amounts of protein.

The diets of most population groups feature one or more foods that are high in carbohydrates. Plant carbohydrate is a good return from the investment of soil, fertilizers, and labor. It is cheap and sustains many people in developing countries. And carbohydrate-rich foods are practically the only ones that can be stored for a reasonably long period without deterioration.

CARBOHYDRATES, HEALTH, AND DISEASES

Just how carbohydrate intake relates to health and disease is currently one of the most debated topics in the field of nutrition. For example, many popular food items with high carbohydrate content, such as soft drinks, candy, potato chips, and french fries, are considered to have only "empty" calories with no nutritive value. Many consumer groups claim that such foods are responsible for a number of human diseases, especially among children. Yet there is no evidence to indicate that these foods are disease causing. Too much sugar will, however, contribute to the development of dental caries (cavities).

Another concern is that dietary carbohydrates, such as spaghetti, rice, potatoes, sugar, bread, and pastries, will make us fat. The fact is, carbohydrates by themselves do not cause obesity. Dietary fat, by contrast, provides nearly twice as many calories per unit weight. The bad habit of overeating carbohydrates (or any food) is responsible for the adding of unwanted pounds.

As already indicated, carbohydrates are important to many body processes, which may not function optimally in their absence. For example, they provide a readily available source of energy and may be used in intravenous feeding.

STUDY QUESTIONS

1. What are our major sources of carbohydrate? What is the basic chemical composition of all carbohydrates? Which foods provide most of the carbohydrates in the American diet?
2. Define monosaccharide. Describe the main functions and sources of glucose, fructose, and galactose. What are pentoses? Identify some six-carbon and five-carbon sugar alcohols.
3. Define oligosaccharide. What are the scientific names for table sugar, milk sugar, and malt sugar? What are the two sweetest carbohydrates?
4. Define polysaccharide. Discuss the characteristics and sources of at least five polysaccharides.
5. What functions does dietary fiber serve in the body?
6. Is carbohydrate an essential nutrient? What happens in the body when insufficient carbohydrates are consumed? Are there disadvantages with an excessive carbohydrate intake? If yes, what are they? Be specific.

REFERENCES

American Medical Association. 1975. Nutrients in processed foods. Fats and carbohydrates, vol. 3. Acton, Mass.: Publishing Science Group.

Dahlqvist, A. 1984. Carbohydrates. In *Present knowledge in nutrition*, 5th ed. Washington, D. C.: The Nutrition Foundation.

Hodges, R. E. 1966. Present knowledge of carbohydrates. *Nutr. Rev.* 24:65.

Macdonald, I., ed. 1967. Symposium on dietary carbohydrates in man. *Amer. J. Clin. Nutr.* 20:65.

Sharon, N. 1980. Carbohydrates. *Sci. Amer.* 243:90.

Sipple, H. L., and McNutt, K. W., eds. 1974. *Sugars in nutrition.* New York: Academic Press.

Southgate, D. A. T., et al. 1978. Free sugars in foods. *J. Human Nutr.* 32:335.

Spiller, G. A., and Amen, R. J. 1978. *Fiber in human nutrition.* New York: Plenum.

Stare, F. J. 1975. Sugar in the diet of man. *World Rev. Nutr. Dietet.* 22:37.

U. S. Department of Agriculture. 1972. *Sugar report.* Agricultural Stabilization and Conservation Service, publ. no. 241. Washington, D. C.: Government Printing Office.

3 FATS

Fats are similar to carbohydrates and proteins in that they are made up of carbon, hydrogen, and oxygen, but in different ratios. Each molecule of fat provides more than twice as many calories as a molecule of carbohydrate or protein, because fat has a lower ratio of oxygen to carbon and hydrogen. Fats are insoluble in water but soluble in organic or fat solvents, such as chloroform, ether, and petroleum.

Some foods, such as butter or oils, are almost pure fat. Other foods combine fat with other nutrients such as protein, carbohydrate, and fiber. Major sources of fat include animal fats and vegetable oils. Fats may be visible, as in meat; or hidden, as in cheese or bakery products. Table 3-1 shows the fat content of representative foods; refer to Table 5 in the appendix for more information on the level of fats in other common foods.

The contribution of fat to health and disease is controversial. Many nutritionists feel that the typical American diet contains too much fat. This chapter discusses the general functions of fat, types of fat, and the relationship of fat intake to certain health problems.

THE FUNCTIONS OF FAT

Some fat is essential in our diets, because it serves a number of important functions. First, fats are carriers of essential nutrients, including fatty acids and the fat-soluble vitamins A, D, E, and K.

TABLE 3-1. Fat Content of Representative Foods*

Food	Serving Size	Fat (g)
Cottage cheese, creamed, large curd	1 c	10
Milk, whole	1 c	8
Ice cream, regular	1 c	14
Eggs, whole	1	6
Butter	1 T	12
Mayonnaise, regular	1 T	6
Fish sticks, breaded, cooked	1 fish stick	3
Ground beef, lean	3 oz	10
Chicken breast, fried	2.8 oz	5
White bread, enriched	1 sl	3
Rice, enriched	1 c	trace
Almonds, shelled	1 c	70
Peanut butter	1 T	8
Honey	1 T	0
Green beans, cooked	1 c	trace
Carrots, cooked	1 c	trace
Tomato, raw	1	trace
Apple, raw	1	1
Grapefruit, raw	½	trace
Beer	12 fl oz	0
Chocolate, baking	1 oz	15
Soup, cream of mushroom	1 c	10

*Adapted from *Nutritive Value of Foods*, Home and Garden Bulletin No. 72 (Washington, D.C.: U.S. Department of Agriculture, 1981).

Second, fats are a concentrated source of energy, providing 9 kcal per gram as compared to 4 for carbohydrate and protein. As a permanent source of energy, stored body fat is especially useful in times of stress such as illness.

Third, fats offer protection from cold and injury. By acting as insulation, stored body fat protects us from cool temperatures. Fat also provides good protection against injury by padding vital parts such as the heart, kidney, breasts, ovaries, hands, and feet.

A fourth important function of fats is their biochemical interrelationship with protein and carbohydrate. Fatty acids enable fat to be converted to protein. Also, the ability of fat to provide energy can spare carbohydrate. Chapter 8 provides more information on fat metabolism.

Fifth, fats contribute to the satisfying feeling of being full. This quality of foods is referred to as their **satiety value.** Fats also improve the taste and desirability of foods.

CHEMICAL CLASSIFICATION OF FATS

The chemical term for **fats** is **lipids,** which are divided into three types: simple, compound, and derived. Simple lipids include **fatty acids** and **glycerides.** Compound lipids include **phospholipids** and **lipoproteins.** Derived lipids include **sterols,** such as cholesterol, and the *fat-soluble vitamin* D. In the following sections fatty acids, triglycerides, cholesterol, phospholipids, and lipoproteins are discussed.

Fatty Acids and Triglycerides

A linear chain of carbon atoms with hydrogen atoms attached and with a special chemical ending makes up a **fatty acid.** Both the number of carbon atoms in the chain and the number of hydrogen atoms that the chain can hold determine the characteristics of each fatty acid.

Beef fat, lard, and corn oil, examples of visible fats or oils, are made up mostly of triglycerides. Sometimes called a *neutral fat,* a triglyceride is made up of glycerol and three fatty acids. A **diglyceride** contains two fatty acids, and a **monoglyceride** contains only one fatty acid.

Glycerol is a neutral substance, but fatty acids are highly active substances that determine the chemical property of simple fat. Whether a fat is long chain or short chain and "saturated" or "unsaturated" are factors that determine whether the fat is hard or liquid at room temperature and the ease with which it can be absorbed by the body.

Saturated vs. unsaturated fatty acids

A **saturated fatty acid** is one in which each carbon joins with four other atoms. Because every carbon in the chain has two hydrogen atoms attached to it—the maximum it can hold—the fatty acid is said to be *saturated.* **Unsaturated fatty acids** are those in which each of the pair of adjacent carbon atoms has only one hydrogen atom. A **polyunsaturated fatty acid** (PUFA) contains at least two double bonds in the chain. Unsaturated fatty acids with only one double bond are sometimes called **monounsaturated fatty acids.**

Table 3-2 lists the most common fatty acids—saturated, monounsaturated, and polyunsaturated. Most of the approximately 40 fatty acids have an even number between 2 and 24 of carbon atoms. Among the few living organisms that contain fatty acids with an odd number of carbon atoms are fish and bacteria.

Solubility, Melting Point, and Absorption

As already indicated, the chemical characteristics of fats are determined by their component fatty acids. For example, fatty acids that

TABLE 3-2. Common Fatty Acids

Name	No. of Carbons	No. of Double Bonds
Saturated fatty acids		
Butyric acid	4	
Caproic acid	6	
Caprylic acid	8	
Capric acid	10	
Lauric acid	12	
Myristic acid	14	
Palmitic acid	16	
Stearic acid	18	
Arachidonic acid	20	
Behenic acid	22	
Monounsaturated fatty acids		
Palmitoleic acid	16	1
Oleic acid	18	1
Erucic acid	22	1
Polyunsaturated fatty acids		
Linoleic acid	18	2
Linolenic acid	18	3
Arachidonic acid	20	4

are fairly soluble in water have very short chains (small number of carbon atoms).

In general, glycerides with more short-chain (fewer than eight carbons) or unsaturated fatty acids are soft fats or oils (liquid at room temperature, with a low melting point). In addition to unsaturated fatty acids, these fats contain mostly oleic acid and linoleic acid. By contrast, fats with long-chain fatty acids are hard fats (solid at room temperature, with a higher melting point). These fats contain mostly palmitic and stearic saturated fatty acids. Such fats melt at temperatures above 50°C (122°F) and are poorly utilized by the body.

Unsaturated fats oxidize more easily than saturated ones. Cooked fats or oils with a higher content of unsaturated fatty acids are therefore more likely to become rancid (from oxidation).

Short- or medium-chain fatty acids are more easily absorbed than long-chain fatty acids. In the same way, fats with PUFAs are absorbed more efficiently than saturated fats with the same number of carbon chains.

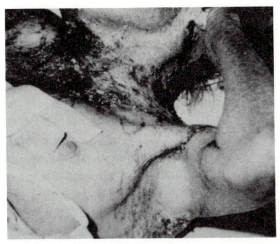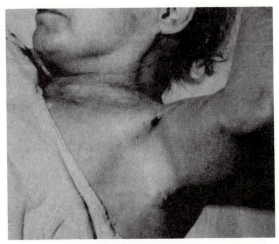

FIGURE 3-1. Relief of dermal symptoms of essential fatty acid deficiency that had been induced by fat-free intravenous alimentation by administration of intravenous fat emulsion. (From M. C. Riella et al., *Annals of Internal Medicine* 83 [1975]: 786). Reprinted by permission.

Essential Fatty Acids

The human body is unable to synthesize (manufacture) two important PUFAs: linoleic acid and linolenic acid (each containing 18 carbons, as shown in Table 3-2). Because these substances must be ingested in the diet, they are called **essential fatty acids.**

Essential fatty acids have several important functions: (1) To aid in the metabolism of cholesterol; (2) to maintain the functions and stability of cell membranes; (3) to serve as precursors for the formation of certain hormonelike substances.

Infants fed nonfat milk for a prolonged period can develop essential fatty acid deficiency. The classic symptom of this deficiency is eczematous dermatitis. Skin lesions respond readily to linoleic acid and/or arachidonic acid therapy.

Because their body storage of fat is high, adults are less likely to develop essential fatty acid deficiency. Figure 3-1 shows the classic deficiency symptoms in an adult after prolonged deprivation of essential fatty acids. Linoleic acid administered orally, topically, or intravenously relieves the deficiency symptoms.

One of the major reasons we require fat in our diet is our need for essential fatty acids. The amount of linoleic acid required is small—about 3 to 4 percent of the total caloric intake for infants and only 1 to 2 percent for adults. The younger the human (or animal), the greater the essential fatty acid requirement. A high intake of saturated fatty acids and cholesterol increases the need.

According to U. S. Department of Agriculture estimates, Americans ingest about 23 grams of linoleic acid per day, an amount considered adequate. The typical American diet, which has 25 to 50 percent calories as fat, provides 5 to 10 percent of the calories as linoleic acid.

Dietary Sources of Fatty Acids

About 90 percent of the daily fatty acids consumed in an American diet are made up of the following four substances: linoleic and oleic acids (unsaturated fatty acids); and stearic acid and palmitic acids (saturated fatty acids).

The two major sources of fatty acids are animal fats and plant oils. Although animal fats tend to be saturated and plant oils unsaturated, there are exceptions. Table 3-3 gives a breakdown of the amounts and ratios of saturated and unsaturated fatty acids in common foods.

The oils of land plant seeds contain mostly oleic and palmitic acids, followed by linoleic acid. Nevertheless, most seed oils contain more linoleic acid than do animal fats. Olive and coconut oils are exceptions. Olive oil has a large amount of oleic acid and only a little linoleic acid. Coconut oil, on the other hand, contains little linoleic or oleic acid, with large amounts of short-chain, saturated fatty acids.

Hydrogenation is a process that changes oils with a high concentration of unsaturated fatty acids into a fat with any desired texture. Foods most commonly hydrogenated are shortening, margarine, and spreads (such as cheese, butter, or cream). Not only does hydrogenation improve the texture of fats but it inhibits the oxidation process, thus preventing fats from becoming rancid even at room temperature.

In addition, hydrogenated margarines, because they contain up to 50 percent PUFAs, may be acceptable for heart patients advised to increase their PUFA intake (see later discussion). Hydrogenated oil can be made from corn, soybean, cottonseed, safflower, peanut, or olive oil.

Animal fats differ according to whether the animal lived on land or in the water. For example, many land-animal fats are made up of mostly oleic and palmitic acids in 16- to 26-carbon-atom chains. These fats are hard, since 20 to 30 percent of the fatty acids are saturated palmitic acids. Fats from cattle are even harder, because they contain more saturated stearic acid instead of unsaturated oleic acid. Milk fats such as butter are unique in that they contain some fatty acids with only 4 to 12 carbons.

By contrast, freshwater animal fats usually contain 16-, 18-, 20-, and 22-carbon fatty acids. Palmitic acid makes up 10 to 18 percent of the total fatty acids in these foods. Fatty acids in saltwater animals have 20 to 22 carbon atoms with up to six double bonds, making them polyunsaturated.

TABLE 3-3. Fat Content and Major Fatty Acid Composition of Selected Foods*

Food	Total fat (%)	Saturated (%)[‡]	Unsaturated Oleic (%)	Unsaturated Linoleic (%)	P/S[§]
Salad and cooking oils					
Safflower	100	10	13	74	7.4/1.0
Sunflower	100	11	14	70	6.4/1.0
Corn	100	13	26	55	4.2/1.0
Cottonseed	100	23	17	54	2.3/1.0
Soybean[‖]	100	14	25	50	3.6/1.0
Sesame	100	14	38	42	3.0/1.0
Soybean, special processed	100	11	29	31	2.8/1.0
Peanut	100	18	47	29	1.6/1.0
Olive	100	11	76	7	0.6/1.0
Coconut	100	80	5	1	0.2/1.0
Margarine, first ingredient on label[¶]					
Safflower oil (liquid)—tub	80	11	18	48	4.4/1.0
Soybean oil (liquid)—tub[#]	80	15	31	33	2.2/1.0
Butter	81	46	27	2	0.4/1.0
Animal fats					
Poultry	100	30	40	20	0.67/1.0
Beef, lamb, pork	100	45	44	2–6	0.04–0.13/1.0
Fish, raw					
Salmon	9	2	2	4	2.0/1.0
Mackerel	13	5	3	4	0.8/1.0
Herring, Pacific	13	4	2	3	0.75/1.0
Tuna	5	2	1	2	1.0/1.0
Nuts					
Walnuts, English	64	4	10	40	10.0/1
Walnuts, black	60	4	21	28	7.0/1
Brazil	67	13	32	17	1.3/1
Peanuts or peanut butter	51	9	25	14	1.6/1
Egg yolk	31	10	13	2	0.2/1
Avocado	16	3	7	2	0.67/1

*Adapted from *Fats in Food and Diet*, U.S. Department of Agriculture Information Bulletin No. 361.

[†]Total is not expected to equal total fat.

[‡]Includes fatty acids with chains containing from 8 to 18 carbon atoms.

[§]P/S = Linoleic acid content/saturated fatty acid content.

[‖]Suitable as salad oil.

[¶]Mean values of selected samples, which may vary with brand name and date of manufacture. Includes small amounts of monounsaturated and diunsaturated fatty acids that are not oleic or linoleic.

[#]Linoleic acid includes higher polyunsaturated fatty acids.

Patients who are advised to avoid red meat because of its high content of saturated fat will most likely be urged to eat more poultry and fish, since they contain higher amounts of unsaturated fatty acids.

Medium-chain Triglycerides in Diet Therapy

Medium-chain triglycerides (MCTs), containing only fatty acids with 6 to 12 carbon atoms, are important in diet therapy because of their special characteristics. First, because of their short chain length and low melting points, they are liquid at room temperature. Second, MCTs are more soluble in water than natural glycerides. Third, MCTs are easily digested and absorbed.

Although MCTs occur rarely in nature, they can be produced synthetically from coconut oil. They are used frequently in the treatment of such digestive disorders as malabsorption, steatorrhea (fatty stools), and pancreatic insufficiency. Further, MCTs provide patients with a ready source of energy and prevent starvation from a lack of absorbed calories. More information about this special dietary product is presented in Chapters 14 and 18.

Cholesterol

Another type of fat occurring in both plant and animal fatty tissues is **sterols.** Plant sterols probably are not absorbed to any great extent by the human body. The animal sterol **cholesterol,** however, found only in animal products such as beef fat and eggs, is significant because of its possible relationship to heart disease. Table 3-4 describes the cholesterol content of selected foods.

Cholesterol is normally found in both blood and tissues, especially bile and nerves. While some cholesterol is supplied by the diet, two or three times more cholesterol is synthesized by the body, mainly in the intestinal mucosa and the liver.

Since the body can make cholesterol, the substance is not essential in our diet. Nevertheless, cholesterol performs a number of important functions. It is one of the basic ingredients of bile salts, vitamin D, and certain hormones. Cholesterol also facilitates the absorption of fatty acids, thus promoting the formation of **esters** (cholesterol + fatty acid). Finally, cholesterol esters transport fatty acids in the blood circulation.

The link between cholesterol and heart disease is discussed in Chapter 17. Although many professionals believe that reducing dietary intake of cholesterol decreases the risk of heart disease, the relationship is a complex and controversial one.

TABLE 3-4. Cholesterol Content of Selected Foods*

Food	Amount	Cholesterol (mg)
Milk, skim, fluid or reconstituted	1 c	5
Cottage cheese, uncreamed	½ c	7
Lard	1 T	12
Cream, light table	1 fl oz	20
Cottage cheese, creamed	½ c	24
Cream, half and half	¼ c	26
Ice cream, regular, approximately 10% fat	½ c	27
Cheese, cheddar	1 oz	28
Milk, whole	1 c	34
Butter	1 T	35
Oysters, salmon; cooked	3 oz	40
Clams, halibut, tuna; cooked	3 oz	55
Chicken, turkey; light meat, cooked	3 oz	67
Beef, pork, lobster; chicken, turkey, dark meat; cooked	3 oz	75
Lamb, veal, crab; cooked	3 oz	85
Shrimp, cooked	3 oz	130
Heart, beef, cooked	3 oz	230
Egg	1 yolk or 1 egg	250
Liver (beef, calf, hog, lamb), cooked	3 oz	370
Kidney, cooked	3 oz	680
Brains, raw	3 oz	1,700+

*Adapted from R. M. Feeley et al., "Cholesterol Content of Foods," *J. Amer. Dietet. Assoc.* 61 (1972):134.

Phospholipids

One example of compound lipid is **phospholipids.** Serving primarily as a structural component of cell membranes, this type of fat can mix with either fat- or water-soluble ingredients. This versatility makes phospholipids especially useful in transporting both water- and fat-soluble substances across membrane barriers. Even if an animal is starved, phospholipids in its cell membranes will not be degraded to provide energy.

Phospholipids occur in all cell membranes and are present in almost everything we eat. Prevented from being absorbed intact, phospholipids are broken down in the small intestine into their chemical components: glycerol, fatty acids, phosphate, and other chemicals. Since these chemicals can be synthesized by the body, phospholipids are not needed in our diet.

A major use of phospholipids is in commercial processing of food. For example, mayonnaise is made by using phospholipids to mix the fat and water ingredients so that they will not separate.

Similar to phospholipids are **lipoproteins,** which contain both a fat and a protein component. Like phospholipids, lipoproteins cannot be absorbed intact but can be synthesized by the body. The important function of transporting fat and protein in the blood is performed by lipoproteins. However, this substance is suspected of playing a significant role in the risk of heart disease (see Chapter 20).

FATS AND HEALTH

Many factors determine how fats are related to our health. Among these factors are methods of storing and cooking fats, individual variations in fat need and intake, how fats interact with the other foods we eat, and a possible link between fat and heart disease.

Cooking and Storage of Fats

Although overheating cooking oils can give food an unpleasant flavor, normal frying does not reduce their nutritional value. Fats are easily oxidized, giving them a *rancid* flavor and destroying their vitamins A and E. Refrigeration of cooked fats, the use of certain antioxidants, and special packaging can inhibit the oxidation process.

Individual Variations

Individuals vary greatly in their ability to use fats. Some factors involved include:

1. **Variations in the endocrine system.** How well an individual uses fats is at least partially determined by the hormonal processes of the thyroid, adrenals, pituitary, ovaries, pancreas, and other organs.
2. **Activity level.** Exercise increases the oxygen supply to tissues, improves circulation, and relieves stress, thus enhancing our metabolic processes.
3. **Emotional health.** One's emotional nature affects the body's utilization of fat.
4. **Age.** Physiological processes slow down with age, affecting the body's ability to handle the food we eat.
5. **Nutritional status.** What we have eaten throughout life and our present nutritional status influence our use of fats.
6. **Specific diseases.** Certain clinical conditions interfere with the absorption and metabolism of fats.

Relationship of Fats to Other Food Eaten

Our utilization of fats is affected by all the nutrients we ingest and their interaction. High dietary fat intake can create abnormally high body levels of fatty chemicals such as fatty acids, glycerides, and cholesterol. Evidence linking high blood levels of cholesterol and triglycerides to atherosclerosis is as yet inconclusive. However, as indicated in Chapter 17, some physicians recommend that cardiovascular patients limit their intake of saturated fats.

Certain nutrients are important in fat utilization, particularly calcium, magnesium, chromium, zinc, vanadium, niacin, biotin, pantothenic acid, vitamin B_6, and vitamin E. The kind of carbohydrate in the diet also influences fat metabolism. A high sucrose intake may produce high levels of lipid in the blood.

Unresolved Issues

The role of fat in our health status is not well understood. For example, how the body utilizes fats is unclear. Not enough is known about how the foods we eat affect our body processes or what influence emotions and stress have on fat metabolism. Finally, no one can say for sure what the limits of polyunsaturated fats, cholesterol, and total fats should be in diets.

STUDY QUESTIONS

1. How are fats chemically similar to carbohydrates and proteins? How do they differ chemically and calorically?
2. Discuss at least four important functions of fats in the body.
3. What is a fatty acid? Distinguish between saturated and unsaturated fatty acids.
4. Which fatty acids are considered essential? What are their functions? Discuss the symptoms of essential fatty acid deficiency. Which four fatty acids are most common in the American diet?
5. What is hydrogenation?
6. Define medium-chain triglycerides. Why are they used in diet therapy?
7. What are the origins and functions of body cholesterol?
8. Define phospholipids and lipoproteins.
9. How can cooking and storage affect the nutritional value of fats?

10. In what ways do individuals vary in the ability to use fats? How do intakes of other nutrients affect the body's use of fats?

REFERENCES

American Medical Association. 1975. Nutrients in processed foods. *Fats and carbohydrates*, vol. 3. Acton, Mass.: Publishing Science Group.

Brisson, G. J. 1981. *Lipids in human nutrition.* Englewood, N. J.: Jack K. Burgess.

Coniglio, J. G. 1984. Fat. In *Present knowledge in nutrition,* 5th ed. Washington, D. C.: The Nutrition Foundation.

Ernst, N. D., and Levy, R. I. 1984. Diet and cardiovascular disease. In *Present knowledge in nutrition,* 5th ed. Washington, D. C.: The Nutrition Foundation.

Hausman, P. 1981. *J. Sprat's legacy: the science and politics of fat and cholesterol.* New York: Richard Marek Publishers.

Rapaport, E., ed. 1980. *Current controversies in cardiovascular disease.* Philadelphia: Saunders.

U. S. Department of Agriculture. Revised 1976. *Fats in food and diet.* USDA Bulletin no. 361. Washington, D. C.

Vergroesen, A. J., ed. 1975. *The role of fats in human nutrition.* New York: Academic Press.

4 ENERGY

From a chemical point of view, the human body is simply a conglomeration of water, fat, and cell mass. To enable this "lump of clay" to move, think, and breathe—and to carry on the many and varied activities of which it is capable—requires energy. This energy comes from the foods we eat.

This chapter discusses the methods of defining and measuring energy, the main dietary sources of energy, and the amount of energy required to support our body processes and physical activities. We will also examine the methods of estimating desirable body weight and individual energy needs.

MEASURING ENERGY INTAKE

Every day we take in energy from foods and expend energy in our activities. This section will examine the unit measurement for energy, sources of our dietary energy, and how energy levels in food can be determined.

Unit Measurement

Energy is defined as the capacity to do work. One way to measure energy is by the heat it produces. For example, the **calorie** is a unit measure of the amount of heat energy required to raise the temperature of 1 g of water from 15°C to 16°C. A larger unit, called the **kilocalorie** (= 1,000 calories) is also commonly used. Various forms and abbreviations of these terms are in current use:

calorie: cal
kilocalorie: Kilocalorie, Calorie, kcal, Cal

Although the kilocalorie is the preferred unit of measurement, many nutritionists simply refer to it as "calorie" or "cal" instead of "Calorie" or "Cal." This practice is convenient and traditional.

Another system of measuring energy is based on mechanical energy. The basic unit in this system is the **joule** or the **Joule.** One Joule (= 1,000 joules) is the amount of mechanical energy required when a force of 1 newton (N) moves 1 kilogram (kg) by a distance of 1 meter (m). Forms of these terms in current use are:

joule = j
Joule = kilojoule, kilojoule, kJ, KJ

Although the joule system is favored by some, calorie units are still widely used in the field of nutrition, and are the units of measure throughout this book. Joule units are given whenever necessary. To convert calories to joules, multiply calorie units by the equivalency factor of 4.18:

1 calorie   = 4.18 joule
1 kilocalorie = 4.18 Joule

Sources of Food Energy

The nutrients protein, carbohydrate, and fat are the primary sources of food energy. In the diet of most Americans, 10 to 15 percent of the total daily caloric intake comes from protein, 50 to 60 percent from carbohydrate, and 35 to 45 percent from fat. However, the proportions of each of these vary from person to person and from country to country.

In contrast to protein, carbohydrate, and fat, alcohol is not a **nutrient** because it is not a nourishing substance. Alcohol does, however, contain calories and can contribute from 0 to 50 percent of a person's daily intake of calories, often at the expense of nutrients from other food sources.

Some experts feel that Americans get too many of their daily calories from fat, especially animal fat, thus increasing the risk of heart disease. Conclusive evidence to substantiate this claim is so far lacking.

Estimating Energy in Foods

In the laboratory, the caloric content of the different foods we eat is analyzed by means of a **bomb calorimeter** (see Figure 4-1). This device measures the heat energy released by burning a food sample under strictly controlled circumstances and noting the rise in water temperature. The amount of heat released depends on the relative contents of carbon and oxygen in the sample.

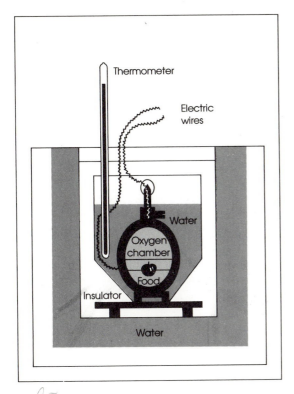

FIGURE 4-1. A simplified diagram of a bomb calorimeter.

A similar process takes place in the human body, especially in muscle tissue and in the liver. The major difference is that the energy produced is greater in the calorimeter than in the human body for three reasons. First, part of the ingested food is digested and absorbed, part eliminated as fecal waste, and the remaining kept as residue in the bowel. Second, some of the food energy is spent on the "work" of ingesting, digesting, and absorbing food. Finally, part of the absorbed nutrient is not completely **oxidized,** or burned.

A comparison of energy values between laboratory and human utilization is made in Table 4-1. For example, the table indicates that 1 g of ingested protein will provide 4 kcal of energy for the body, 1 g of carbohydrate 4 kcal, and 1 g of fat 9 kcal.

These approximate energy values can be used to determine the energy content of a food sample whose protein, carbohydrate, and fat content is known. (See the appendix for more information.) The contents of protein, carbohydrate, and fat can then be multiplied in grams by the appropriate factor (4, 4, and 9, respectively—refer to Table 4-1), and the results totaled. Table 4-2 lists the energy contents of some representative foods.

TABLE 4-1. Energy Values of Food and Alcohol

Substance (1 g)	Energy Content		
	In bomb calorimeter	In human body	
	kcal	kcal	kJ*
Protein	5.65	4	17
Carbohydrate	4.1	4	17
Fat	9.45	9	38
Alcohol (ethanol)	7.1	7	29

*The numbers are rounded for easy reference.

TABLE 4-2. The Caloric Contents of Some Common American Foods*

Food Item	Serving Size	kcal
Cheese, natural blue	1 oz	100
Milk, fluid, whole	1 c	150
Egg, scrambled in butter, milk added	1	95
Butter	1 pat	35
Beef, rib roast, lean and fat	3 oz	375
Salmon, pink, canned, solids and liquid	3 oz	120
Banana	1	100
Raisins, seedless	1 c	420
Bread, French, enriched	1 sl	100
Rice, white, cooked, long-grain	1 c	225
Beans, lima, dry, cooked, drained	1 c	260
Peas, split, dry, cooked	1 c	230
Honey, strained or extracted	1 T	65
Sugar, white, granulated	1 T	45
Broccoli, raw, cooked, drained	1 stalk	45
Potato, baked	1	145
Vegetables, mixed, frozen, cooked	1 c	115
Beer	12 fl oz	150
Cola beverage	12 fl oz	145
Yeast, brewer's, dry	1 T	25

*Adapted from *Nutritive Value of Foods*, Home and Garden Bulletin No. 72 (Washington, D.C.: U.S. Department of Agriculture, 1981).

INDIVIDUAL ENERGY REQUIREMENTS

The amount of energy we need every day depends upon the amount we expend both in a resting state and to power our physical activities.

Estimating Energy Expenditures

There are two methods of determining how much energy we expend: direct and indirect calorimetry.

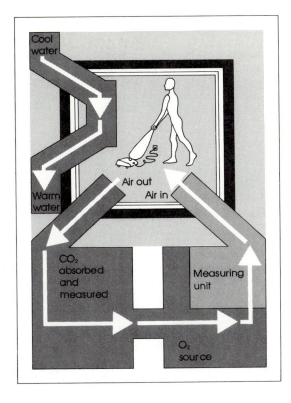

FIGURE 4-2. Measuring the human body's heat production by direct calorimetry.

In *direct calorimetry* a person is placed in an insulated chamber that is equipped to detect any slight rise in temperature due to heat released by the person. The amount of heat released indicates the approximate energy expenditure. See Figure 4-2.

The *indirect calorimeter* method requires only a simple measurement of the amount of oxygen consumed by the person over a specific period. This measurement may be made in one of two ways: (1) The subject breathes pure oxygen from a respirometer and the exhaled carbon dioxide is collected and measured; (2) the amount of oxygen in a room is calculated before and after the subject has spent a specific period in the room. The amount of energy spent by the individual can be calculated easily, since the relationship of 1 L of oxygen to 4.82 kcal of energy released is well known.

Basal Metabolism

Calorimetry may be used to determine energy expenditure when the body is either resting or physically active. The amount of energy used at rest is known as the **basal metabolism rate,** or BMR—the least amount

TABLE 4-3. Effect of Specific Dynamic Action of Food on BMR

Status of Basal Metabolism	Hypothetical Value of Basal Metabolism (kcal)	Increase over Normal (%)
After an overnight fast (i.e., normal basal metabolism)	1,500	0
Within 7 hr after eating a meal	1,575–1,950	5–30

of energy required by the resting human body to keep the most important life processes functioning properly. Such processes include heartbeat, brain activity, respiration, hormonal activity, and the activity of the muscular and nervous systems.

Basal metabolic rates differ among individuals. The BMR can be determined only when the subject is at complete physical and mental rest, free from worry and emotional excitement, and in normal health. The subject must not have eaten for 12 hours.

After a meal is eaten, the basal metabolic rate increases 5 to 30 percent. Scientists explain this increase by a very complicated physiological process known as *specific dynamic action*. An average meal produces an average rise of about 10 percent within 5 hours of eating. This increase drops to about 0 to 5 percent above BMR 24 hours after eating. This effect is shown in Table 4-3.

The exact reason for the rise in BMR after eating is not fully known. Part of the increase is due to the work and energy used in ingesting, digesting, absorbing, and oxidizing food. Large increases (15 to 30 percent) in BMR after eating are usually attributable to a high-protein diet. The formation of uric acid and urea from protein also uses a lot of energy.

The basal metabolic rate of an "average" adult is about 1 kcal/kg body weight/hr, but BMRs vary considerably among individuals because of several factors, including:

1. **Age.** The BMR of a person varies from birth to adulthood, as shown in Table 4-4. In general, the fluctuation is the same for males and females. The need for energy for growth decreases after age 21.
2. **Pregnancy.** The BMR of a pregnant woman increases by about 20 percent.
3. **Undernourishment.** In circumstances of undernourishment, as in

TABLE 4-4. Changes in BMR with Age

Age Range (yr)	BMR
0–2	Increases
2–puberty	Drops
Puberty–20	Rises slowly
21–old age	Falls

Age (yr)	Average BMR (kcal/m²/h)*
6	53
20	41
60	34

*Basal metabolic rate is more accurately reflected in the kilocalories needed per square meter of body surface area per hour than in kilocalories needed per kilogram body weight per hour.

starvation, the body responds to a reduction in caloric intake by decreasing the BMR.

4. **Body composition.** A person with greater muscle mass has a higher BMR than a person of comparable weight but with more body fat.
5. **Sexual difference.** Because females have less muscle and more body fat, their BMR is about 5 percent lower than that of males.
6. **Hormones.** Certain glands have an effect on body metabolism. For example, a person with *hypothyroidism* (subnormal secretion of thyroid hormone) will have a decreased BMR, whereas a person with *hyperthyroidism* (elevated secretion of thyroid hormone) usually has a higher BMR.
    If adrenal glands are stimulated by extreme emotions such as fright or excitement, they secrete *epinephrine* (adrenaline), which can cause a temporary but intense increase in BMR.
7. **Body temperature.** For each degree Fahrenheit rise in body temperature, BMR increases by 7 percent.
8. **Environmental temperature.** An increase in the environmental temperature produces a corresponding increase in the BMR.

Energy Requirements for Physical Activities

In addition to basal metabolic energy requirements, physical activity also places energy demands on the body. Obviously an active person needs more energy than an inactive person, but energy need also is determined by such factors as body build and the type, intensity, and duration of the physical activities performed.

TABLE 4-5. Approximate Energy Cost of Different Forms of Activities for a 70-kg Man*

Activity	kcal/min
Basketball	9.0–10.0
Boxing	9.0–10.0
Cleaning	4.0– 4.5
Coal mining	6.0– 8.0
Cooking	3.0– 3.5
Dancing	3.5–12.5
Eating	1.0– 2.0
Fishing	4.0– 5.0
Gardening	3.5– 9.0
Horse riding	3.0–10.0
Painting	2.0– 6.0
Piano playing	2.5– 3.0
Running	9.0–21.0
Scrubbing floors	7.0– 8.0
Standing	1.5– 2.0
Swimming	4.0–12.0
Typing, electric	1.5– 2.0
Walking	1.5– 6.0
Writing	2.0– 2.5

*The data in this table have been collected from many sources. Because of large variations among the results of different investigators, ranges of values are used so as to give a general idea of the relationship between types of activity and the energy cost.

Table 4-5 describes the *approximate* energy cost of different forms of activity for a man weighing 70 kg. Human activities may be described as very light, light, moderate, and heavy. Very light activities—ironing, sewing, driving a car, walking slowly—will increase a person's total energy need to 130 percent of his or her BMR. Light activities—waiting on tables or repairing cars—will increase energy need to 150 percent of the BMR. Moderate activities—gardening, dancing, riding a bicycle—will increase energy need to 175 percent. And heavy activities—playing football, chopping wood, moving pianos—will increase energy need to 200 percent or more of the BMR.

Total Energy Needs

Both our BMR and our level of physical activities determine our energy needs. Together they influence our total energy needs in several general ways.

1. **Age.** Because of a decrease in both physical activity and BMR with age, the total energy need of the adult is less than that of a child.
2. **Body size.** A larger person's combined BMR and activity energy need is greater than that of a smaller person.
3. **Climate.** Room temperatures below 20°C/68°F increase energy need, as do hot temperatures. However, if a hot climate reduces the amount of work done, then total energy need may actually decrease.
4. **Pregnancy and lactation.** Pregnancy increases a woman's BMR; she also needs more energy to power her larger body's physical activities. A nursing mother needs more energy because part of it is transferred to the infant. See Chapter 11 for more information.

Taking all of these factors into consideration, we can arrive at an average energy need for a "standard" man or woman who is 23 years old, moderately active, and living in a moderate climate 20°C/68°F. This reference person's total need would be:

	Weight		Daily caloric need
Person	lb	Kg	(kcal)
Man	154	70	2700
Woman	128	58	2000

The above reference standards have been established by the National Research Council of the National Academy of Sciences. More information on individual caloric needs is presented in Part II of this book.

ESTIMATING DESIRABLE BODY WEIGHT

As used in this book, *ideal* and *desirable body weight* are interchangeable terms to refer to the optimal weight for good health. There are four general methods for determining ideal weight: standard tables, the sex-frame-height rule of thumb, standard growth charts for children, and various widely used methods of measurement.

Standard Tables

The Metropolitan Life Insurance Company, the Society of Actuaries, and the Association of Life Insurance Medical Directors of America as well as the National Academy of Sciences and the U. S. Public Health Service all have issued tables that are currently in wide use. Two examples are given in Table 4-6.

Although the use of standard tables to determine standard weight is

TABLE 4-6. Desirable Weights by Height and Body Frame for Adults (Issued by the Metropolitan Life Insurance Company of New York and Derived from the Build and Blood Pressure Survey of 1980 by the Society of Actuaries)

	Desirable Weight (lb)		
	Small frame	Medium frame	Large frame
Man, 5'10" with shoes on 1" heels*	144-154	151-163	158-180
Woman, 5'7" with shoes on 2" heels*	123-136	133-147	143-163

Note: The complete tables are located in Table 9 of the appendix.

*Dressed in indoor clothing.

TABLE 4-7. Layman's Method to Determine Body Frame

A. Encircle the wrist bone with index finger and thumb.

If the fingers do not touch or overlap, the body frame is large.

If the fingers just touch or overlap, the body frame is medium.

If the fingers overlap, the body frame is small.

B. Measure the circumference of the wrist bone.

Men

If the circumference is less than 6 in., the body frame is small.

If the circumference is 6 to 7 in., the body frame is medium.

If the circumference is more than 7 in., the body frame is large.

Women

If the circumference is less than 6 in., the body frame is small.

If the circumference is between 6 and 6½ in., the body frame is medium.

If the circumference is more than 6½ in., the body frame is large.

common in the United States, the practice has some drawbacks. First, the tables can be misleading because they do not indicate the proportion of body fat. Excess weight can be fluid, muscle, or bone, and not fat. Second, ideal weights for certain segments of the population have not been determined, thus decreasing the reliability of such "standard" tables. Third, the body frame classification—for example, "small," "medium," and "large"—used in most standard tables does not allow for the general public's limited access to scientific measurement techniques. Table 4-7 presents two lay methods for estimating body frame. Though not scientifically sound, these methods provide some guidance to the general public.

Sex–Frame–Height Method

Table 4-8 describes the procedure of determining body weight based on sex, frame, and height. This method only approximates ideal body weight, and it has many of the same drawbacks as the standard tables:

TABLE 4-8. Ideal Body Weights Using the Height-Frame Rule

Frame Size	Height Data	Weight (lb) Men	Women
Medium	First 5 feet	106	100
	Each inch above 5 feet	6	5
Large	Each inch above 5 feet	$\frac{110}{100}$ × weight calculated for medium-frame person	
Small	Each inch above 5 feet	$\frac{90}{100}$ × weight calculated for medium-frame person	

(1) It does not distinguish between fat and other forms of extra weight; (2) it requires the lay person's judgment of body frame.

Growth Charts for Children

Standard growth (height-weight) charts, such as those developed by Wetzel, Iowa, Stuart, or the U. S. Public Health Service, are useful in evaluating the growth rate of infants, children, and adolescents. Some are reproduced in the appendix.

Popular Physical Measurements

An obvious way of determining whether one is overweight is visual inspection. Another is the "pinch test," where an area such as the abdomen is pinched to determine the amount of skinfold fat. If more than 1 inch of fat is pinched, one is probably overweight. More information on assessing a person's nutritional status, including the extent of overweight, may be obtained from references at the end of this chapter.

METHODS OF ESTIMATING INDIVIDUAL ENERGY NEED

The number of calories each of us needs daily to maintain ideal body weight may be determined either by using a general standard or by figuring basal metabolic needs plus the calories needed to support one's daily activities.

TABLE 4-9. American Diabetes Association Method of Calculating Daily Caloric Needs According to Basal Metabolism, Body Weight, and Activity Level

Physical Activity	Total Calories Needed Daily*
Sedentary	Basal calories + (desirable body weight × 3)
Moderate	Basal calories + (desirable body weight × 5)
Strenuous	Basal calories + (desirable body weight × 10)

*Note that only numbers are used since the units of calories and weight do not mix. This is not a mathematical formula; it is an estimation.

Standard Caloric Approximations

The daily calorie allowances included in the 1980 Recommended Dietary Allowance (RDA; also see Chapter 13) are based on age, height, and sex. For example, for a man 23 to 50 years of age, weighing 154 lb (70 kg) and 5'10" in height, the daily caloric need is 2,700 kcal. Similarly, for a woman in the same age range, 120 lb (55 kg) and 5'4", the daily caloric need is 2,000 kcal (see earlier discussion). These standards assume a moderate amount of physical activity. See the appendix for more information.

For children, either the RDA or the age rule can be used to determine daily caloric need. In general, the age rule allows 1,000 kcal per day for a 1-year-old, and 100 kcal more for each year above one. This method is used until age 13 for girls and 16 to 18 for boys.

Basal Metabolism Plus Activity Level

The second general way to determine the calories needed to support ideal body weight involves adding basal metabolic needs to the calories used in physical activity. This can be done in a number of ways:

1. Adding the basal calories needed to the desirable body weight that has been multiplied by a factor keyed to the person's activity level. See Table 4-9.
2. Using basal caloric need and degree of activity. See Table 4-10.
3. Using known caloric need per pound of ideal body weight according to activity level. See Table 4-11.
4. Using the USDA rule of thumb for calculating daily caloric needs according to daily activity. See Table 4-12.

TABLE 4-10. One Method of Calculating Daily Caloric Needs According to Basal Metabolism and Activity Level

Physical Activity	Total Calories Needed Daily
Sedentary to light	$\frac{130}{100} \times$ basal caloric need
Moderate	$\frac{150}{100} \times$ basal caloric need
Strenuous	$\frac{175-200}{100} \times$ basal caloric need

TABLE 4-11. Daily Caloric Needs According to Activity Level and Ideal Body Weight by Using Approximations of Caloric Expenditure per Pound Body Weight

Physical Activity	kcal/lb Ideal Body Weight
Sedentary	11–12
Light	13–14
Moderate	15–16
Strenuous	18–19

TABLE 4-12. USDA Rule of Thumb for Calculating Daily Caloric Needs

Physical Activity	Total Calories Needed Daily*	
	Women	Men
Sedentary	Ideal body weight × 14	Ideal body weight × 16
Moderate	Ideal body weight × 18	Ideal body weight × 21
Strenuous	Ideal body weight × 22	Ideal body weight × 26

*All ideal body weights expressed in pounds.

All these methods have one problem in common: defining the degree of activity. There are standard tables that state the amount of calories needed for various occupations. These tables are available in standard textbooks.

STUDY QUESTIONS

1. What is one calorie? One joule?
2. How is the energy in food samples measured in the laboratory? How does this method differ from the actual utilization of food energy in the body? What numerical values are used to account for this difference?

3. Discuss the two methods of determining individual energy expenditure.
4. Define basal metabolic rate (BMR). What is the average BMR? What variables influence individual differences in BMR? How?
5. How is a person's total energy need calculated?
6. Describe at least three ways of estimating desirable body weight.
7. Do some library research and obtain another set of growth charts for children that are different from those provided in the appendix of the book.

REFERENCES

Bradfield, R. B., ed. 1971. Symposium: assessment of typical daily energy expenditure. *Amer. J. Clin. Nutr.* 24:1111, 1405.

Dairy Council Digest. 1980. Energy balance throughout the life cycle. 51:19.

Dauncey, M. J. 1979. Energy metabolism in man and the influence of diet and temperature: a review. *J. Human Nutr.* 33:259.

Grande, F. 1984. Body weight, composition and energy balance. In *Present knowledge in nutrition*, 5th ed. Washington, D. C.: The Nutrition Foundation.

Griffith, W. H., and Dyer, H. M. 1967. Present knowledge of specific dynamic action. In *Present knowledge in nutrition*, 3rd ed., chap. 7. New York: The Nutrition Foundation.

Hegsted, D. M. 1984. Energy requirements. In *Present knowledge in nutrition*, 5th ed. Washington, D. C.: The Nutrition Foundation.

Johnston, F. E., et al., eds. 1980. *Human physical growth and maturation: methodologies and factors.* New York: Plenum Press.

Proc. Nutr. Soc. 1978. The application of human and animal calorimetry. 37:1.

Society of Actuaries and Association of Life Insurance Medical Directors of America. 1980. *Build study*, 1979, vols. 1–2. Chicago.

5 PROTEIN

All living substances, including viruses and plants, contain protein. Distributed through blood, fat, skin, bones, and muscles, protein makes up from 18 to 20 percent of a living person, as shown in Table 5-1. Our bodies can make protein predictably and systematically. This body protein is in a constant state of change—either being broken down (degraded) or built up (resynthesized). Certain basic ingredients of protein must come from the foods we eat, since the body cannot synthesize them.

The first section of this chapter discusses the elements of protein biochemistry: essential and nonessential amino acids, the components of protein, and the relationship between nitrogen and protein. Also examined are the functions of protein as well as protein quantity and quality. The digestion, absorption, and metabolism of protein are discussed in Chapter 8, protein malnutrition is discussed in Chapter 9, and a diet adequate in protein in Chapter 10.

ELEMENTS OF PROTEIN BIOCHEMISTRY

Carbon, hydrogen, oxygen, and nitrogen occur in all protein substances. Each of the many types of protein contained in the body is made up of numerous individual units called **amino acids.**

TABLE 5-1. Distribution of Protein in the Body*

Tissue	% of Body Protein (approx.)
Blood proteins (albumin and hemoglobin)	10
Fat cells of adipose tissues	3–4
Body skin	9–9.5
Bones	18–19
Muscles	46–47

*The values have been obtained from different investigators and are presented in ranges to emphasize their variability in human bodies.

Essential and Nonessential Amino Acids

The human body can systematically synthesize most amino acids from nutrients such as carbohydrates, fats, and nitrogen sources. In general, **essential** is a term applied to nutrients that the body needs but is unable to manufacture. Instead, dietary sources must provide these substances. An **essential amino acid,** therefore, is one of the eight to ten amino acids, necessary to proper body function, that must be consumed in the diet because the body cannot manufacture them. By contrast, **nonessential amino acids** can be made by the body so long as the necessary ingredients are available.

It should be emphasized that both essential and nonessential amino acids are necessary to protein manufacture and use. First, essential amino acids must be present in the diet in the "right" ratio—that is, in a specific proportion. Second, nonessential amino acids must be available to provide sources of nitrogen for the body's work of maintenance and repair.

Table 5-2 lists the amino acids that occur in nature, both essential and nonessential. All adults need the same essential amino acids.

Protein Components

Protein substances come in all sizes, shapes, and molecular weights. When amino acids exist singly or in free form, they are known as **free amino acids.** Larger molecules with a larger number of amino acids (100 or more) linked together are known as **proteins.**

Free amino acids are most easily absorbed by the body. Larger molecules must be digested, or **hydrolyzed,** into free amino acid forms for

TABLE 5-2. Amino Acids Occurring in Nature

Essential for Adults and Infants	Essential for Infants Only	Nonessential	Questionable[1]
Isoleucine	Arginine*	Alanine	Hydroxyproline
Leucine	Histidine*	Asparagine	Norleucine
Lysine		Aspartic acid	Thyroxine
Methionine		Cysteine	
Phenylalanine		Cystine	
Threonine		Glutamic acid	
Tryptophan		Glutamine	
Valine		Glycine	
		Proline	
		Serine	
		Tyrosine	

*Preliminary evidence suggests that histidine is also an essential amino acid for adults. Some scientists question the essentiality of arginine.

[1] These substances are sometimes called amino acids.

maximum absorption. This digestive function is performed by substances called **enzymes,** which are released from the intestinal wall.

Protein substances differ in the following ways: (1) The number of amino acids present, (2) the specific amino acids present, (3) the frequency with which natural amino acids appear, (4) the possible combinations of amino acids, and (5) the shape of the protein molecules.

Nitrogen and Protein

Protein molecules contain nitrogen. One common method of estimating the level of protein in food is to measure the amount of nitrogen. Although the level of nitrogen may directly reflect the quantity of protein present, there is one major drawback to this method of estimating the protein content of foods: Many nonprotein substances in food contain nitrogen. For example, free amino acids, purines, ammonia, urea, and creatine all contain nitrogen but are not protein. The functional contributions of both protein and nonprotein nitrogen sources are summarized in Table 5-3.

Nitrogen estimation is still widely used to estimate the amount of protein present. Table 5-4 lists the approximate protein content of some common foods.

TABLE 5-3. Functional Contributions by Different Sources of Nitrogen to the Human Body

Nitrogen Source	Functional Contribution
Essential amino acids (protein and nonprotein substances)	Most needed by the human body both quantitatively and qualitatively.
Nonessential amino acids (protein and nonprotein substances)	Needed by the human body in quantity. No specific need for any of the particular amino acids.
Other nonprotein substances	Because the body can make them, they are not needed for any specific function. However, when present in a normal and nonpathological condition, they may facilitate different aspects of body metabolism.

FUNCTIONS OF PROTEINS

Proteins serve many essential purposes in the body, including the following:

1. **Building blocks** for many important substances, such as hormones, plasma proteins, antibodies, and chromosomes. For example, the hormone insulin, also a protein, is very important in controlling the physiological usage of glucose. Plasma proteins include such substances as hemoglobin and albumin, which maintain proper blood chemistry.
2. **Body development.** Protein is essential for the growth, repair, and maintenance of most body structures.
3. **Body metabolism.** As enzymes, proteins trigger and participate in many biological and chemical reactions.
4. **Body fluids and acid-base balance.** Proteins help to maintain proper pressure within the body's compartment partitions. Protein molecules also serve as an effective buffer system, controlling body acid-base balance.
5. **Source of energy.** Part of the protein we eat contributes to our caloric intake.
6. **Body detoxification.** Protein helps to regulate the body's ability to detoxify ingested foreign substances.

DIETARY REQUIREMENTS FOR PROTEIN

Although there is no real agreement about the exact amount of protein required for adults, the National Research Council of the National Academy of Sciences suggests about 0.8 g/kg of body weight per day. This

TABLE 5-4. Protein Content of Some Common American Foods*

Food Product	Serving Size	Protein (g)
Cheese, natural, cheddar	1 oz	7
Milk, whole, 3.3% fat	1 c	28
Ice cream, regular, hardened	1 c	5
Egg, cooked in any form	1	6
Butter	1 T	trace
Beef, ground, lean, broiled	3 oz	18
Tuna, canned in oil, drained	3 oz	24
Apple	1	trace
Grapefruit	½	1
Bread, white, enriched	1 sl	2
Breakfast cereal, hot, cooked (oatmeal or rolled oats)	1 c	5
Spaghetti, tomato sauce with cheese	1 c	6
Beans, cooked, drained	1 c	15
Peanut butter	1 T	4
Walnuts, English, chopped	1 c	18
Cabbage, raw, shredded	1 c	1
Corn, canned, cream style	1 c	5
Potatoes, cooked, baked (2/lb)	1	4
Beer	12 fl oz	1
Gelatin, dry	7 oz	6
Yeast, brewer's, dry	1 T	3

*Adapted from *Nutritive Value of Foods*, Home and Garden Bulletin No. 72 (Washington, D.C.: U.S. Department of Agriculture, 1981).

TABLE 5-5. 1980 Recommended Daily Allowance (RDA) for Protein for Different Age Groups and During Pregnancy and Lactation

Age (years) or Condition	RDA (g protein/day)
0.0–0.5	body weight (kg) × 2.2
0.5–1.0	body weight (kg) × 2.0
1–3	23
4–6	30
7–10	34
11–14, male	45
15–51+, male	56
11–18, female	46
19–51+, female	44
Pregnancy	+30
Lactation	+20

amount is an allowance for mixed proteins—that is, those of both animal and plant origin. Table 5-5 lists the daily protein need given in the 1980 Recommended Dietary Allowances (RDA).

Protein need refers to: (1) adequate intake of 8 to 10 essential amino acids, (2) a good source of nitrogen, and (3) sufficient calories. The minimum daily intake of the essential amino acids recommended in Table 5-6 is slightly lower than the actual intake of most Americans.

TABLE 5-6. Estimated Amino Acid Requirements of Humans*

Amino Acid	Requirement, mg/kg Body Weight/Day			Amino Acid Pattern for High-Quality Proteins, mg/g of Protein[1]
	Infant (4–6 months)	Child (10–12 years)	Adult	
Histidine	33	?	?	17
Isoleucine	83	28	12	42
Leucine	135	42	16	70
Lysine	99	44	12	51
Total *S*-containing amino acids (methionine and cystine)	49	22	10	26
Total aromatic amino acids (phenylalanine and tyrosine)	141	22	16	73
Threonine	68	28	8	35
Tryptophan	21	4	3	11
Valine	92	25	14	48

*Source: *Recommended Dietary Allowances* (Washington, D.C.: Food and Nutrition Board, National Research Council, National Academy of Sciences, 1980). The essentiality of arginine is undetermined.

[1] 2 g/kg/day of protein of the quality listed will meet the amino acid needs of infants.

Tests of Protein Need

There are several techniques for determining whether a person's protein intake is adequate. For children, the test is based on growth measurements. An adult's protein need is usually determined by a technique known as *nitrogen balance study*, which requires careful measurement of the amount of nitrogen consumed and excreted. A normal, healthy adult is in **nitrogen equilibrium** if he is eating an appropriate amount of protein for his individual needs. Table 5-7 gives some hypothetical examples of nitrogen balance studies. Table 5-8 presents some common clues to nitrogen balance that are not dependent on nitrogen measurements.

Individual Factors

The individual need for protein may differ from the RDA average for a number of reasons. These include:

1. **Body size.** All other factors being equal, more protein is required by a larger person.
2. **Age.** Protein need during the growing years is two to three times higher than during the adult years. During puberty the increased need for protein stabilizes. It is estimated that protein need during old age is similar to that of a 25-year-old adult.

TABLE 5-7. Hypothetical Examples of Nitrogen Balance in the Human after Ingesting 90-95 g Protein

Nitrogen Status	Example				
	1	2	3	4	5
Nitrogen ingested (g)	15	15	15	15	15
Nitrogen in feces (g)	1.5	2.0	1.5	1.5	1.8
Nitrogen in urine (g)	10	16	13.8	13.5	13.0
Nitrogen retained by body (g)	3.5	0	0	0	0.2
Total nitrogen lost by body (g)	0	3.0	0.3	0	0
Nitrogen balance	Positive	Negative	Equilibrium	Equilibrium	Equilibrium

Note. All values are approximations.

TABLE 5-8. Some Common Examples for the Different Types of Nitrogen Balance

Nitrogen Balance	Most Likely Situation	Remark
Positive	Growing child Pregnant woman Person recovering from an illness Person's diet changed from low to high protein	Growth and development
Negative	Person receiving surgery or crush injury Person suffering starvation Person immobilized Person receiving a low fat and carbohydrate diet Person's diet changed from high to low protein Elderly*	Body wasting
In equilibrium	A normal, healthy adult 21–40 years old† Subject in a human nitrogen balance experiment	Maintenance; repair of body

*This is not necessarily true in all elderly individuals.

†This is theoretically true and the exact age limit is not yet defined.

3. **Sex.** Because of greater body fat and less muscle mass in a woman, her protein need is slightly less than that of a man of the same age and weight. However, the stated protein requirement of 0.8 g per kg of body weight applies to both adult men and women.
4. **Nutritional status.** Substandard nutrition increases protein need.
5. **Pregnancy and lactation.** A pregnant woman needs more protein for the developing fetus, while a nursing mother requires more protein for milk production. See Table 5-5 and Chapter 11 for information.

6. **Climate.** High temperatures can lead to a significant loss of nitrogen, thus increasing the need for dietary protein.
7. **Activity.** In general, heavy physical activity does not require additional protein. However, inactivity for a prolonged period may require more protein to repair wasted muscles.
8. **Conditioning.** The human body is able to adjust to a subnormal amount of essential amino acids by decreasing the protein requirement for maintenance, repairs, and life processes. On the other hand, when a person *starts* athletic training, an increased amount of protein is needed to build up the muscles. Once the athletic routine has been established, only a normal amount of protein is needed.
9. **Dietary components.** The relative amount of carbohydrate and fat in the diet affects the protein requirement. Also, the quality of protein available determines the amount required.
10. **Emotional status.** Fear, anxiety, and depression may increase protein need by causing the body to excrete more nitrogen.
11. **Disease.** Both injury and illness generally increase the need for protein: injury, because tissue loss requires protein replacement; and illness, because processes such as the manufacture of antibodies increases protein need.

EVALUATION OF PROTEIN QUALITY

Quality as well as quantity is important to our protein requirement. Three common techniques for determining the quality of a protein substance are described below. Some comments on the value of different kinds of protein follow.

Biological Value

One method of evaluating protein quality is to measure its **biological value**—that is, determine whether the protein contains all the essential amino acids in the appropriate proportions needed by the body. A protein is said to have good biological value if most of its nitrogen—70 percent or more—is retained by the body after ingestion. Table 5-9 shows the biological values of a number of protein foods.

Net Protein Utilization

A second technique, *net protein utilization*, was developed to take into account the *digestibility* of various proteins. Table 5-9 provides the net protein utilization (amount of protein available to the body) of some common foods.

TABLE 5-9. Biological Value, Net Protein Utilization, and Protein Efficiency Ratio of Various Food Products*

Food Category	Example	Biological Value (%)	Net Protein Utilization (%)	Protein Efficiency Ratio (Using Rats)
Meat and equivalent	Beef, Fish	70–75	70–75	2.1–2.5
		80–85	80–85	3.3–3.7
Dairy products	Milk	80–85	80–85	2.8–3.4
Egg	Egg	90–95	90–95	3.7–4.1
Grains	Whole wheat	60–65	55–60	1.5–2.0
Beans	Soybeans	70–75	65–70	2.1–2.5
Nuts	Peanuts	50–55	45–50	1.4–1.8

*These data have been obtained from the results of a number of investigators. Because of highly variable results, ranges are provided to serve as a general guide only.

Protein Efficiency Ratio

The **protein efficiency ratio** is the simplest method of determining protein quality. This method involves feeding a specific amount of protein food to a group of animals daily and observing their growth over a given period. The protein efficiency ratio of a particular protein food is the gram of body weight gained by the animals per gram of protein food eaten. Examples for some food products are shown in Table 5-9.

Defining Protein Quality

A good-quality protein is one in which the eight to ten essential amino acids exist in a proportion that meets our minimal needs. Such a protein is usually made up of half essential and half nonessential amino acids. Most animal protein, therefore, is high-quality protein. Most vegetable protein, on the other hand, contains only some of the essential amino acids and will not support growth in maintenance of an animal when fed as the only protein source. Vegetable protein is usually low-quality protein. Table 5-10 indicates the different categories of vegetable proteins and the amino acid(s) that are most likely to be low or deficient in them.

Protein deficiency in the United States and Canada is insignificant compared with that in many developing countries. However, insufficient protein intake does occur among low-income individuals, especially elderly and ethnic populations. Vegetarianism also can lead to protein deficiency.

TABLE 5-10. Limiting Amino Acids in Categories of Vegetable Protein Foods

Category	Limiting Amino Acid(s)
Most grain products	Lysine, threonine (sometimes tryptophan)
Most legumes or pulses	Methionine, tryptophan
Nuts and oil seeds	Lysine
Green leafy vegetables	Methionine
Leaves and grasses	Methionine

STUDY QUESTIONS

1. What are the four major elements found in all proteins?
2. Define amino acid, essential amino acid, and nonessential amino acid. Why is regular consumption of nonessential amino acids important?
3. Discuss at least five important functions of protein.
4. When we talk of protein need, we imply three important premises. What are they?
5. Discuss at least eight factors involved in determining individual need for protein.
6. What are the three most common methods of determining the quality of proteins? Which kinds of foods are considered complete proteins? Incomplete proteins? What are complementary protein foods?

REFERENCES

Chopra, J. G., et al. 1978. Protein in the U. S. diet. *J. Amer. Dietet. Assoc.* 72:253.

Crim, M. C., and Munro, H. N. 1984. Protein. In *Present knowledge in nutrition*, 5th ed. Washington, D. C.: The Nutrition Foundation.

Harper, A. E., et al. 1973. Human protein needs. *Lancet* 1:1518.

Hegsted, D. M. 1965. Variation in requirements of nutrients—amino acids. *Fed. Proc.* 22:1424.

Irwin, M. I., and Hegsted, D. M. 1971. A conspectus of research on amino acid requirements of man. *J. Nutr.* 101:539.

Palombo, J. D., and Blackburn, G. L. 1980. Human protein requirements. *Contemp. Nutr.* 5 (January): 1.

Porter, J. W. G., and Rolls, B. A. 1973. *Proteins in human nutrition.* New York: Academic Press.

Scrimshaw, N. S. 1976a. An analysis of past and present recommended dietary allowances for protein in health and disease. Part one. *N. Engl. J. Med.* 294:136.

———. 1976b. An analysis of past and present recommended dietary allowances for protein in health and disease. Part two. *N. Engl. J. Med.* 294:198.

6 VITAMINS

Like carbohydrates, proteins, and fats, vitamins are **organic** compounds—that is, substances that contain carbon and hydrogen, and often oxygen, nitrogen, and/or sulfur. But unlike these other organic compounds, which must be present in fairly large quantities in the diet, vitamins are required in very small amounts to perform the functions essential for life. Little is known about the biochemical functions of vitamins, except for their role as coenzymes in biological reactions (see Chapter 8). The human body can synthesize at least 3 of the 13 known vitamins, although the amount varies with circumstances. All known vitamins are therefore considered essential nutrients and must be supplied to the body as needed.

In this chapter, we will discuss the vitamins according to their functions, sources, requirements, symptoms of deficiency, and possible toxic reactions.

VITAMIN GROUPS

Certain vitamins are similar to each other in several ways. First, all known vitamins can be divided into two major categories according to whether they are soluble in water or oil (fat). The main characteristics of the water-soluble vitamins are summarized in Table 6-1, and those of the fat-soluble ones in Table 6-2.

Second, vitamin D, vitamin A, and niacin share the unique characteristic of being capable of synthesis by the body if the appropriate ingredients are available. Certain starting materials, called **precursors** or

TABLE 6-1. Major Characteristics of Water-Soluble Vitamins*

Vitamin	Human Deficiency Symptoms	Major Functions	Food Sources	RDA† Established	Remarks
Vitamin C	Scurvy: loose teeth, bleeding gums, painful joints, bruising, skin hemorrhage.	Healing wounds, collagen formation, utilization of other nutrients, body metabolism.	Citrus fruits, strawberries, cantaloupes, kale, broccoli, sweet peppers, parsley, turnip greens, potatoes.	Yes	Undesirable effects from excess dose. Very unstable substance.
Vitamin B₁	Beriberi: fatigue, mental depression, poor appetite, polyneuritis, decreased muscle tone.	As coenzyme. Metabolism of carbohydrate, fat, and protein.	Pork, liver and other organ meats, grain (whole or enriched), nuts, legumes, milk, eggs.	Yes	Unstable in food processing.
Vitamin B₂	Cheilosis: cracked lips, scaly skin, burning/itching eyes. Glossitis: smooth, red, sore tongue, with atrophy.	As coenzyme. Metabolism of fat, carbohydrate, and protein.	Liver, milk, meat, eggs, enriched cereal products, green leafy vegetables.	Yes	Very susceptible to UV or visible rays of sunlight.
Vitamin B₆	In infants: convulsion, irritability. In adults: microcytic hypochromic anemia, irritability, skin lesions, and other nonspecific signs.	As coenzyme. Metabolism of protein.	Pork, beef, liver, bananas, ham, egg yolks.	Yes	Pharmacological dose occasionally relieves morning sickness.
Niacin	Pellagra (the 4 D's): dermatitis, diarrhea, dementia, death. Also sore mouth, delirium, darkened teeth and skin. Hyperpigmentation.	As a coenzyme in the metabolism of fat, carbohydrate, and protein.	Meat, fish, liver, poultry, dark green leafy vegetables, whole or enriched grain products.	Yes	May be synthesized from tryptophan in body.
Folic acid	Megaloblastic anemia.	Formation of nucleic acids (DNA, RNA). Metabolism of methyl (CH_3) groups. Rapid turnover of cells, e.g., red blood cells.	Pork, liver and other organ meats, peanuts, green leafy vegetables, yeast, orange juice.	Yes	Deficiency probably most prevalent in Western societies.

TABLE 6-1. (continued)

Vitamin	Human Deficiency Symptoms	Major Functions	Food Sources	RDA[†] Estab- lished	Remarks
Vitamin B$_{12}$	Megaloblastic anemia; neurodegeneration.	Same as above.	Animal products: meat, poultry, fish, eggs, etc. Not found in edible plant products.	Yes	Pernicious anemia infers a lack of the intrinsic factor (see text).
Pantothenic acid	Nonspecific symptoms: weight loss, irritability, intestinal disturbances, nervous disorders, burning sensation of feet.	As a coenzyme in the metabolism of fat, protein, and carbohydrate.	Widespread in nature. Meat, poultry, fish, grains, some fruits and vegetables.	No	Sensitive to dry heat.
Biotin	In infants: dermatitis. In adults: anorexia, nausea, muscle pain, depression, anemia, dermatitis, and other non-specific symptoms.	As a coenzyme in metabolism of fat, carbohydrate, and protein.	Organ meats (liver, kidney), egg yolk, milk, cheese.	No	Antagonist, avidin, found in egg white.

*Only an overview is provided. For details and explanations, consult the sections on the individual vitamins in text.
†RDA = Recommended Dietary Allowance, established by the National Research Council of the National Academy of Sciences.

provitamins, eventually become activated vitamins by a complex conversion process. On the other hand, vitamin D, vitamin A, and niacin also occur in food as the vitamins and will be ingested as ready-made vitamins. In this case, they are referred to as **preformed** vitamins.

Third, at least two vitamins remain biologically inactive until activated: vitamin D and folic acid. Once *activated*, the vitamins can be utilized by the body.

VITAMIN DEFICIENCY

Individual requirements of specific vitamins depend on many factors. The most common cause of human vitamin deficiency is inadequate intake. Other factors include any interference with the body's ability to absorb or synthesize vitamins and increased need due to stress, drugs, or excess excretion.

TABLE 6-2. Major Characteristics of Fat-Soluble Vitamins*

Vitamin	Human Deficiency Symptoms	Major Functions	Food Sources	RDA[†] Established	Remarks
Vitamin A	Eye: night blindness, Bitot's spot, partial and total blindness. Skin: dryness, scaliness, hardening and epithelial changes (affecting body surface), mucosa along respiratory, gastrointestinal, and genitourinary tracts.	In the eye: synthesis of rhodopsin, visual pigment. In the epithelium: differentiation. In the bones and teeth: proper development.	Carotene: dark green and yellow leafy vegetables. Dark yellow fruits. Vitamin A: liver, butter, whole-milk and other fortified dairy products.	Yes	Large doses may be toxic.
Vitamin D	Infancy and childhood: rickets. Adults: osteomalacia.	Calcium metabolism, especially its absorption from the intestine and mobilization from bones.	Fish, especially liver and oil; liver and fortified whole milk.	Yes	Large doses may be toxic.
Vitamin E	Uncommon in adults. Infants (especially premature): RBC susceptibility to hemolysis.	Not known. An antioxidant in food industry.	Wheat germ, vegetable oils, nuts, legumes, green leafy vegetables.	Yes	Therapeutic effects of large doses not substantiated.
Vitamin K	Prolonged blood-clotting time. Hemorrhage. Delayed wound healings.	Responsible for prothrombin synthesis in liver.	Dark green leafy vegetables; alfalfa.	No	Synthesized by intestinal bacteria.

*Only an overview is provided. For details and explanations, consult the sections on the individual vitamins in text.
[†]RDA = Recommended Dietary Allowance, established by the National Research Council of the National Academy of Sciences.

A combination of methods can be used to confirm vitamin deficiency. One is the observance of clinical symptoms. A second is blood and urine analysis to check the level of the vitamin and its accumulated metabolites. The third and most common method of determining vitamin deficiency is the administration of a large amount of the vitamin. A normal person will then show increased levels of the vitamin and its metabolites in the blood and urine, whereas a person deficient in the vitamin usually will show decreased levels.

VITAMIN SOURCES

Under normal circumstances, we ingest vitamins from many foods and, as already indicated, synthesize a few of them in our bodies. How nearly we meet our daily requirements, however, depends on a number of variables.

First, the true values of some food vitamin contents are uncertain. The retention of vitamins in commercially processed food products varies with the type of food, processing, and storage. Even fresh foods vary widely in vitamin content.

Second, the body's ability to absorb (and synthesize) needed vitamins is highly individualized. Everyone harbors bacteria in the large intestine, but the numbers and types of bacteria are largely determined by diet. These bacteria are a necessary part of the process of vitamin absorption and synthesis; however, certain dietary factors can destroy the bacteria or inhibit their vitamin synthesis. Drugs such as antibiotics also can reduce the contribution of this source of vitamins.

A third factor in vitamin intake is the common practice of eating foods with vitamins added and taking vitamin supplements. Food companies are increasingly enriching or fortifying food products with vitamins. The general public may be taking more vitamins than they need, both in the form of food additives and as dietary vitamin supplements. Guidelines for safe enrichment and fortification are currently being determined.

WATER-SOLUBLE VITAMINS

Vitamins C, B_1, B_2, and B_6, niacin, folic acid, vitamin B_{12}, pantothenic acid, and biotin are known as water-soluble vitamins. The term **vitamin B complex** usually includes all known water-soluble vitamins except C. The abbreviation RDA refers to the Recommended Dietary Allowances for healthy persons established by the National Research Council of the National Academy of Sciences (see Chapter 10).

Vitamin C

Vitamin C, also known as ascorbic acid, was discovered in 1932, although its importance was recognized much earlier in association with scurvy and the lack of citrus fruits among British sailors. It is a white crystal, stable in acid, fairly stable in light, but sensitive to heat, air, and alkali. When a vitamin can be destroyed easily, it is said to be *labile*.

The human body stores enough vitamin C, mainly in the adrenal cortex, to exist normally without dietary intake for only 90 days. After this period, symptoms of scurvy appear. Any excess is excreted in the urine or converted to oxalic acid, which is also excreted. Certain drugs such as oral contraceptives can influence the excretion and utilization of vitamin C.

Functions

Vitamin C plays an important role in many body processes. As the most active reducing agent in living substances, it serves important functions in food processing. It increases the absorption of iron and calcium, thus promoting the proper formation of teeth and bones.

Vitamin C is needed as a catalyst to transfer nerve impulses between cells. It is also important in the synthesis of corticosterone.

The role of vitamin C in collagen synthesis is of major importance. **Collagen,** an insoluble protein in connective tissue, is found in skin, cartilage, tendons, ligaments, bone, teeth, and blood vessels. The organized way in which cells and tissues are held together is due to the presence of collagen.

Requirements and Deficiency Symptoms

Because humans are unable to synthesize vitamin C, they must consume it in their diets. A vitamin C deficiency causes the syndrome known as **scurvy.** Blood vessels become fragile, causing bruising and bleeding of the tissues, especially the joints and gums. Wound healing is also adversely affected by the lack of vitamin C. Table 6-3 shows the 1980 RDA for persons of varying age groups.

Infant Scurvy. Between 1960 and 1970, infant scurvy was directly related to the use of cow's milk. Pasteurization and the lack of orange juice or a vitamin C supplement resulted in a deficiency uncommon among breast-fed babies. Afflicted children with classic deficiency develop hemorrhaging, fever, and anemia, and cannot move their legs. Bones show distinct changes. One preventive measure is to avoid using unfortified formula as the only food for a prolonged period.

A child with scurvy is given 25 mg of vitamin C, which is usually added to milk, four times a day (100 mg total). Some pediatricians prescribe 50 to 100 mg four times daily; after 1 week on this regimen, the dose may be reduced to 30 mg per day, which may be obtained from orange juice or a supplement.

Adult Scurvy. Adult scurvy is uncommon except among alcoholics, mental patients, and those who avoid vegetables and fruits. Early symptoms include loss of appetite, fatigue, irritability, muscle and joint pain, and

TABLE 6-3. 1980 RDA for Vitamin C for Different Age Groups and During Pregnancy and Lactation

Population Group	Vitamin C RDA (mg)
Infants	
0−12 months	35
Children	
1−10	45
11−14 years	50
Males and females	
15+ years	60
Pregnancy	+20
Lactation	+40

skin lesions. More advanced vitamin C deficiency is characterized by a marked tendency toward hemorrhaging, delayed wound healing, and infection. Bone joints become painful and swollen, limiting motion. As the disease progresses, mucous membranes bleed and gums become red, swollen, and ulcerated, causing loose teeth to fall out. Anemia may occur. Sudden death or heart failure may result from internal hemorrhage. See Figures 6-1, 6-2, and 6-3.

Food Sources

The richest sources of vitamin C are citrus fruits, tomatoes, and green vegetables. Potatoes and root vegetables, although low in vitamin C content, contribute to the American intake because of the large amount consumed. Animal products are not good sources, since the vitamin is destroyed during food preparation.

Vitamin C is one of the most unstable vitamins. During food preparation, it is important to remember that vitamin C is sensitive to air, cooking temperature, pressure, and light and that it can be leached by water. For example, normal home cooking processes can destroy 50 to 90 percent of the vitamin C in foods.

In food processing, vitamin C serves as an additive in juices, fruit cocktail, white flour, jams and jellies, and wine and beer. This extensive use of vitamin C in commercial foods greatly increases the American intake.

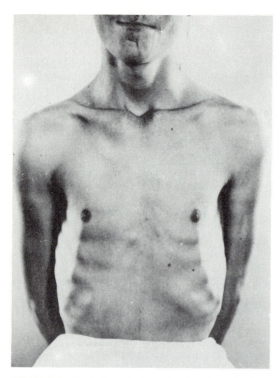

FIGURE 6-1. Healed scorbutic rosary in a boy who had had scurvy off and on since infancy. The sharp edges of the costochondral junctions are easily visible. (From R. W. Vilter, "Effect of Ascorbic Acid in Man," in *The Vitamins: Chemistry, Physiology, Pathology, Methods,* ed. W. H. Sebrell and R. S. Harris [New York: Academic Press, 1967, p. 468]. With permission of Academic Press.)

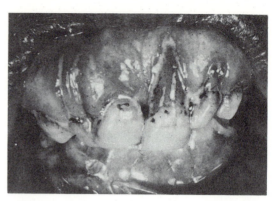

FIGURE 6-2. Scorbutic gingivitis. (From S. Dreizen, *Geriatrics* 29 [1974]: 97. By permission of *Geriatrics*)

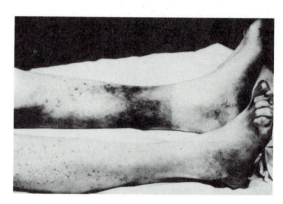

FIGURE 6-3. Ecchymosis and petechiae from vitamin C deficiency. (From S. Driezen, *Geriatrics* 29 [1974]: 97. By permission of *Geriatrics.)*

Vitamin B$_1$

Thiamine is another name for vitamin B$_1$. It was discovered in 1921 and synthesized in 1936. It is made up of white crystals that are water soluble and highly unstable to oxidation and temperatures above 100°C.

Functions and Requirements

Vitamin B$_1$ plays an essential role in metabolism, especially of carbohydrates. Nerve cell membranes also require vitamin B$_1$ to transmit high-frequency impulses. Interference with the basic functions of thiamine can lead to symptoms of beriberi.

A person's requirement for vitamin B$_1$ is directly related to caloric intake. That is, the more carbohydrate one eats, the more thiamine

TABLE 6-4. 1980 RDA for Vitamin B₁ for Different Age Groups and During Pregnancy and Lactation

Population Group	Thiamine RDA (mg)
Infants	
0– 6 months	0.3
6–12 months	0.5
Children	
1– 3 years	0.7
7–10 years	1.2
Adolescents (11–18 years)	
Male	1.4
Female	1.1
Adults	
Male	
19–22 years	1.5
23–50 years	1.4
51+ years	1.2
Female	
19–22 years	1.1
23+ years	1.0
Pregnancy	+0.4
Lactation	+0.5

is needed. Small amounts of thiamine are stored in heart and brain tissues, and any excess is excreted in the urine. Table 6-4 provides the average 1980 RDA for different age groups.

Deficiency

Thiamine deficiency can be caused by a number of factors: (1) low intake of vitamin-rich foods, calories, carbohydrates, or folic acid; (2) excess carbohydrate intake; (3) alcoholism; (4) clinical stresses such as drug therapy. Most patients also are deficient in other B vitamins.

Pronounced thiamine deficiency results in the disease **beriberi,** which literally means "I can't, I can't" (a good description of this weakness-inducing condition). Damage to the central nervous system, heart, circulation, and alimentary tract is common.

Adult Beriberi. Symptoms of beriberi include loss of appetite, fatigue, nausea and vomiting, irritability, weak and heavy extremities, depression, cardiac disturbance, and abnormal gait. As the condition pro-

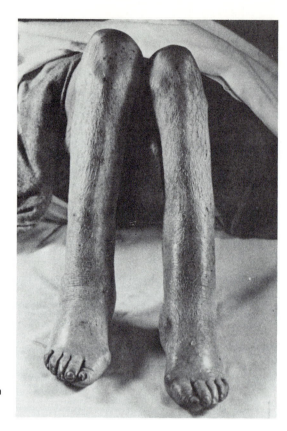

FIGURE 6-4. Wet beriberi with edema of the legs. (From S. Dreizen, *Geriatrics* 29 [1974]: 97. By permission of *Geriatrics*)

gresses, patients become emaciated and unable to walk properly. They suffer mental deterioration, confusion, and apathy. In some patients, the heart swells and eye muscles become paralyzed. Without treatment most patients die from sudden heart failure. Figure 6-4 illustrates one classic symptom of B_1 deficiency.

Infant Beriberi. In developing countries, infantile beriberi is still common, especially in breast-fed babies. The infant is pale, restless, and unable to sleep. Edema, diarrhea, muscle wasting, breathing difficulty, and crying weakness are characteristic. Without treatment, death from acute heart failure may result in 1 to 2 days after symptoms appear.

Food Sources

Whole and enriched grains, pork, and legumes are the richest sources of thiamine. Good sources include kidney, liver, beef, eggs, fish, milk, green vegetables, and some fruits.

Vitamin B_1 is easily destroyed, especially during home food preparation. Boiling, stirring, and soaking eliminate a great deal of thiamine as does alkali, sulfite, and irradiation.

Vitamin B_2

Vitamin B_2, or **riboflavin,** consists of yellow-orange crystals that are water soluble and stable to heat, acid, and oxidation. Of all known vitamins, however, riboflavin is the most unstable to sunlight. The vitamin was discovered in 1932 and synthesized in 1935.

Very little riboflavin is stored in the body; the liver and kidneys are the main storage sites. Any excess is excreted in the urine. Large doses of B_2 have so far proved to be nontoxic.

Functions

Riboflavin performs a very important function in the body by making many biological reactions possible, including: (1) energy metabolism; (2) indirect regulation of DNA and protein synthesis; (3) breakdown of fatty acids; (4) glycogen formation; (5) conversion of tryptophan to niacin; (6) production of red blood cells; (7) synthesis of corticosteroids in the adrenal gland.

Deficiency

Table 6-5 shows the 1980 RDA for riboflavin according to age group. Riboflavin deficiency is uncommon in the United States, except for female adolescents, alcoholics, and the elderly. A lack of riboflavin usually is combined with a niacin deficiency.

The major causes of riboflavin deficiency are inadequate dietary intake, malabsorption, and clinical stresses such as diabetes or surgery. Although a lack of the vitamin causes some unique symptoms, there is no known associated specific disease.

Patients with riboflavin deficiency may elicit such symptoms as oral lesions; dry, scaly skin; and serious eye defects. Since these symptoms also may result from other vitamin B deficiencies, specific riboflavin deficiency is sometimes difficult to diagnose.

Food Sources

The wide distribution of riboflavin in food makes a deficiency less likely. The best sources are meat—especially liver, kidney, and heart—milk, eggs, certain vegetables, and enriched cereals and bread. Food preparation and processing can deplete riboflavin, however.

TABLE 6-5. 1980 RDA for Riboflavin for Different Age Groups and During Pregnancy and Lactation

Population Group	Riboflavin RDA (mg)
Infants	
0– 6 months	0.4
6–12 months	0.6
Children	
1– 3 years	0.8
7–10 years	1.4
11–14 years	
Male	1.6
Female	1.3
Adolescents (15–18 years)	
Male	1.7
Female	1.3
Adults	
Male	
19–22 years	1.7
23–50 years	1.6
50+ years	1.4
Female	
19–22 years	1.3
23+ years	1.2
Pregnancy	+0.3
Lactation	+0.5

Vitamin B_6

Vitamin B_6, sometimes called **pyridoxine,** was discovered in 1934 and synthesized in 1939. It is water soluble and unstable to light, alkali, and oxidation, but stable to heat and acid. The body stores very little B_6, and the substance is relatively nontoxic.

Functions

The most important biological function of vitamin B_6 is to serve as a coenzyme in certain metabolic processes. B_6 is involved in the production of antibodies and reactions within the central nervous system. It is also important to the development of the myelin sheath surrounding nerve fibers.

TABLE 6-6. 1980 RDA for Vitamin B$_6$ for Different Age Groups and During Pregnancy and Lactation

Population Group	Vitamin B$_6$ RDA (mg)
Infants	
0– 6 months	0.3
6–12 months	0.6
Children	
1– 3 years	0.9
7–10 years	1.6
11–14 years	1.8
Adolescents (15–18 years)	2.0
Adults (19+ years)	
Male	2.2
Female	2.0
Pregnancy	+0.6
Lactation	+0.5

Deficiency

Healthy adults are rarely deficient in vitamin B$_6$, because it occurs widely in nature and the body's requirements for it are small. Table 6-6 gives the 1980 RDA of B$_6$ for different age groups. Besides the problems of inadequate intake, intestinal malabsorption, and clinical stresses— for example, alcoholism or hyperthyroidism—the practice of eating a low-carbohydrate, high-protein diet may increase the vitamin B$_6$ requirement. Drugs such as penicillin and oral contraceptives also may increase the need for vitamin B$_6$.

Symptoms of B$_6$ deficiency include irritability, depression, and drowsiness. Skin lesions, weight loss, and increased susceptibility to infection are also present. Patients may develop anemia and an increased risk of kidney stones. The severity of these symptoms is magnified when protein intake is high.

Food Sources

Vitamin B$_6$ is widespread in nature, with good sources including meat (especially liver and kidney), egg yolk, yeast, and whole grain cereals. Despite their low B$_6$ content, vegetables contribute more B$_6$ to the American diet than many other foods because the vitamin in vegetables resists being destroyed during processing and storage. For example, from 20 to 30 percent of B_6 is lost in the freezing of vegetables while milling grains results in 90 percent loss.

Niacin

The vitamin **niacin** is unlike most other vitamins in that it is moderately stable to heat, light, acid, alkali, and oxidation. As a result, very little of the vitamin is lost during food preparation. The substance has been known since 1867 but was first recognized as a vitamin in 1936.

Found in forms slightly different in plant products than in animal products, niacin is readily absorbed by the body. Very little is stored, however, since any excess is excreted in the urine.

Functions

Niacin is required by all living cells. As a coenzyme the vitamin can release energy from carbohydrate, fat, and protein as well as making oxidation possible. This oxidation of food releases energy that is stored by the body.

A unique characteristic of niacin is that it is the only water-soluble vitamin capable of being synthesized by the body. This transformation, however, cannot occur in the absence of certain B vitamins and other substances.

Deficiency

A significant lack of niacin causes **pellagra,** which means literally "rough skin." Once common in the southern United States, pellagra still is widespread in places where corn is the major cereal, such as Yugoslavia, Africa, and India. In this country, pellagra is usually associated with diabetes, alcoholism, and other kinds of clinical stress. Table 6-7 shows the 1980 RDA for niacin for different age groups.

Early symptoms of pellagra include loss of appetite, apathy, weakness, irritability, anxiety, depression, numbness, insomnia, and gastrointestinal problems. The classic clinical manifestations of the disease are frequently termed the "4 D's": dermatitis, diarrhea, depression, and, if untreated, death.

Skin lesions initially resemble ordinary sunburn, but they occur in a typically symmetrical pattern. That is, both hands, both feet, and/or both sides of the face are affected. See Figure 6-5.

Oral lesions and infection are common, making eating or drinking difficult to impossible. Common intestinal complaints include indigestion, pain, and diarrhea. Involvement of the central nervous system can lead to delirium, coma, and death.

TABLE 6-7. 1980 RDA for Niacin for Different Age Groups and During Pregnancy and Lactation

Population Group	Niacin Equivalent (mg)
Infants	
0– 6 months	6
6–12 months	8
Children	
1– 3 years	9
7–10 years	16
11–14 years	
Male	18
Female	15
Adolescents (15–18 years)	
Male	18
Female	14
Adults	
Male	
19–22 years	19
23–50 years	18
51+ years	16
Female	
19–22 years	14
23+ years	13
Pregnancy	+2
Lactation	+5

Food Sources

Foods rich in niacin include lean meat, kidney and liver, poultry, fish, yeasts, and peanut butter. Whole grain products, potatoes, and some green vegetables contain moderate amounts of niacin.

Folic Acid

Discovered and synthesized in 1945, **folic acid** consists of yellow crystals that are slightly soluble in water and stable in acid solution. It is rapidly destroyed in neutral or alkaline solution and can be lost during food preparation. The compound is essential for humans and is relatively nontoxic.

Although folic acid is fairly readily absorbed, vitamin C and some antibiotics facilitate the process. Enough of the active vitamin can be

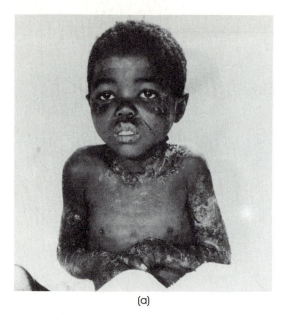
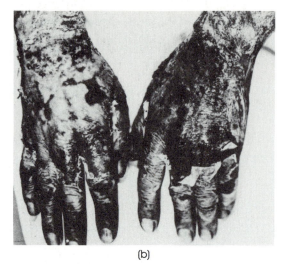

(a)   (b)

FIGURE 6-5. Classic symptoms of pellagra. Note symmetrical dermatitis in these South African patients. (a) (Courtesy of Dr. J.G. Prinsloo). Skin dermatitis in an American patient. (b) (From S. Dreizen, *Geriatrics* 29 [1974]: 97. By permission of *Geriatrics*)

stored in the liver to last the host from 4 to 5 months. Absorption is decreased by alcohol and by drugs such as oral contraceptive pills and anticonvulsants. Such drugs also may interfere with the utilization and metabolism of the vitamin, further increasing the host's requirement.

Functions

Folic acid indirectly contributes to the formation of DNA; that is, the formation or turnover of body cells. In the absence of folic acid, replenishment of cells, especially red blood cells, will be defective. **Megaloblastosis** (failure of red blood cells to mature) occurs in the bone marrow. Folic acid is necessary to the synthesis of enzymes and other protein molecules.

Deficiency

The classic symptom of folic acid deficiency is macrocytic or megaloblastic anemia. Other symptoms include diarrhea, weight loss, and inflammation of the tongue. Anemia and the low supply of oxygen to tissues results in fatigue, weakness, fainting, and pallor. Cardiac enlargement with occasional congestive heart failure is not uncommon.

TABLE 6-8. 1980 RDA for Folacin for Different Age Groups and During Pregnancy and Lactation

Population Group	Folacin RDA (μg)
Infants	
0– 6 months	30
6–12 months	45
Children	
1– 3 years	100
7–10 years	200
Adolescents and adults (11+ years)	400
Pregnancy	+400
Lactation	+100

Deficiency of folic acid is widespread in all parts of the world, especially the tropical zones. It is probably the most prevalent of all vitamin deficiencies, even in the United States. Most American diets, in fact, provide less than the RDA for adults shown in Table 6-8. Causes of deficiency include inadequate intake, reduced absorption, increased demands and/or losses, and metabolic disorders. Human storage of the vitamin is minimal.

Infants, adolescents, and pregnant women are vulnerable to folic acid deficiency, since they require rapid cell division for growth, thus creating a large demand for DNA, and, consequently, folic acid. Dietary intake is often insufficient to meet this need.

In poor countries, folic acid deficiency is common and often associated with vitamin B_{12} deficiency. From 20 to 30 percent of the populations in poor countries suffer folic acid deficiency. Affected infants and children in these countries usually suffer malabsorption, caused in part by megaloblastic anemia. The malabsorption further aggravates folic acid deficiency, which intensifies anemia further. It is a vicious cycle.

In the Western world, folic acid deficiency is also common among the old, the poor, and others with irregular eating habits such as alcoholics. An imbalanced diet, defective absorption, liver failure, excess excretion, and disturbed metabolism and utilization of folic acid lead to deficiency in more than half the alcoholics. Low income individuals often show biochemical deficiency of the vitamin. About 10 to 20 percent of pregnant women may have folic acid deficiency, usually because of inadequate intake.

Elderly patients with rheumatoid arthritis and other clinical problems are especially susceptible to folic acid deficiency. Parasitic infection also can cause deficiency. Anticonvulsants and oral contraceptive pills can interfere with the absorption, utilization, and metabolism of the vitamin. Ascorbic acid, on the other hand, can enhance the absorption of folic acid.

The treatment of folic acid deficiency is fairly simple. Synthetic folic acid appears to be well assimilated by the body, and a dose of 0.1 mg can prevent deficiency. Infants with folic acid deficiency usually are given 5 mg daily of oral folic acid. Affected adults usually receive 5 mg orally two to three times a day. Patient response is rapid. Within a few days after treatment begins, patients have better appetites and signs of general well-being; their blood profiles gradually return to normal.

Food Sources

The richest food sources of folic acid are green leafy vegetables, asparagus, liver, kidney, yeast, and wheat germ. Good sources are beef, whole grain cereals, nuts, lima beans, legumes, green vegetables, and fruits such as cantaloupe, lemons, strawberries, and bananas.

Folic acid is highly susceptible to destruction during food preparation. High temperatures and excess water in cooking can be responsible for nearly 100 percent loss. Light is also responsible for some destruction.

Vitamin B$_{12}$

Cobalamin is the general chemical term for vitamin B$_{12}$. The chemical was discovered in 1948 and synthesized in 1974.

Much of the B$_{12}$ in the body is not in free form. Instead, B$_{12}$ molecules attach themselves to large protein molecules, which transport the vitamin from one part of the body to the next. Any excess B$_{12}$ is stored in the liver, which can accumulate enough vitamin to last the host for 5 to 6 years without any intake.

Absorption and Functions

Vitamin B$_{12}$ plays an important role in the metabolism of all cells, in tissue growth, and the maintenance of the central nervous system. It is, however, essential to all cells.

The absorption of cobalamin occurs mainly in the lower ileum and, unlike the absorption of other water-soluble vitamins, requires the presence of **intrinsic factor,** a mucoprotein normally present in gastric juices. Combining with ingested vitamin B$_{12}$, intrinsic factor transports the vitamin into the mucosal wall at the absorption site, where the vitamin is released and transferred into the blood. If intrinsic factor is absent for any reason, little or no B$_{12}$ is absorbed.

The higher the intake of vitamin B_{12}, the lower the percentage of it is absorbed. Absorption is decreased by old age, iron or pyridoxine deficiency, or hypothyroidism.

Deficiency

People who eat animal products rarely suffer dietary vitamin B_{12} deficiency. The body can store enough B_{12} to last a person 5 to 6 years before deficiency develops.

Inadequate supply of cobalamin causes megaloblastic anemia. If the intestinal absorption of cobalamin is defective, the resulting deficiency also causes megaloblastic anemia. However, if the absorption defect results from a lack of intrinsic factor, the megaloblastic anemia is commonly referred to as **pernicious anemia.**

Other symptoms of vitamin B_{12} deficiency include *glossitis* (inflammation of the tongue), tiredness, headache, breathing difficulty, and low-grade fever. Pernicious anemia patients may show lemon yellow pallor, hyperpigmentation, weight loss, and various gastrointestinal problems.

Degeneration of the central nervous system occurs in patients with a prolonged B_{12} deficiency. Loss of sensation of the extremities, muscle weakness and atrophy, and mood changes such as irritability and depression are present. Whatever the cause of B_{12} deficiency, it must be diagnosed early to prevent permanent damage to the nervous system.

Requirements and Sources

The exact requirement for vitamin B_{12} has not been determined, but it is known that a person's need increases during illness and hyperthyroidism. Table 6-9 presents the 1980 RDA for vitamin B_{12} for different age groups.

The best sources of vitamin B_{12} are chicken, pork, beef, liver, kidney, eggs, whole milk, and fresh shrimp and oysters.

Pantothenic Acid

Once called vitamin B_3, **pantothenic acid** was discovered in 1933 and synthesized in 1940. It is widely distributed in nature and recognized as essential to most living things.

Functions and Deficiency

Nutrient metabolism is the primary function of pantothenic acid. It combines with other substances to form **coenzyme A** (CoA), which is important in the metabolism of fat, protein, and carbohydrate. As discussed in Chapter 8, CoA participates in the citric acid cycle and permits

TABLE 6-9. 1980 RDA for Vitamin B$_{12}$ for Different Age Groups and During Pregnancy and Lactation

Population Group	Vitamin B$_{12}$ RDA (μg)
Infants	
0– 6 months	0.5
6–12 months	1.5
Children	
1– 3 years	2.0
7–10 years	3.0
Adolescents and adults (11+ years)	3.0
Pregnancy	+1.0
Lactation	+1.0

the release of energy. CoA is, therefore, essential to all cells that require energy.

No cases of pantothenic acid deficiency from natural causes have been documented. Laboratory-induced symptoms include fatigue, insomnia, nausea, intestinal disturbances, muscle cramps, and upper respiratory infections.

Requirements and Sources

The human body needs from 5 to 10 mg of pantothenic acid per day. Of the 10 to 20 mg consumed by most adults daily, about 50 percent is excreted in urine.

Although the vitamin is widely distributed in nature, the best food sources are liver and kidney, fish, egg yolk, fresh vegetables, yeast, and wheat bran. Fair amounts are also found in lean beef, skim milk, sweet potatoes, and molasses.

Since pantothenic acid is stable to moist heat, normal cooking temperatures destroy very little of the vitamin. Dry-heat cooking or processing, however, will cause a large loss. Canning of both animal and vegetable products is accompanied by a significant loss of the vitamin. The milling of grain results in about a 50 percent loss of pantothenic acid.

Biotin

Biotin occurs in many foods and is essential for humans. There are five different forms of this vitamin, which was discovered in 1935 and synthesized in 1942. Biotin in food may be free or bound to a protein. The bound form, found mostly in animal products, is fat soluble. Plants contain mainly the free form, which is water soluble.

Functions and Deficiency

Occurring as a coenzyme in the human body, biotin participates in many important biological reactions, including the oxidation of fatty acids and carbohydrates and the conversion of tryptophan to niacin. It plays a major role in adding a carbon unit to other chemicals.

Although spontaneous deficiency of biotin is uncommon, experimentally induced deficiency produces symptoms that include loss of appetite, nausea, muscle pain, depression, anemia, pallor, dermatitis, glossitis, and increased skin sensitivity. Dry, scaly skin, especially around the eyes, is characteristic of the disorder.

Food Sources

Normally associated with other B vitamins, biotin is found in greatest quantity in liver and kidney, egg yolk, milk, and yeast. Legumes, nuts, chocolate, and certain vegetables (cauliflower, for example) contain fair amounts of biotin. The vitamin is stable to heat used in the cooking and processing of food, but unstable to alkali and oxidation. It can be leached from food by water.

Intestinal bacteria synthesize biotin for our daily use. Certain antibiotics can inhibit bacterial activity and reduce the availability of this vitamin, possibly causing human deficiency.

FAT-SOLUBLE VITAMINS

Vitamins A, D, E, and K are the four remaining substances classified as vitamins. They are the currently known fat-soluble vitamins and have several characteristics in common: solubility medium, body storage capacity, body disposal route, body absorption, urgency of dietary intake, rapidity of symptom appearance if deficient, and chemical constituents. See Table 6-2. In certain other factors, including functions and sources, they differ considerably.

Vitamin A

Vitamin A, discovered in 1915 and synthesized in 1946, is almost colorless and is soluble in fat. Although relatively stable, the vitamin is sensitive to light and is destroyed by oxidation at high temperatures. Large doses of vitamin A can be toxic.

Food Sources

Plant foods that contain vitamin A include many that are orange or yellow; for example, carrots, peaches, and sweet potatoes.

Preformed vitamin A is found in kidney and liver, egg yolk, and butter. The provitamin A is found in green and yellow vegetables and fruits such as sweet potatoes, squash, carrots, apricots, cabbage, broccoli, spinach, collard, and other dark green vegetables. Provitamin A is β-carotene.

Functions

Vitamin A is currently believed to have four functions important to humans. These include biochemical reactions necessary to: (1) night vision, (2) bone growth, (3) nervous system development, (4) cell membrane metabolism and structure.

Deficiency

Dietary abundance and ample body storage make vitamin A deficiency uncommon in Western countries. See Table 6-10 for the 1980 RDA for vitamin A. The body stores enough vitamin A in the liver to last for several years without an external supply, and body storage must be depleted before deficiency symptoms appear. In many underdeveloped areas of the world, however, vitamin A deficiency is the major cause of blindness.

Vitamin A deficiency results mainly from a low-fat diet, malabsorption of fat, lack of pancreatic juice, gallbladder diseases, intestinal disorders, and loss of utilization of the vitamin.

Another cause of deficiency is when carotene (provitamin A) is not converted to vitamin A in the intestinal walls. Also associated with vitamin A deficiency are such disorders as liver cirrhosis, kidney disease, tuberculosis, pneumonia, and cancer.

Although such symptoms as arrested growth and abnormal bones and teeth have been attributed to vitamin A deficiency, the classic signs are disorders of the eyes and skin.

Eye Symptoms. Deterioration of the eyes begins with night blindness (see Figure 6-6). Lesions of the eye appear, and the patient becomes seriously ill. Total blindness in one or both eyes eventually will result if treatment is not administered before the advanced stage. Figures 6-7 and 6-8 show the classic eye lesions of vitamin A deficiency.

Skin Symptoms. In addition to pathological conditions in the eyes, vitamin A deficiency causes problems in the *epithelial cells* that make up

TABLE 6-10. 1980 RDA for Vitamin A for Different Age Groups and During Pregnancy and Lactation

Population Group	Vitamin A RDA	
	μg RE	IU
Infants		
0– 6 months	420	1,390
6–12 months	400	1,320
Children		
1– 3 years	400	1,320
7–10 years	700	2,310
Males (11+ years)	1,000	3,300
Females (11+ years)	800	2,640
Pregnancy	+200	+660
Lactation	+400	+1,320

the skin. The skin becomes dry, rough, and cracked. Skin lesions are usually related to combined deficiencies of vitamin A, linoleic acid, ascorbic acid, and other nutrients. Figure 6-9 shows the classic signs of skin lesions resulting from vitamin A deficiency.

Damage to mucous membranes is another symptom of vitamin A deficiency. Such damage can cause susceptibility to respiratory infections, gastrointestinal disorders, and genitourinary infections.

Toxicity

Large doses of vitamin A can cause toxic side effects. The higher the dose, the more rapid the onset of toxicity. Ingesting vitamin A in excess of 20,000 IU per day for 1 or 2 months is hazardous. However, a single large dose (200 times the RDA) also can produce toxicity. For example, some of the earliest documented cases of vitamin A poisoning involved the accidental ingestion of the livers of large animals such as polar bears and seals. Just 1 oz of polar bear liver contains 600,000 IU vitamin A.

Other cases of vitamin A poisoning have resulted from mothers giving their children vitamin A supplements (cod liver oil) in addition to the amount they ingested in foods. Some individuals precipitate a toxic reaction by consuming large doses of vitamin A in the belief that it will cure acne or improve their general health.

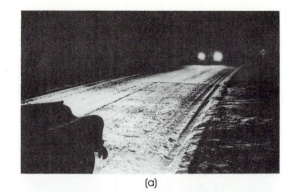

(a)

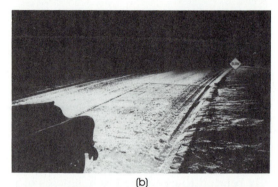

(b)

FIGURE 6-6. Night blindness caused by vitamin A deficiency. (Courtesy of the Upjohn Company) Night blindness is a useful and early diagnostic sign of vitamin A deficiency. This loss of visual acuity in dim light following exposure to bright light is illustrated here. Both the normal individual and the vitamin-A–deficient subject see the headlights of an approaching car as shown in (a). After the car has passed, the normal individual sees a wide stretch of road, as it appears in (b). The vitamin-A–deficient subject, whose view of the road is shown in (c), can barely see a few feet ahead and cannot see the road sign at all.

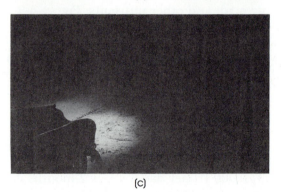

(c)

FIGURE 6-7. (a) Conjunctival xerosis in a 4-year-old child. (Courtesy of the World Health Organization and Dr. D. S. McLaren) (b) Bitot's spot in a 2-year-old child. (Courtesy of the World Health Organization and Dr. D. S. McLaren) (c) Bitot's spot with conjunctival xerosis. (Courtesy of the World Health Organization and Dr. A. Sommer) (d) Conjunctival and corneal xerosis. (Courtesy of the World Health Organization and Dr. A. Sommer) (e) Corneal ulceration with xerosis. (Courtesy of the World Health Organization and Dr. A Sommer) (f) Keratomalacia. (Courtesy of the World Health Organization and Dr. D. S. McLaren) (From *Control of Vitamin A Xerophthalmia* [Geneva: World Health Organization, 1982])

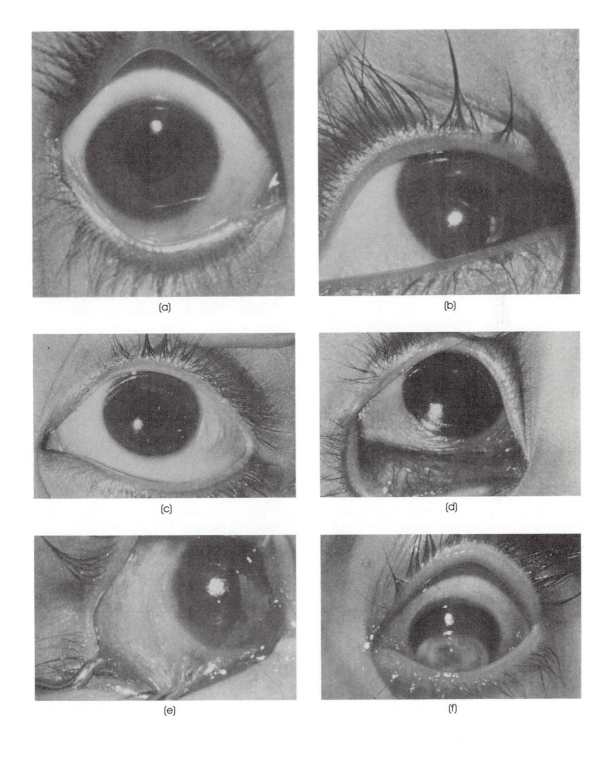

(a) (b)

(c) (d)

(e) (f)

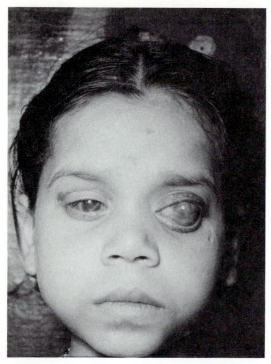

FIGURE 6-8. Blindness in one eye due to keratomalacia. (From G. Venkataswamy, *Israel J. Med. Sci.* 8 [1972]: 1190)

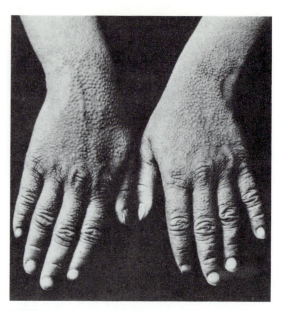

FIGURE 6-9. Classic skin lesions of follicular hyperkeratosis due to vitamin A deficiency, which resembles gooseflesh but can be distinguished from it because it does not disappear when the skin is rubbed. (From S. Dreizen, *Geriatrics* 29 [1974]: 97. By permission of *Geriatrics*)

The only therapy for vitamin A poisoning is to stop taking the vitamin, either through vitamin A–rich foods or tablets. Usually the symptoms are reversed within 72 hours, except in extreme cases.

Vitamin D

Vitamin D is fat soluble and very stable. It exists in both plant form (vitamin D_2) and animal form (vitamin D_3). Known as the "sunshine vitamin," vitamin D was discovered in 1918 and synthesized in 1936.

The body can transform ordinary metabolites into vitamin D with the help of sunlight. Ingested vitamin D, however, must be activated to be utilized.

Vitamin D is absorbed mainly in the duodenum and jejunum, from which it is transported to the blood. Fat malabsorption or gallbladder disease severely limit the amount of vitamin D absorbed.

TABLE 6-11. 1980 RDA for Vitamin D for Different Age Groups and During Pregnancy and Lactation

Population Group	Vitamin D RDA	
	μg	IU
Infants, children, adolescents (under 18 years old)	10	400
Adults		
19–22 years	7.5	300
23+ years	5	250
Pregnancy	+5	+250
Lactation	+5	+250

Functions and Requirements

The main function of vitamin D is to regulate the calcification of bones by increasing the absorption of calcium. From 30 to 35 percent of ingested calcium is absorbed if adequate amounts of vitamin D are present. Table 6-11 shows the 1980 RDA for vitamin D for different age groups.

Food Sources

Only animal products—milk, butter, eggs, and cod liver oil—are rich food sources of vitamin D. Most American diets supply less than half the vitamin required, thus making the fortification of foods, especially milk, an essential process.

Deficiency

Deficiency of vitamin D in adults is uncommon, since most people are exposed to the sun. There are documented cases of vitamin D deficiency, however. The most likely causes include: (1) decreased absorption of the vitamin due to a large reduction in fat, (2) strict vegetarianism, (3) premature birth, and (4) clinical stress.

Vitamin D deficiency can cause **rickets.** Once common throughout the world, rickets is now confined to underdeveloped countries.

Infantile Rickets. Rickets in newborns may be the result of the mother failing to eat an adequate amount of vitamin D. A baby born without rickets may develop the condition later because of an imbalanced diet or no exposure to sunlight.

Early symptoms of rickets in children include *tetany* (muscle spasms and rigidity) and convulsion. Skeletal deformities and growth retardation occur, such as bowleggedness or knock-knee. See Figure 6-10. Teeth erupt late and have defective enamel. Bone malformation is compounded by crawling, standing, and walking. Curvature of the spine (scoliosis) may result from sitting.

Adult Rickets. Adult rickets, which is called **osteomalacia,** is characterized by softening of the bones due to impaired mineralization. Intestinal malabsorption of fat is the usual cause of this disease.

Patients with osteomalacia suffer muscular weakness and back pain. Bones are highly sensitive to pressure. In severe cases, bones may be bent, and the patient develops a waddling gait.

Toxicity

Large amounts of vitamin D can be toxic, causing growth retardation, weight loss, loss of appetite, nausea, and failure to thrive in children. During World War II excess vitamin D fortification resulted in an intake of 3,000 to 4,000 IU of vitamin D per day among many children in England. Since then, a daily intake of less than 1,500 IU/day has been shown to be adequate for children.

Adult symptoms of toxicity include: (1) abnormal calcium metabolism; (2) kidney malfunction; (3) other clinical signs such as nausea, vomiting, and hypertension. Even more pronounced symptoms, such as severe hypercalcemia, drowsiness, and coma, can be induced if the serum calcium level exceeds 12 mg/100 mL blood.

Treatment for vitamin D poisoning includes correcting the fluid and electrolyte imbalance and administering cortisone continuously until the serum calcium level decreases and symptoms begin to subside.

Vitamin E

Vitamin E was discovered in 1922 and synthesized in 1937. Sometimes referred to as the "antisterility factor," this vitamin is known to be essential for about 20 animal species, including humans.

Although vitamin E deficiency is known to cause sterility in rats, no evidence has been found that links a lack of vitamin E to any abnormal reproductive capacity in humans. In fact, the role of this vitamin is still largely unknown. Research is presently being conducted to identify the role of vitamin E in clinical nutrition.

The body absorbs about 20 to 30 percent of ingested vitamin E, most

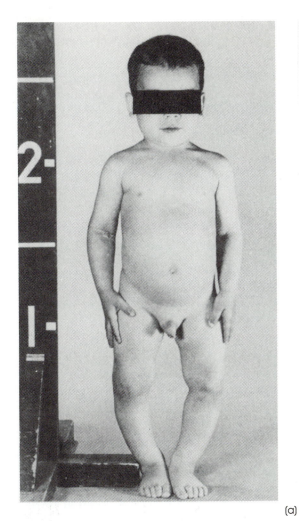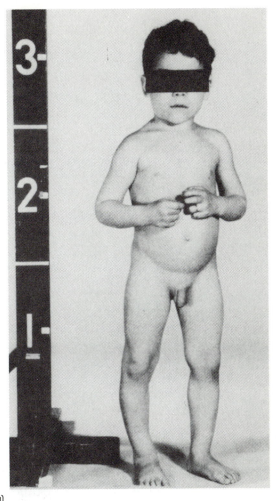

(a)

FIGURE 6-10. Classic signs of rickets. (a) Left: bowlegs in a 2½-year-old child with rickets. Right: normal bone development at 4½ years of age after treatment with vitamin D and phosphate. (Courtesy of Dr. C. R. Scriver. Reproduced with permission of *Nutrition Today* magazine, P.O. Box 1829, Annapolis, Maryland 21404 © September/October 1974) (b) Typical enamel hypoplasia in the permanent dentition of a child with hereditary vitamin-D-dependency rickets. (From G. Nikiforuk and D. Fraser, "The Etiology of Enamel Hypoplasia: A Unifying Concept," *J. Pediatr.* 98 [1981]: 888)

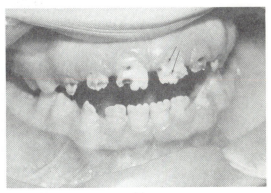

(b)

TABLE 6-12. 1980 RDA for Vitamin E for Different Age Groups and During Pregnancy and Lactation

Population Group	Vitamin E RDA (mg α-TE)*
Infants	
0– 6 months	3
6–12 months	4
Children	
1– 3 years	5
7–10 years	7
Males (11+ years)	10
Females (11+ years)	8
Pregnancy	+2
Lactation	+3

*α-Tocopherol equivalents.

of which enters the blood and attaches itself to lipoproteins. Major storage sites are muscle and fat tissue and the liver. Most of the excess is excreted in the urine.

Functions and Requirements

Five major roles have been identified for vitamin E in animals and plants. First, it protects certain substances from oxidation. Since aging may be due to the oxidation of cells, vitamin E may be related to the process of aging.

Second, vitamin E assists with biochemical processes within the respiratory chain. Third, vitamin E is necessary for synthesizing other essential body substances.

Fourth, vitamin E is essential in synthesis of heme, a component of hemoglobin. Finally, vitamin E is required for the maintenance of cell membranes. See Table 6-12 for the 1980 RDA for vitamin E (tocopherol) for different age groups.

Deficiency

Most healthy adults do not develop vitamin E deficiency. The condition can occur, however, in individuals with certain clinical disorders, such as gallbladder disease, and in premature infants.

Cystic fibrosis in a child is frequently associated with vitamin E deficiency. Premature infants develop such symptoms as anemia, edema, skin lesions, and the destruction (hemolysis) of red blood cells. The major symptom in adults is increased hemolysis.

Food Sources

Vegetable oils probably contain the greatest concentration of vitamin E. Ordinary cooking temperatures cause very little vitamin E loss, but boiling or frying may destroy the small amount in cooking oil.

Whole grains, especially wheat germ, contain ample amounts of vitamin E. Without refrigeration, most of the vitamin will be destroyed by oxidation.

Toxicity

Though vitamin E seems to have a low toxicity, large amounts can interfere with the body's utilization of both vitamins A and K. The requirements of these vitamins are increased when large amounts of vitamin E are ingested. A tendency toward bleeding and intestinal disturbances also may develop.

Vitamin K

Vitamin K was discovered in 1934 and synthesized in 1949. Vitamin K is stable to heat and reducing agents but sensitive to acid, alkali, alcohol, light, and oxidizing agents. Various forms of the vitamin are shown in Table 6-13, which also lists their usage under different clinical conditions.

Absorption of vitamin K requires fat. Normally only about 10 percent of ingested vitamin K is absorbed in the upper part of the intestinal tract. Certain clinical conditions such as jaundice, pancreatic disorder, and liver failure interfere with its absorption. Unused vitamin K is excreted in the bile and urine.

Functions

The primary role of vitamin K is in the clotting of blood. It is currently believed that vitamin K is directly or indirectly responsible for the liver synthesis of prothrombin, one of the many body agents responsible for blood clotting.

TABLE 6-13. Some Characteristics of Vitamin K

Natural or Synthetic*	Name†	Solubility	Natural Analogue	Routes of Administration	Clinical Usage	Safety
Natural (from green plants, e.g., alfalfa)	Vitamin K₁ (phyllo-quinone)	Fat soluble	None	Oral (not recommended for infants); intravenous or subcutaneous injection	Pregnancy; surgery; countering anticoagulants. (see text)	Acceptable in appropriate doses.
Natural (from bacteria)	Vitamin K₂ (mena-quinone)	Fat soluble	None	Same as above	Same as above	Same as above
Synthetic	Menadione (formerly vitamin K₃)	Fat soluble	Mena-quinone	Intramuscular or subcutaneous injection	Hemorrhage of infancy and labor; obstructive jaundice	Relatively safe for adults; safe for infants more than a few weeks old if recommended doses are complied with. Effects of large doses in infants: hemolytic anemia, hyper-bilirubinemia, kernicterus.
Synthetic	Mephyton Konakion	Water miscible	Phyllo-quinone	Oral; intramuscular, intravenous, or subcutaneous injection	Newborn infants	Acceptable in appropriate doses.
Synthetic	Mono-Kay	Water miscible	Phyllo-quinone	Same as above	Same as above	Same as above

*Vitamin K is also located in purified fish meal.
†Other analogues not mentioned are Hykinone, Synkavite, and Kappadione of menaquinone and menadione.

Sources

Green and yellow vegetables and synthesis in the colon usually supply our required vitamin K. Drugs such as aspirin and antibiotics can inhibit or reduce synthesis by intestinal bacteria. No RDA has been established for this vitamin.

Deficiency

Newborns fed only milk with no chemical supplement can become vitamin K deficient, resulting in bleeding or long blood clotting time. Children who suffer starvation, diarrhea, cystic fibrosis, malabsorption, or exposure to antibiotics may develop vitamin K deficiency.

Vitamin K deficiency in a normal adult is uncommon, although the prolonged use of anticoagulants can result in a deficiency and cause bleeding problems.

Toxicity

Large doses of vitamin K are toxic under various circumstances. In infants, any amount of the vitamin in excess of 10 mg is likely to cause a toxic reaction. If the infant is premature and deficient in vitamin E, the toxic effects of vitamin K are increased.

Adults can tolerate 10 to 40 mg for several weeks without suffering ill effects, although vomiting may be precipitated if the dosage is larger. Dosages of one or more grams may cause increased excretion of albumin and porphyrin.

STUDY QUESTIONS

1. What is a vitamin? How do vitamins differ from other organic compounds?
2. What three methods are used in diagnosing vitamin deficiency?
3. Describe the functions of vitamin C and symptoms of its deficiency.
4. What condition is associated with moderate to severe vitamin B_1 deficiency?
5. Describe the symptoms of vitamin B_2 deficiency.
6. What factors may cause vitamin B_6 deficiency?
7. What deficiency disease is classically characterized by the 4 D's? What are they?
8. What is an intrinsic factor?
9. Is pantothenic acid deficiency common? Why?

10. What characteristics do vitamins A, D, E, and K have in common?
11. Summarize the symptoms of vitamin A deficiency.
12. What is the chief function of vitamin D? Which foods contain this vitamin? What condition is created by its deficiency?
13. What is known about the role of vitamin E in human health? What are the richest food sources of this vitamin?
14. Is vitamin K deficiency more common in breast-fed or formula-fed infants? What problem may this deficiency cause?

REFERENCES

Bieri, J. G., and Farrell, P. M. 1976. Vitamin E. *Vit. Horm.* 34:31.

Darby, W. J., et al. 1975. Niacin. *Nutr. Rev.* 33:289.

Gubler, C. J., et al., eds. 1976. *Thiamine.* N. Y.: Wiley-Interscience.

National Research Council. 1980. *Recommended daily dietary allowances.* FNB/NRC, National Academy of Sciences.

Norman, A. W. 1979. *Vitamin D.* New York: Academic Press.

Nutrition Review. 1984. *Present knowledge in nutrition,* 5th ed. Washington, D. C.: The Nutrition Foundation.

Phelps, D. L. 1979. Vitamin E: where do we stand? *Pediatrics* 63:933.

Rivlin, R. S. 1975. *Riboflavin.* New York: Plenum Press.

Srikanitia, S. G. 1975. Human vitamin A deficiency. *World Rev. Nutr. Dietet.* 20:184.

7   MINERALS

The **inorganic elements** known as **minerals** are among the body's essential nutrients. When we eat vegetables (such as cabbage, lettuce, and spinach) and meat (beef, chicken) we take in minerals. The plants have obtained these substances from the soil, and the beef cattle and chickens have been fed plant feeds. Few of the inorganic elements we consume exist alone but instead are bound with organic substances.

Sometimes the term **ash** is used in place of minerals. Ash actually refers to the residue left after a substance has been oxidized (or burned). This residue contains the minerals originally present in the substance.

CLASSIFICATION AND FUNCTIONS

Mineral elements make up about 4 percent of our body weight. These elements are divided into two groups: **macroelements,** which are needed in relatively large amounts; and **microelements,** which are needed in very small amounts. Table 7-1 shows their classification and approximate daily body need. Figure 7-1 shows the approximate distribution of organic and inorganic elements in the body.

Despite the fact that they are far outweighed by organic elements, mineral elements serve two important purposes for the body. First, minerals act as structural components of parts of the body, as shown in Table 7-2. Second, minerals regulate normal body functions, including: (1) transmission of nerve impulses, (2) control of acid-base balance, (3) proper distribution of fluid and osmotic pressure, (4) digestion of certain foods, (5) normal muscle contractions, (6) the triggering of important chemical and biological reactions.

TABLE 7-1. Approximate Distribution of Mineral Elements in the Body*

Elements	% of Body Weight	Amount Needed in the Daily Diet (mg/day/element)
Macroelements (calcium, phosphorus, potassium, sodium, sulfur, magnesium, chlorine)	3.2–3.8	100+
Microelements (iron, copper, cobalt, zinc, manganese, iodine, molybdenum, selenium, fluorine, chromium)	less than 0.1	0.05–5

*Although RDAs have not been established for sodium, potassium, chloride, copper, manganese, fluoride, chromium, selenium, and molybdenum, the National Academy of Sciences has estimated the safe and adequate daily dietary intakes of these elements.

MACROELEMENTS

Those mineral elements needed in relatively large amounts by the body are sodium, potassium, calcium, phosphorus, magnesium, chlorine, and sulfur. Found primarily in fruits and vegetables, sodium, potassium, calcium, and magnesium are basic, or alkaline, in solution. Phosphorus, chlorine, and sulfur are acid in solution and more commonly found in protein foods (other than milk) and cereal products. Chapter 22 discusses the effects of acid- and alkaline-forming foods on body chemistry.

Sodium

Sodium may be obtained from many foods but is most familiar to us as sodium chloride, or table salt. As indicated in Table 7-3, the body loses from 40 to 220 mg of sodium a day. Although the exact amount needed per day is uncertain, a daily intake of 500 mg (0.5 g) should be sufficient for most adults. Individual need varies according to occupation, climate, and area of residence, since these factors contribute to perspiration and resulting sodium loss. It is estimated that many adults eat from 3 to 7 g of sodium per day, or roughly 5 to 15 times more than they need.

Among the important functions of sodium are: (1) maintaining proper osmotic pressure and fluid balance; (2) maintaining pH or acid-base balance; (3) regulating cell permeability, muscle function, and the transmission of nerve impulses; (4) absorbing and transporting certain nutrients.

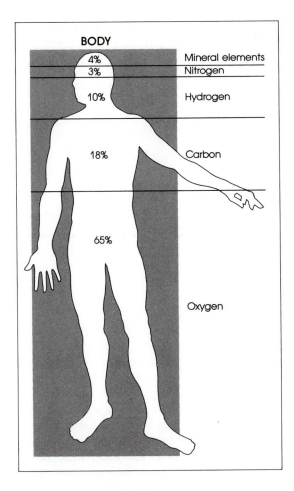

FIGURE 7-1. Approximate distribution of organic and in-organic elements in the body.

TABLE 7-2. Mineral Elements that are Components of Important Body Structures

Element(s)	Chemical Substance(s)	Body Structures
Calcium, phosphorus, magnesium	Hydroxyapatite	Teeth, bones
Sulfur	Cystine, cysteine, methionine	Protein of skin, hair, nails
Iron	Hemoglobin, myoglobin	Blood components
Iron, copper	Cofactors of enzymes	Enzyme complexes
Iodine	Thyroxine	Hormone of thyroid gland
Cobalt	Cobalamin	Water-soluble vitamin B_{12}

TABLE 7-3. Approximate Daily Loss of Sodium

Source of Loss	Amount (mg)
Skin	
Perspiration	15–25
Desquamation (sloughing of skin), hair loss	10–25
Urine	5–40
Stool	10–130
Menstrual fluid	trace
Approximate daily loss of sodium	40–220

Sodium balance in the body is rigidly controlled by the hormonal and kidney (renal) systems. The body can adapt to a wide range of sodium intake by varying the excretion of sodium. However, certain clinical conditions may lead to body sodium excess or deficiency. These conditions include heart or kidney failure (see Chapters 17 and 19), adrenal insufficiency, and diarrhea or vomiting.

As already indicated, table salt is a major source of sodium in the American diet. Sodium also occurs naturally in other foods, especially animal products. The sodium content of drinking water varies, with soft water containing more sodium than hard water. Table 7-4 lists the sodium content of some common foods. More information on the sodium content of food is presented in Chapters 17 and 19.

Potassium

Potassium, also an essential element, occurs in a wide variety of foods. A normal American diet provides 2 to 5 g of potassium, but the exact daily need of the body is unknown. Washing foods with water during preparation causes some potassium to be lost. Table 7-5 presents the potassium content of some common foods.

Some major body functions in which potassium is involved are: (1) fluid distribution and osmotic pressure balance in the different body compartments, (2) transmission of nerve impulses, (3) maintenance of body acid-base balance, (4) catalyzing of major chemical and biological reactions in the body, (5) normal muscular relaxation, (6) regulation of the release of insulin from the pancreas.

Although the kidney can excrete any excess intake of potassium, it is

TABLE 7-4. Sodium Content of Representative Foods*

Food	Serving Size	Sodium (mg)
Cheese, cheddar	1 oz	168
Ice cream, 10% fat	1 c	84
Milk, whole, fluid	1 c	122
Egg, whole, raw, large	1	61
Butter or margarine	1 T	140
Beef, ground	1 c	55
Chicken, fried	1¾ oz	34
Pork, roasted	4½ oz	74
Turkey	3 oz	111
Apples	1	1
Juice, cranberry, cocktail	1 c	3
Raisins, seedless	1 c	39
Bread, white	1 sl	142
Cake, no icing	1 in³	12
Beans, dry	1 c	34
Peanut butter	1 T	97
Jam or preserves	1 T	2
Sugar, white, granulated	1 c	2
Asparagus, cooked	1 c	1
Potato, baked, no skin	1	6
Squash or zucchini, cooked, drained	1 c	2
Brewer's yeast, dried	1 T	10
Baking powder, sodium aluminum sulfate	1 T	1,205
Soy sauce	1 fl oz	2,666

*Adapted from *Nutritive Value of American Foods*, Agriculture Handbook No. 456 (Washington, D.C.: U.S. Department of Agriculture, 1975).

unable to store potassium when the body is deficient. For example, if the body is deprived of potassium, the kidney still excretes between 100 and 500 mg per day. Only a small amount of potassium is excreted in the sweat and stool; urine is the major disposal route.

Few normal people have a dietary deficiency of potassium. However, clinical conditions such as long-term intravenous feeding and malnutrition can result in potassium deficiency.

Calcium

Most (99 percent) of the adult body's 1,200 g of calcium exists in salt forms, providing hardness to bones and teeth. The remaining 1 percent, or 10 to 12 g, of body calcium is distributed in the compartments of the body. Plasma calcium is kept within a narrow range. Bone serves as a reservoir that stores and releases calcium to the blood to maintain this equilibrium.

TABLE 7-5. Potassium Content of Representative Foods*

Food	Serving Size	Potassium (mg)
Cottage cheese, small curd	1 c	179
Milk, fluid, whole	1 c	301
Ice cream, regular	1 c	313
Egg, raw, large	1	65
Apricots, dried, large	10 halves	470
Avocado	1	1,303
Grapefruit, raw	1	265
Mayonnaise, commercial, regular	1 T	5
Beef, round steak	3 oz	272
Ham, baked, some fat	3 oz	199
Salmon, fresh, baked	1 oz	126
Bread, cracked wheat	1 sl	34
Cashew nuts, roasted in oil	1 oz	132
Peanuts, roasted, salted	1 oz	191
Beans, navy, cooked, drained	1 c	790
Sugar, brown, packed	1 c	757
Molasses, cane, light	1 T	183
Broccoli, fresh, cooked, drained	1 c	414
Carrots, raw, whole	1	246
Potato, baked in skin	1	782
Onion, mature, raw	1 T	16
Brewer's yeast, dry, debittered	1 T	152
Soy sauce	1 T	66

*Adapted from *Nutritive Value of American Foods*, Agriculture Handbook No. 456 (Washington, D.C.: U.S. Department of Agriculture, 1975).

Functions

The major functions of calcium are: (1) serving as a component of bone and teeth, (2) participating in the blood clotting process, (3) assisting in the transmission of messages (nerve impulses) through the nervous system, (4) regulating the contraction and relaxation of muscle fibers, (5) protecting the body against absorption of certain radioactive chemicals, (6) maintaining proper heart muscle functioning, and (7) activating certain enzymes.

For normal adults the current recommended daily intake is 800 mg, although that amount is subject to controversy. Pregnant and nursing mothers need more; calcium needs according to age group are listed in the appendix.

TABLE 7-6. Calcium Content of Some Common Foods*

Food	Serving Size	Calcium (mg)
Sardines	1 oz	115
Cheese, cheddar	1 oz	220
Biscuit, 2" diam	1	40
Beans, dry, cooked	½ c	45
Milk, whole	1 c	290
Milk, skim, powdered, dry	½ c	350
Orange, medium size	1	40
Broccoli	½ c	90
Collards	½ c	190
Turnip greens	½ c	185
Artichokes	½ c	50
Kale	½ c	190
Custard, baked	⅓ c	110
Ice cream	½ c	110
Sherbet	⅓ c	25

*Adapted from *Nutritive Value of Foods*, Home and Garden Bulletin No. 72 (Washington, D.C.: U.S. Department of Agriculture, 1981).

Food Sources and Absorption

As the richest source of calcium, cow's milk contains four times more calcium than breast milk does. Another excellent source of calcium is canned fish, especially those with dissolved bones. Good sources of calcium are whole grains, nuts, legumes, and leafy vegetables. Table 7-6 provides the calcium content of some common foods.

The amount of calcium available to the body is determined largely by the amount absorbed. Factors or conditions that may increase the absorption of calcium include: (1) adequate vitamin D intake; (2) the presence of lactose; (3) a balance of dietary calcium and phosphorus in the ratio of 1:1; (4) conditions such as pregnancy, growing years, bone fractures, and starvation; and (5) acidic conditions that may promote the solubility of calcium.

On the other hand, certain factors may decrease the absorption of calcium. These include: (1) excess dietary roughage or fiber; (2) a dietary calcium to phosphorus ratio that deviates from 1:1; (3) excessive use of laxatives; (4) diarrhea; (5) an excessive amount of magnesium, albumin, or iron; (6) an alkaline intestinal medium; (7) lack of physical activity.

An eighth factor that may decrease absorption of calcium is excessive consumption of oxalic and phytic acid in the diet. **Oxalic acid** occurs in some vegetables such as chard and spinach. The ingestion of a small quantity of oxalic acid poses no problem, but excess consumption may interfere with calcium absorption. **Phytic acid,** found in the outer husks of cereals, also can make calcium unavailable for absorption. In countries where unleavened bread is a staple, calcium deficiency is a problem. The leavening process decreases phytic acid availability.

Deficiency or Excess

A number of clinical disorders may result from calcium deficiency. Among them are rickets, osteoporosis, and tetany. **Hypercalcemia,** on the other hand, is excess calcium in the blood.

In infancy and childhood, rickets may result from a lack of dietary calcium (vitamin D deficiency and/or phosphorus imbalance also may produce the disorder). The growth and structure of teeth also may be affected (see Chapter 6).

In adults, nutritional **osteomalacia,** or adult rickets, is a disorder characterized by a softening of the bone. The total amount of bone remains unchanged. This condition may be caused by any circumstance that reduces the absorption of calcium—inadequate calcium intake, deficiency of vitamin D, or inappropriate intake of phosphorus.

Osteoporosis is a clinical disorder in which the total quantity of bone is reduced. Aging, hormonal imbalance, lifetime calcium deficit, overconsumption of phosphorus, and limited exercise also are believed to contribute to osteoporosis. Older people, especially women, are susceptible to the disease. Treatment includes administration of oral calcium salt, estrogen, and sodium fluoride (see Chapter 13).

Even when dietary intake of calcium is adequate, a *secondary deficiency* may result from other disorders. These include renal malfunction, malabsorption, dietary magnesium deficiency, and immobilization. A secondary deficiency of calcium also results in bone disorders.

Tetany results from low blood calcium, or **hypocalcemia,** which may be preceded by hypoproteinemia, hypoparathyroidism, vitamin D deficiency, defective calcium absorption, or magnesium deficiency. In addition to nervous excitability, muscular twitching and contractions, instability, confusion, uncontrolled seizures, cramps, and convulsions, tetany may cause hair loss and skin dryness.

Emergency treatment is required when tetany occurs, usually with calcium glucomate given intravenously. Acute hypocalcemia resulting from hypoparathyroidism requires restriction of dietary phosphorus and, in some cases, the administration of parathyroid extract and vitamins. Long-term management to increase intestinal absorption of calcium is required for patients with chronic hypoglycemia.

Among the causes of **hypercalcemia,** an excessive level of calcium in the blood, are: Cancer, excess intake of vitamin D, hyperparathyroidism, thyroid disease, and hypophosphatemia. Symptoms of high blood calcium include nausea, vomiting, anorexia, abdominal pain, constipation, increased thirst and urination, mental disorder, dullness, calcium stones, and soft-tissue calcification. Coma, even death, may result from hypercalcemia. Rehydration is the major treatment, accompanied by drugs to lower blood calcium. An ongoing calcium-restricted diet is recommended.

Phosphorus

The body contains approximately 600 to 700 g of phosphorus, 80 to 90 percent of which is concentrated in the bones and teeth. The rest is distributed in various compartments of the body.

Functions

The major functions of phosphorus are: (1) formation and maintenance of bones and teeth; (2) regulation of body acid-base balance; (3) control of energy; (4) serving as a structural component of nucleic acid, enzymes, and certain lipids; (5) regulation of hormonal activities; and (6) participation in nutrient metabolism, including nutrient absorption, transportation, and utilization.

Food Sources and Deficiency

The adult RDA for phosphorus is 800 mg/day. Phosphorus deficiency in humans is rare because this nutrient occurs so widely in foods. Most protein foods are rich in phosphorus, with beef, poultry, and fish the major sources in the American diet. However, drugs such as antacids may lead to phosphorus deficiency by interfering with phosphorus absorption. Symptoms of depletion include anorexia, fatigue, and bone demineralization.

Calcium:Phosphorus Relationships

Calcium and phosphorus are similar in many aspects, including the following: (1) important in the development of bone and teeth; (2) regulated by the parathyroid gland; (3) presence of vitamin D increases absorption; (4) bones store and release these elements; (5) overall absorption of both elements is similarly regulated. Table 7-7 shows the body distribution of calcium and phosphorus.

Most authorities suggest that for the best absorption levels of both elements the ideal ratio of calcium:phosphorus (Ca:P) is 1:1. There is some evidence, however, that the typical American diet may pro-

TABLE 7-7. Approximate Body Distribution of Calcium and Phosphorus

	% of Body Content		
Mineral	Bones, teeth	Soft tissues, organs	Blood, extra-cellular tissues
Calcium	99	trace	1
Phosphorus	80	19	1

TABLE 7-8. Ratios of Phosphorus to Calcium Contents of Natural Food Products

Food	Phosphorus: Calcium Ratio
Meats, poultry, fish	15–20:1
Organ meats, such as liver	25–50:1
Eggs, grains, nuts, dry beans, peas, lentils	3–10:1
Milk, natural cheese, green vegetables	0.1–0.8:1

vide more phosphorus than calcium. One reason for a low Ca:P ratio is that phosphorus is naturally more abundant than calcium in foods; also, phosphorus is frequently added as an additive during food processing. Table 7-8 shows the calcium:phosphorus ratio of some common types of natural foods. Table 7-9 shows the calcium and phosphorus content of common natural and processed foods (more examples may be obtained from the appendix). At present no conclusions can be made about whether Americans eat more phosphorus than is necessary and desirable.

Magnesium

Another macroelement with close relationships to calcium is magnesium. Of the 20 to 30 g of magnesium in the body, 10 percent is present on the bone surface, 30 percent is bound with phosphate, and about 50 to 60 percent occurs as a component of bones and teeth.

Functions

Magnesium is involved in several important functions in the body. These include: (1) muscular relaxation, a function opposite to that of calcium; (2) protein synthesis; (3) cellular respiration; (4) catalyzing some important chemical and biological reactions involving ATP and ADP (see Chapter 8).

Food Sources and Absorption

The latest RDA indicates that the adult requirement is 300 to 350 mg per day. The average American diet contains about 120 mg per 1,000 kcal, which is believed to satisfy the body's need. As a component of chlorophyll, magnesium is contained in green leafy vegetables as well as

TABLE 7-9. Calcium and Phosphorus Content of Representative Foods*

Food	Serving Size	Calcium (mg)	Phosphorus (mg)
Dairy products			
Milk, whole	1 c	285	227
Milk, skim	1 c	296	233
Meat and equivalents			
Beef, rib roast	3 oz	8	158
Frankfurter	1	4	76
Luncheon meat	½ lb	25	377
Roast chicken, light meat	½ lb	25	617
Grain and equivalents			
Bread, enriched, white	1 sl	26	28
Rice, white, enriched, cooked	1 c	21	57
Potatoes, french fried	10 strips	5	39
Fruits			
Grapefruit, medium size	1	16	16
Apple	1	10	15
Figs dried, small	2	40	25
Vegetables			
Beans, green, cooked	½ c	63	46
Corn, sweet, yellow, fresh	½ c	2	75
Peppers, sweet, raw, green, chopped	½ c	5	15
Nuts			
Almonds, roasted	1 oz	67	143
Peanuts, roasted, salted	1 oz	20	115
Miscellaneous			
Shake, vanilla, McDonald's	1	126	105
Soft drink	8 oz	0	500
Pie, baked, sector	1	3	7
Pretzels, thin	10	13	79

*Adapted from *Nutritive Value of Foods*, Home and Garden Bulletin No. 72 (Washington, D.C.: U.S. Department of Agriculture, 1981).

many other foods. Although milk provides an adequate amount of magnesium for both bottle- and breast-fed infants, milk is a poor source for adults. Table 7-10 presents the magnesium content of some common foods.

Certain dietary factors affect our absorption of magnesium, with the result that only 40 to 50 percent of ingested magnesium is absorbed. As the amount of magnesium consumed increases, the amount absorbed decreases. Calcium and magnesium absorption is competitive and mutually exclusive—that is, if a large amount of magnesium is present, less calcium is absorbed. The phytic and oxalic acids present in fruits and vegetables also can reduce the absorption of magnesium.

TABLE 7-10. Magnesium Content of Some Common Foods*

Food	Serving Size	Magnesium (mg)
Dairy products		
Milk, whole, fluid	1 c	30
Milk, skim	1 c	3
Cheese, cheddar	1 oz	8
Ice cream, vanilla, plain	½ c	10
Eggs		
Whole, hard boiled, large	1	6
Grain products		
Bread, white, enriched	1 sl	5
Granola, ready-to-eat	½ c	60
Oatmeal	½ c	30
Noodles	⅔ c	25
Rice, white, cooked	⅔ c	10
Meat, fish, poultry		
Beef, chuck roast	3 oz	20
Chicken, fried, breast	½	10
Cod, steak, sauteed	4 oz	30
Pork chop, medium size	1	15
Lobster, Northern, meat	⅔ c	20
Fruits		
Apple, medium size	1	10
Avocado	½	55
Cherries, raw, sweet	10	10
Plum, raw, medium size	1	6
Strawberries, whole, fresh	⅔ c	12
Vegetables		
Asparagus, fresh	½ c	15
Beans, lima, boiled	½ c	55
Cauliflower, cooked	½ c	8
Mushrooms, raw	½ c	5

*Data have been adapted from published results of a number of reports.

Deficiency

Magnesium deficiency produces characteristic symptoms such as: (1) tetany similar to that of hypocalcemia; (2) loss of muscular control; (3) nervousness, irritability, and tremors sometimes leading to confusion; (4) induction of calcium deficiency; (5) other changes affecting the cardiovascular and renal systems.

Because the bone surface stores and releases magnesium, severe deficiency is uncommon. The kidney tubules offer additional protection through their ability to reabsorb magnesium. However, it is suspected that the average American may consume a barely adequate amount of the element. Magnesium deficiency may occur in individuals under stress or receiving medications. A person deprived of magnesium for 1 to 3 months may experience severe deficiency. The deficiency is magnified by a diet high in calcium or fluoride, since both can increase the excretion of magnesium.

Also, a number of clinical situations can produce magnesium deficiency, such as: (1) gastrointestinal disorders, including malabsorption, steatorrhea, vomiting, nausea, and diarrhea; (2) drugs, including diuretics; (3) alcoholism; (4) kwashiorkor, a deficiency disease related to a lack of protein in severely malnourished infants and children; (5) long-term parenteral feeding.

Chlorine

Of the 100 g of chlorine contained in the body, most exists in the form of chloride, as in sodium chloride. Extracellular fluid contains most of the chloride. The functions of chloride in the body are: (1) assisting in maintaining fluid, electrolyte, acid-base, and osmotic pressure balance in the compartments of the body; (2) serving as a component of hydrochloric acid in the stomach; (3) regulating certain enzyme activities; (4) facilitating the transfer of carbon dioxide from blood to the lungs.

Because all foods contain some chloride, especially fruits and vegetables, and because table salt contains sodium chloride, deficiency of chlorine is rare. In addition, the kidney excretes and reabsorbs the chloride ion. Although chloride is an essential element, the human requirement for it is unknown.

Some clinical conditions can produce chlorine deficiency. These include vomiting, diarrhea, fistula (artificial) drainage of the intestinal system, alkalosis, and excessive perspiration.

Sulfur

As a component of amino acids (methionine and cystine), sulfur is found in nucleic acids and all animal protein. It is present in every cell. **Methionine** and **cystine** are especially abundant in hair, skin, and nails. In the inorganic form, sulfur exists in the form of sulfate in fruits and vegetables.

Some major functions of sulfur in the body are: (1) storage and release of energy; (2) serving as a structural component of nucleic acid and vitamins (thiamine, biotin, and pantothenic and lipotic acids); (3) promotion of certain enzyme reactions; (4) serving as a component of body substances needed for the detoxification process; (5) collagen synthesis; (6) promotion of blood clotting.

The human requirement for this element is unknown, and no known deficiency symptoms have been associated with a reduced intake of sulfur.

MICROELEMENTS

The elements iron, iodine, fluorine, copper, and other trace elements exist in much smaller quantities in the human body than the macroelements. Nevertheless, their presence in these small amounts is essential to body structures and processes.

Iron

The importance of iron in human nutrition cannot be overemphasized. Despite extensive research and public health efforts, iron deficiency remains a serious problem among certain population groups. The following discussion reviews the functions and distribution of iron in the body, requirements of different population groups, factors influencing the absorption of iron, food sources of iron, symptoms of and treatment for iron depletion, iron supplements, and iron toxicity.

Body Functions and Distribution

Iron serves two major functions in the body. First, iron is involved in cellular respiration. As part of **hemoglobin** and myoglobin, iron makes possible the transportation of oxygen and carbon dioxide to and from the cells. Second, iron regulates many important biological and chemical reactions in the body. Many reactions would not be possible without the presence of iron. For example, iron is needed to synthesize vitamins, purines, and antibodies.

About 70 percent of the body's 3 to 5 g of iron is in the blood, with most of the remainder in the liver, spleen, bone marrow, and intestine. Iron is found in every living cell, usually in combination with some form of protein:

> *Blood:* For respiration process, **hemoglobin**
> For transport purposes, **transferrin**
> *Organs:* For storage purposes, **ferritin**

The overall body content of iron depends on the amount absorbed. Although the body cannot regulate excretion of iron, there are other very efficient release and storage mechanisms to retain iron. All iron-containing substances are recycled in the body, and all iron released from body catabolism is also recycled and for the most part retained.

TABLE 7-11. Approximate Iron Requirements of Certain Population Groups

Population Group	Iron Needed Each Day (mg)				
	Obligatory loss	Loss from menstruation	Need for growth	Need for pregnancy	Total need
Postmenopausal females and adult males	0.7–1.0	0	0	0	0.7–1.0
Menstruating females	0.7–1.0	0.5–1.0	0	0	1.2–2.0
Pregnant females, over 17 years	0.7–1.0	0	0	1.0–2.0	1.7–3.0
Nonpregnant females 12–17-year-old	0.7–1.0	0.5–1.0	0.4–0.8	0	1.6–2.8
Pregnant females 12–17-year-old	0.7–1.0	0	0.4–0.8	1.0–2.0	2.1–3.8
0–3-year-olds	0.2–0.3	0	0.3–0.6	0	0.5–0.9
3–10-year-olds	0.3–0.4	0	0.4–0.5	0	0.7–0.9
10–17-year-olds*	0.5–0.8	0	0.1–0.9	0	0.6–1.7
Nursing mothers	0.7–1.0	0–1.0	0.5–1.0[†]	0	1.2–2.0

*Excluding 12 to 17-year-old females.
[†]Amount in milk for infant growth.

Requirements of Different Population Groups

A normal blood profile requires a certain amount of iron. Of the approximately 5 L of blood in the body, there are about 15 g hemoglobin per 100 mL blood in the adult male and about 13.6 g in the female.

Iron is lost daily in skin, hair, feces, urine, nails, intestinal linings, and sweat. Additional iron is lost in menstrual fluids. An average iron loss is from 0.7 to 1 mg per day, while menstruation accounts for an additional loss of 0.5 to 1 mg. Children and infants need extra iron to support their growth.

Table 7-11 gives the iron requirements of different population groups. More information is presented in the appendix.

Absorption Rate

The absorption of iron is accomplished primarily in the first part of the small intestine, though the stomach and the entire small intestine also permit absorption. Only about 2 to 10 percent of the 10 to 20 g of iron ingested in the typical American diet is absorbed within 5 to 24 hours.

Certain needs of the body—growth, iron deficiency, pregnancy, surgery, and hemorrhage—may increase this absorption rate. Under such stressful circumstances, from 50 to 60 percent of the ingested iron may be absorbed.

Some foods increase iron absorption. For example, meat and citrus fruits eaten together improve iron absorption. From 30 to 40 percent of the iron in meat is absorbed; ascorbic acid (vitamin C) in large amounts facilitates iron absorption. Amino acids such as methionine and cystine also enhance absorption.

Other foods reduce the absorption of iron. Only 5 to 10 percent of the iron in egg yolk is absorbed. Fruits and vegetables, because of their bulk, interfere with iron absorption. Both phytic acid, found in oatmeal and other whole grain cereals, and oxalic acid in vegetables such as rhubarb and spinach reduce absorption. In general, the more iron consumed at one time, the less absorbed. Antacids also can hinder the absorption of iron.

Food Sources

Iron intake must be considerably higher than iron needs, since only a portion of the iron ingested is actually absorbed. Nevertheless, the amount of iron needed daily is relatively small.

The 6 mg of iron per 1,000 kcal in the average American diet provides an adequate amount for most adult males. However, the 15 to 20 mg of iron needed by adult women would require a consumption of 3,000 kcal or more per day.

Table 7-12 lists the iron content of some representative foods. However, no food is a significant source of iron unless it is consumed in large enough amounts and the iron it contains is available for absorption. Other factors can affect the absorption and availability of iron, such as whether the food is eaten alone and the methods used in its preparation.

Liver is one of the richest sources of iron, while milk and milk products are the lowest. Vegetables have 2 to 4 times more iron than fruits and juices. Good sources of iron are potatoes and the stalks and leaves of green vegetables. Most bread and flour and some prepared and dry cereals have high concentrations of iron because of enrichment. Such products as raisins, blackstrap molasses, oysters, clams, and cocoa have high iron contents but are usually consumed in small quantities.

Iron Depletion Symptoms and Treatment

Anemia, the deficiency of oxygen-carrying components in the blood, is a severe disorder. Simple iron deficiency does not necessarily lead to anemia. Table 7-13 describes the different stages of iron depletion and indicates how each stage is diagnosed. Characteristic symptoms include:

TABLE 7-12. Iron Content of Some Representative Foods*

Foods	Serving Size	Iron (mg)
Dairy products		
Milk, whole, fluid	8 oz	0.10
Cheese, cheddar or Swiss	1 oz	0.30
Meat and alternates		
Liver, calf or lamb	2 sl	13.4
Liver, beef or chicken	¼–½ c	5.0
Beef, lamb, pork, veal; cooked	3 oz	2.5
Fish	3 oz	1.0
Grain products		
Bread, enriched or whole grain	3 sl	1.7
Cereals, enriched, ready-to-eat	1 oz	1.3
Spaghetti, noodles, macaroni, cooked	3 oz	1.0
Vegetables		
Spinach, cooked	½ c	2.0
Beet greens, cooked	½ c	1.9
Chard, cooked	½ c	1.8
Potato, white, medium size	1	0.7
Soybeans, cooked	½ c	2.5
Beans, lima, cooked	½ c	2.0
Peas, green, cooked	½ c	1.4
Fruits		
Figs, dried, small	2	0.9
Raisins	2 T	0.6
Peach, raw, medium size	1	0.6
Grapes, average size	22–24	0.4
Cherries, small	20–25	0.4

*Adapted from *Nutritive Value of Foods,* Home and Garden Bulletin No. 72
(Washington, D.C.: U.S. Department of Agriculture, 1981).

pallor, weakness, palpitation, coldness, and extreme fatigue. Other symptoms also may be present, such as oral and intestinal lesions, constipation or diarrhea, and heartburn. Thin, brittle nails are symptomatic of long-term deficiency; severe clinical disorders, such as heart trouble and visual abnormalities, are rare. See Figure 7-2.

Causes of iron deficiency are: (1) loss of blood; (2) inadequate intake; (3) drug use, especially antibiotics, laxatives, and aspirin. Certain population groups are more vulnerable to iron deficiency (see Table 7-11). Premature and low birth-weight infants and women with one or two babies are among the most susceptible to iron depletion.

Treatment of iron deficiency or anemia is twofold: correctly diagnosing the cause and eliminating the symptoms. The patient is given 50 mg of oral iron per day—for example, 0.2 g of ferrous sulfate or 0.3 g of ferrous gluconate three times daily after meals. A rise of at least 2 g

TABLE 7-13. Progressively Reduced Body Iron Nutriture

Iron Nutriture	Clinical Observations							
	Iron storage in bone marrow	Tissue iron content	Red blood cell iron content	Iron absorption	Anemia	Transferrin* saturation (%)	Hematocrit[†] (%)	Hemoglobin[‡] (g/100 mL)
Normal body iron content	Normal	Normal	Normal	Normal	No	>16	>38	>12
Latent iron deficiency or iron depletion	Reduced	Normal	Normal	Slightly elevated	No	10–16	>38	10–12
Iron-deficient erythropoiesis or reduced red blood corpuscle formation due to iron deficiency	Empty	Normal	Slightly reduced	Greatly elevated	Maybe	10–16	31–37	10–12
Body iron deficiency anemia	Empty	Slightly reduced	Reduced by half	Greatly elevated	Microcytic hypochromic	<10	<31	<10
Body tissue iron deficiency	Empty	Reduced by half	Reduced by half	Greatly elevated	Microcytic hypochromic	<10	<30	<10

*In the presence of carbon dioxide, the iron from the plasma forms a complex with a metal-binding β-globulin known as transferrin. The extent to which transferrin is saturated with iron indicates the amount of iron (ferric) available for the bone marrow.

[†]When blood with anticoagulant is centrifuged, the cell solids settle to the bottom of the tube. A straw-colored liquid, the plasma, stays on top. Normally the cells comprise about 45% of the total volume. This reading (45%) is a normal hematocrit, or packed-cell volume, for males; for females, the figure is 41%.

[‡]The concentration of hemoglobin is usually measured by the grams of the substance per 100 mL of blood.

of hemoglobin/100 mL every three weeks is considered an adequate response.

Possible side effects include gastric pain, nausea, heartburn, diarrhea, and constipation. Such results may be avoided by taking the tablets with food or starting with low doses and slowly progressing to higher ones.

Iron Supplements

Supplemental iron is taken orally with or without prescription. Ferrous sulfate is the most widely used iron supplement. It is cheap, palatable, has minimal side effects, and is as effective as other more expensive preparations. Table 7-14 shows the appropriate form of iron supplement

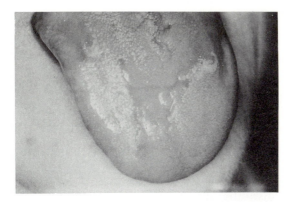

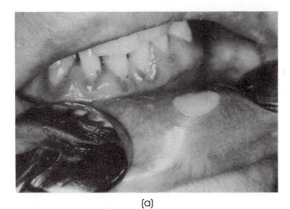

(a)

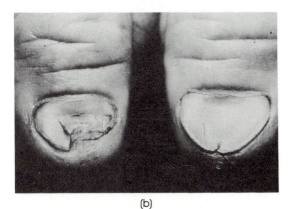

(b)

FIGURE 7-2. Signs of iron deficiency. (a) Top: patchy depapillation of tongue (latent iron deficiency). Bottom: generalized stomatitis, ulceration, and gingivitis (malabsorption syndrome). (From W. R. Tyldesley, *Brit. Dent. J.* 139 [1975]: 232) (b) Iron deficiency koilonychia. (From S. Dreizen, *Geriatrics* 29 [1974]: 97. By permission of *Geriatrics*)

TABLE 7-14. Quantities of Elemental Iron Contained in Iron Compounds or Supplements

Iron Compound or Supplement	Iron per Tablet (mg)	No. of Tablets Daily per Adult*
Ferrous sulfate (hydrated or dehydrated)	55–65	4
Ferrous fumarate (small tablet)	65	4
Ferrous gluconate	40	5–6
Ferroglycine sulfate	40	5–6

*To provide 240 mg of iron.

and the necessary number of tablets a day for a patient for whom 200 to 250 mg of iron a day has been prescribed.

Iron Toxicity

Iron toxicity—in the form of either an increased blood level of iron or disturbed iron metabolism—may result from numerous causes. Among these causes are: (1) hereditary disease leading to excess storage of iron; (2) excess consumption; (3) excess blood transfusion, leading to iron deposition in the liver; (4) clinical disorders, such as alcoholism or hepatitis; (5) accidental ingestion.

Symptoms of acute iron poisoning are severe gastrointestinal reactions such as cramps, pain, vomiting, and nausea, leading to shock, convulsions, and coma. Treatment includes gastric aspiration and lavage.

Iodine

Iodine is an essential element found in the thyroid gland. A component of the thyroid hormone *thyroxine,* iodine helps regulate basal metabolic rate.

Deficiency

Simple goiter results from a lack of iodine, causing a reduction of the thyroid hormone in circulation, which in turn stimulates the gland to make more of the hormone. This fruitless attempt results in the enlargement of the gland (Figure 7-3). Goiter is more prevalent among women than men and is intensified during cold weather.

Iodine deficiency in children is particularly harmful, since growth and development may be impaired. Serious depletion may cause **cretinism,** a disorder of infancy or childhood that retards physical and mental development.

Geographical areas with little iodine in the soil and drinking water are more likely to produce iodine deficiency and goiter. In the United States, the Rocky Mountain states and areas around the Great Lakes still have problems with iodine deficiency. By contrast, coastal areas do not have trouble with iodine deficiency, since the air, soil, and water all have a high level of this element.

Requirements and Food Sources

The RDA for iodine is about 100 to 130 μg per day. As already mentioned, geographic area helps to determine the level of iodine intake from plant and animal foods.

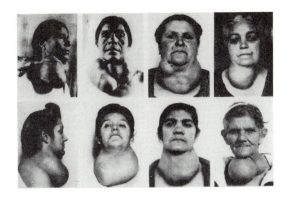

FIGURE 7-3. Iodine deficiency and goiter. Severe endemic goiter in Mendoza Province, Argentina, as seen between 1930 and 1950. (From H. Perinetti and L. N. Staneloni, *Environ. Res.* 3 [1970]: 463)

Iodized salt is such an excellent source of iodine that its regular use makes iodine depletion unlikely. Seafood is the next best source of iodine. Fresh fruits and grains contain little iodine, while the iodine content of vegetables, eggs, and milk is determined by the types of soil and animal feed.

Toxicity

From 1 to 50 mg of iodine consumed daily over a long period can result in poisoning. Iodine toxicity can result from doses of iodine for treatment of goiter or from ingestion of kelp or sea salt.

Zinc

Zinc is an important element that is located in almost every part of the body but concentration is highest in the bones, followed by the hair, skin, and (in men) the prostate.

Requirements and Food Sources

The adult requirement for zinc is about 15 to 25 mg per day. An average American diet provides from 10 to 15 mg of utilizable zinc per day. Only about 15 to 35 percent of ingested zinc is absorbed.

Rich amounts of zinc are found in expensive foods such as meat and oysters. As a result, low-income people may tend to have a low zinc intake. Fruits and vegetables contain very little zinc; cow's milk contains more zinc than breast milk does. The zinc contribution of grains is complex; zinc absorption is limited by phytic acid in outer husks.

Table 7-15 describes the zinc content of some common foods.

TABLE 7-15. Zinc Content of Some Representative Foods*

Food	Serving Size	Zinc (mg)
Dairy products		
Milk, whole	1 c	1.0
Cheese, American, pasteurized, processed	1 oz	0.8
Egg, whole, large	1	0.7
Cereals and equivalents		
Bread, white, enriched	1 sl	0.2
Bran, flakes, ready-to-eat	1 c	1.3
Grain and equivalents		
Rice, brown	⅔ c	0.8
Noodle, enriched, cooked	½ c	0.6
Potato, baked, large	1	0.4
Beans, peas, nuts		
Soybeans, cooked	½ c	0.6
Peas, split, dry, cooked	½ c	1.1
Peanut butter	1 T	0.4
Meat, fish, poultry		
Beef, roast, chuck	3 oz	3.7
Chicken, roast, light meat, no skin	3 oz	0.9
Salmon, steak, broiled	1	2.4
Oysters, Eastern, raw	6	90.0
Fruits		
Apricots, fresh, medium size	2–3	0.04
Orange, raw, medium	1	0.3
Pineapple, raw, crushed	1 c	0.3
Raisins	¼ c	0.06
Vegetables		
Broccoli, fresh, boiled	½ c	0.2
Carrot, raw	1	0.3
Onions, green, raw, bulb and top, chopped	¼ c	0.07
Tomato, raw, medium size	1	0.3

*Adapted from E. W. Murphy et al., "The Provisional Zinc Contents of Food," *J. Amer. Dietet. Assoc.* 66 (1975): 345. Also see Table 12 of the appendix.

Functions and Deficiency

Normal serum zinc level is about 6 to 13 mg per 100 mL. However, stresses such as infection, hormonal imbalance, anemia, pregnancy, and the use of certain drugs can decrease the level, whereas conditions such as tissue catabolism may cause the level to rise.

Zinc is important to many body processes. Among these functions are: (1) component of enzymes and of DNA and RNA; (2) metabolism of proteins, fats, carbohydrates, and nucleic acids; (3) sexual development, growth, and reproductive ability; (4) wound healing and skin health;

and (5) sensations of taste and smell. Severe deficiency of zinc leads to a skin disorder called **acrodermatitis enteropathica**.

Some causes of zinc deficiency include: (1) low dietary supply; (2) interference with absorption; (3) inborn error of metabolism; (4) increased body zinc demand, as in pregnancy; (5) presence of a clinical disorder, such as sickle cell anemia.

Zinc supplementation is usually prescribed for symptoms of zinc deficiency. In some patients, especially those with acrodermatitis enteropathica and other skin lesions, supplementation results in dramatic improvement.

Fluorine

Fluorine, more commonly known as fluoride, has been publicized because of its role in tooth decay. Although fluoride is one of the most abundant elements, little is known about its metabolic functions.

Because of its important role in the formation and development of bones and teeth, fluoride is added to water in many parts of the country, thus raising the dietary contribution to about 3.0 mg.

In addition to its effect on teeth, fluoride may protect against magnesium deficiency, osteoporosis, and certain periodontal diseases.

Copper and Other Trace Elements

The body contains about 100 mg of copper. Its major functions are: (1) synthesis of hormonelike substances; (2) serving as a component of important proteins, including enzymes; (3) synthesis of connective tissue; (4) maintenance of functions of the nervous system and normal blood chemistry.

Although copper is an essential element, the amount needed by the body is unknown. It is estimated that the American diet contributes about 2 mg of copper per day. The richest sources of copper are kidney, liver, shellfish, legumes, and raisins, with breast milk providing 0.15 to 1.0 mg of copper in an infant's daily intake.

Copper deficiency is uncommon in adults who eat a normal diet. However, certain disorders such as severe malabsorption can result in copper deficiency. Copper administration can reverse any clinical manifestations.

Infants with copper deficiency may eventually experience abnormal blood cell development and bone demineralization, even death. Causes of copper deficiency include: (1) long-term feeding of cow's milk; (2) chronic malnutrition and diarrhea; (3) Menke's kinky hair syndrome, a defect of copper absorption. Copper given intravenously results in some improvements.

TABLE 7-16. Some Relevant Information on Manganese, Chromium, Cobalt, Molybdenum, and Selenium

Mineral	Functions in the Body	Metabolism and Deficiency	Food Sources	RDA*
Manganese	Component of bone and some enzymes; major role in the intermediate metabolism of carbohydrate; protein synthesis	Not much known	Whole grains, nuts, legumes, fruit and selected vegetables	Not known
Chromium	Suspected to regulate glucose tolerance; associated with enzymes in the intermediate metabolism of carbohydrate and protein synthesis	Not much known	Whole-grain cereals, meat	None
Cobalt	Component of vitamin B_{12}, which plays a major role in body metabolism and physiology (see Chapter 6)	Assumed to be closely related to that of vitamin B_{12}	Associated with vitamin B_{12}	None unless vitamin B_{12} is considered
Molybdenum	Component of xanthine oxidase and flavoprotein, which is very important in body metabolism	Not much known	Whole grains, legumes, organ meats	None
Selenium	Component of enzyme; related to functions of vitamin E and metabolism of fat	Not much known	Grains, meats, vegetables, milk	None

*See footnote to Table 7-1.

Excess copper also can produce severe acute symptoms: headache, dizziness, heartburn, weakness, vomiting, nausea, and diarrhea. Such conditions as pregnancy, use of oral contraceptives, anemia, liver diseases, and rheumatoid arthritis can lead to high blood copper.

Other trace elements, including manganese, chromium, cobalt, molybdenum, and selenium, are described in Table 7-16. More details on these and other trace minerals may be obtained from references at the end of this chapter.

STUDY QUESTIONS

1. Discuss the use of the terms *minerals, inorganic elements,* and *ash.*
2. In what six body processes are minerals important?
3. What distinguishes macroelements from microelements?
4. What can be said about the average person's sodium consumption?

5. What effect do calcium and potassium have on muscles?
6. How do oxalic and phytic acids influence the absorption of calcium and magnesium?
7. What three nutrients may be involved in rickets?
8. Discuss the relationships between calcium and phosphorus.
9. Under what conditions may borderline magnesium deficiency become serious?
10. Are iron deficiency and anemia inevitably linked?
11. Discuss causes and treatment of iron deficiency.
12. Discuss the history of iodine deficiency. Do some library research to support your analysis.
13. Discuss the functions of zinc in the body.
14. Describe the symptoms of copper poisoning.

REFERENCES

Brewer, G. J., and Prasad, A. S., eds. 1977. *Zinc metabolism: current aspects in health and disease.* New York: Alan R. Liss.

Darby, W. J. 1980. Why salt? How much? *Contemporary Nutrition.* 5:1, June.

DeMaeyer, E. M. et al., 1979. Control of endemic goitre. Geneva: World Health Organization.

Finch, C. 1981. Iron nutrition. *West. J. Med.* 134:532.

Horn, B. 1981. Magnesium—it's about time. *West. J. Med.* 134:72.

Hui, Y. H. 1983. *Human nutrition and diet therapy.* Monterey, Calif.: Wadsworth Health Sciences.

Karcioglu, Z. A., and Sarper, R. M. 1980. Zinc and copper in medicine. Springfield, Ill.: C. C. Thomas.

Massry, S. G., et al., eds. 1980. *Phosphates and minerals in health and disease.* New York: Plenum.

Nutrition Review. 1984. *Present knowledge in nutrition,* 5th ed. Washington, D. C.: The Nutrition Foundation.

Randolph, P. M., and Dennison, C. 1980. *Diet, nutrition, and dentistry.* St. Louis: C. V. Mosby.

8

THE PHYSIOLOGY OF INGESTED FOODSTUFFS

THE DIGESTIVE SYSTEM
The Food Path
Enzymes and Coenzymes

CARBOHYDRATES
Digestion and Absorption
Energy Formation and Storage
Cellular Metabolism Processes
Regulation of Blood Glucose

PROTEIN
Digestion
Absorption
Metabolism

FATS
Digestion, Absorption, and Transportation
Metabolism
Ketone Bodies
Cholesterol Metabolism

NUCLEIC ACIDS

WATER, VITAMINS, AND MINERALS
Functions, Distribution, and Balance of Body Water

ost of us take the process of eating for granted, knowing that the body will take care of itself. But after we have eaten, hundreds of thousands of metabolic processes must take place before our cells can utilize the nutrients in our food. Food must first be **digested,** or broken down into particles of a size and chemical composition that the body can readily absorb.

Absorption takes place mostly in the small intestine, where specialized cells transfer digested nutrients into the blood and the lymph vessels. In some cases, special changes are needed so that the nutrients can be *transported* to the cells where they are to be used or further processed. Within the cells, the nutrients are either stored, or they undergo metabolism; that is, they are broken down into simpler components for energy or excretion (**catabolism**), or used to synthesize new materials for cellular growth, maintenance, or repair (*anabolism*).

THE DIGESTIVE SYSTEM

The **alimentary canal,** the principal part of the **digestive system,** is the long tube whose parts include the mouth or oral cavity; the esophagus; the stomach; the small intestine, including the duodenum; the various parts of the colon, or large intestine; the rectum; and the anus. Some important accessory organs connected with the digestive tract are the salivary glands, the gallbladder, the pancreas, and the liver. Along this tract, foods are broken down into small units, both physically and chemically, and then absorbed for use by the body. Figure 8-1 illustrates the digestive tract.

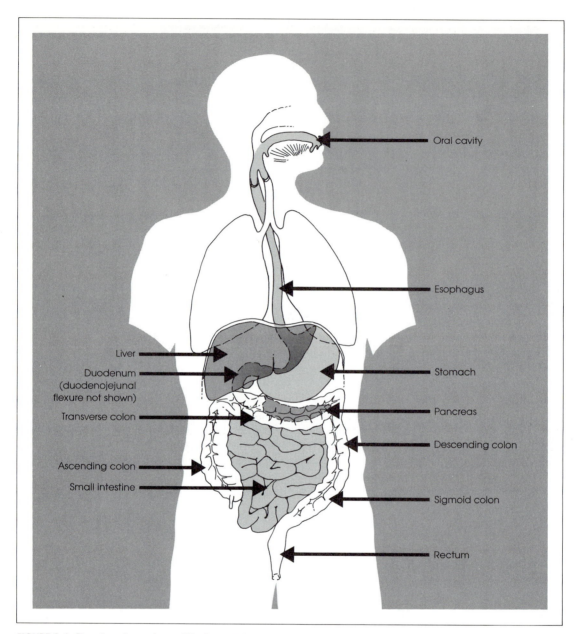

FIGURE 8-1. The digestive system of the human body.

The Food Path

The food placed in your mouth is chewed, softened, and swallowed; in the stomach, it is churned, propelled into the small intestine, and mixed with the bile from the gallbladder and with digestive enzymes from the intestinal walls. The products of this digestion are partly or completely absorbed into either the portal vein (blood vessel leading to the liver) or the **lacteal system** (a special system of lymphatic vessels that transport fat).

In the mouth, chewing (mastication) reduces large food lumps into smaller pieces and mixes them with saliva. This wetting and homogenizing facilitates later digestion. Individuals without teeth or with reduced saliva secretion have trouble eating dry foods and require a soft, moist diet.

Saliva facilitates swallowing and movements of the tongue and lips, keeps the mouth moist and clean, serves as an oral buffer, provides some antibiotic activity, and inhibits loss of calcium from the teeth by maintaining a neutral pH (not overly acidic or alkaline). Saliva contains a digestive enzyme (*ptyalin* or salivary *amylase*) and a special protein called "mucin." **Mucin** lubricates food, and the enzyme digests carbohydrates to a small extent. Each day the "salivary glands" make about 5½ to 6 cups (1,500 mL) of saliva.

The bolus of food is propelled forward by rhythmic contractions of the entire intestinal system (peristalsis). These peristaltic waves move the food from the mouth, through the esophagus, and into the stomach. Certain individuals, especially nervous people, tend to swallow air when eating. When part of the air is expelled through the mouth, belching results; the remaining air is expelled as flatus (gas). If too much air is swallowed, there will be abdominal discomfort.

Food travels through different parts of the stomach (cardiac, body, greater curvature, the pylorus, and the duodenum; see Figure 8-2) and is well mixed there. The acid, mucus, and pepsin (another digestive enzyme) secreted cause partial digestion, and peristalsis (rhythmic movement of the entire gastrointestinal system) mixes up the food. It is then released gradually through the end of the stomach (pylorus) into the beginning of the small intestine (duodenum).

The digestive system breaks down complex carbohydrates, proteins, and fats into absorbable units, mainly in the small intestine. Vitamins, minerals, fluids, and most nonessential nutrients are also digested and absorbed to varying degrees. Foods are digested by enzymes secreted by different parts of the intestine. For reference purposes, Table 8-1 summarizes the major digestive enzymes and their actions. After the digestive process is complete, nutrients are ready for absorption, which occurs mainly at the small intestine. The absorption of each nutrient is discussed later.

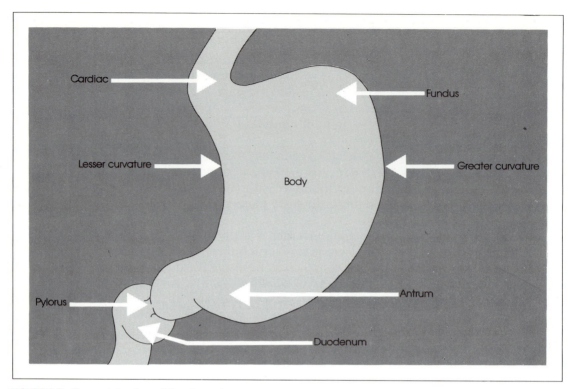

FIGURE 8-2. General structure of the stomach.

After the nutrients have been absorbed, they enter the circulation in two ways. Most fat-soluble nutrients enter the **lacteal** or **lymphatic system** and eventually into the **systemic blood circulation.** Other nutrients enter the *hepatic portal vein* and are received by the liver, which eventually releases them to the blood stream.

Enzymes and Coenzymes

After digestion and absorption, the nutrients exist as hexoses (mainly glucose and fructose; see Chapter 2), fatty acids, and glycerols (see Chapter 3), and amino acids (see Chapter 5) and are then metabolized in various fashions. Many of the metabolic processes require the presence of a *catalyst,* a substance that can facilitate a chemical reaction. Although participating in the process, the catalyst may or may not undergo physical, chemical, or other modification itself. Nonetheless, the catalyst usually returns to its original form after the reaction.

In the body, most biological reactions require a special class of catalysts—**enzymes.** All enzymes are made of protein. Each enzyme cata-

TABLE 8-1. Characteristics of the Enzymatic System of Digestion

Location	Food or Substrate	Products of Digestion	Enzyme(s) Involved for Digestion		
			Name(s)	Source(s)	Active in acid/base (pH)
Mouth	Starch	Maltose, dextrins, di-saccharides, mono-saccharides, branched oligosaccharides	Ptyalin, or salivary amylase	Salivary glands	Slightly acidic (6.7)
Stomach	Protein	Proteoses, peptones, polypeptides, di-peptides, amino acids	Pepsin	Peptic or chief cells of stomach	Acidic (1.6–2.4)
	Milk casein	Milk coagulation	Rennin	Stomach mucosa	Acidic (4.0); re-quires calcium for activity
	Fat	Triglycerides; some mono- and di-glycerides, glycerol, fatty acids	Gastric lipase	Stomach mucosa	Acidic
Small intestine (mainly duodenum and jejunum)*	Protein Proteoses, peptones, etc.	Polypeptides, di-peptides, etc.	Trypsin (activated trypsinogen)	Exocrine gland of pancreas	Alkaline (7.9)
	Proteoses, peptones, etc.	Polypeptides, di-peptides, etc.	Chymotrypsin (activated chymo-trypsinogen)	Exocrine gland of pancreas	Alkaline (8.0)
	Polypeptides with free carboxyl groups	Lower peptides, free amino acids	Carboxypeptidase	Exocrine gland of pancreas	
	Fibrous protein	Peptides, amino acids	Elastase	Exocrine gland of pancreas	
	Carbohydrate Starch, dextrins	Maltose, isomaltose, monosaccharides, dextrins	α-amylase (amylopsin)	Exocrine gland of pancreas	Slightly alkaline (7.1)
	Fat Triglycerides	Mono- and di-glycerides, glycerol, fatty acids	Lipase (steapsin)	Exocrine gland of pancreas	Alkaline (8.0)

TABLE 8-1. (continued)

Location	Food or Substrate	Products of Digestion	Enzyme(s) Involved for Digestion Name(s)	Source(s)	Active in acid/base (pH)
	Cholesterol	Cholesterol esters	Cholesterol esterase	Exocrine gland of pancreas	
	Nucleic acids Ribonucleic acid	Nucleotides Ribonucleotides	Ribonuclease	Exocrine gland of pancreas	
	Deoxyribonucleic acid	Deoxyribonucleotides	Deoxyribonuclease	Exocrine gland of pancreas	
Small intestine (mainly jejunum and ileum)	Protein Polypeptides	Amino acids	Carboxypeptidase, aminopeptidase, dipeptidase	Brush border of the small intestine	
	Carbohydrate Sucrose	Glucose, fructose	Sucrase	Brush border of the small intestine	Acidic/alkaline (5.0–7.0)
	Dextrin (isomaltose)	Glucose	α-dextrinase (isomaltase)	Brush border of the small intestine	
	Maltose	Glucose	Maltase	Brush border of the small intestine	Acidic (5.8–6.2)
	Lactose	Glucose, galactose	Lactase	Brush border of the small intestine	Acidic (5.4–6.0)
	Fat Monoglycerides	Glycerol, fatty acids	Lipase (enteric),	Brush border of the small intestine	
	Lecithin	Glycerol, fatty acids	Lecithinase	Brush border of the small intestine	
	Nucleotides	Nucleosides, phosphate	Nucleotidase	Brush border of the small intestine	
	Nucleosides	Purines, pyrimidines, pentose	Nucleosidase	Brush border of the small intestine	
	Organic phosphates	Free phosphates	Phosphatase	Brush border of the small intestine	Alkaline (8.6)

*The food is not grouped together, e.g., all fat, all proteins, etc. Instead the food is placed in an order that follows the sequence of digestion along the duodenum to jejunum. This attempts to present the digestive enzymes in their expected sequence of action.

lyzes only one or a small number of reactions, so there are many enzymes, each with a specific responsibility. Without enzymes, most biological reactions would proceed at too slow a pace.

Coenzymes are accessory substances that facilitate the effect of an enzyme, mainly by acting as carriers for products of the reaction. In fact, most enzymes contain a coenzyme. Further, many coenzymes contain vitamins or their slightly modified forms as their major ingredient. A coenzyme can catalyze many types of reactions; for example, some coenzymes transfer hydrogens. Other coenzymes transfer groups other than hydrogens.

Because most of the metabolic reactions discussed in this chapter involve coenzymes, the role of vitamins as the major ingredient of coenzymes is important.

CARBOHYDRATE

As discussed in Chapter 2, starch and cellulose are the only polysaccharides consumed to any extent by humans. Major simple sugars include both monosaccharides (such as glucose and fructose in honey and fruit juices) and disaccharides (such as maltose in beer, lactose in milk, and sucrose in table sugar). Also ingested are dextrins, sugar alcohol, and very small quantities of tri- and tetrasaccharides. Discussed briefly in the following sections are the digestion and absorption pathways of carbohydrates, the involvement of carbohydrates in energy formation and storage, the general processes by which carbohydrates are degraded and synthesized, and the regulation of glucose levels in the blood.

Digestion and Absorption

Starch is partially hydrolyzed in the mouth (see Table 8-1) by ptyalin; the action of ptyalin is terminated by the acid in the stomach. In the small intestine, all digestible carbohydrates are reduced to monosaccharides—glucose, fructose, galactose, mannose, and pentoses. The final *hydrolysis*, or digestion, of disaccharides to monosaccharides is believed to occur in the intestinal walls. All nondigestible carbohydrates, such as cellulose, are passed into the colon, where they are fermented to release gas.

Most of the monosaccharides are absorbed before the food residue reaches the end of the ileum. Although absorption is carried out mainly by active transport (requiring energy), diffusion (passive movement) also occurs.

The monosaccharides travel through the intestinal and portal veins to reach the liver, where they may be released into the bloodstream. In the liver, most of the fructose and galactose are converted to glucose, the main simple sugar in the blood.

Of the glucose converted in the liver, part is released to the circulation, part changed to other essential substances, part converted to **glycogen** for storage, and part oxidized to energy. A peak plasma glucose level of 120 to 140 mg/100 mL is normally reached within 60 minutes after a mixed meal.

Once glucose has reached the bloodstream, some enters cells to give energy, and some is converted to glycogen in tissues such as muscle. Most of the glucose is used to provide energy through a three-stage process: glycolysis, the citric acid cycle, and the respiratory chain.

Energy Formation and Storage

Because everything a body does requires energy, nature has provided several methods of permitting energy either to be released or stored for use when needed. Five different energy systems are known to operate in animal cells. The most important one is the direct release of energy, mainly as heat (illustrated below):

$$\text{Glucose, fat, or protein} + \text{oxygen} \xrightarrow{\text{oxidation}}$$
$$\text{carbon dioxide} + \text{water} + \text{energy to be stored} + \text{heat}$$

Substances called high-energy phosphate compounds allow energy to be stored and released when needed. The most important of these compounds is probably **adenosine triphosphate** (ATP), considered the energy powerhouse of the body. It releases its energy in the following reactions:

$$\text{ATP} + \text{H}_2\text{O} \rightarrow \text{ADP} + \text{P} + 7.5 \text{ kcal}$$
$$\text{ADP} + \text{H}_2\text{O} \rightarrow \text{AMP} + \text{P} + 7.5 \text{ kcal}$$
where: P = inorganic phosphate, AMP = adenosine
monophosphate, and ADP = adenosine diphosphate

The energy released from this process can be used for such work as organ building, heart beat, transportation across cell membranes, and muscle contraction. Figure 8-3 summarizes the role of ATP in body energy metabolism.

The topic of how energy is stored in creatine phosphate, "active acetate," and low-energy phosphate compounds will not be discussed here.

Cellular Metabolism

Before glucose (carbohydrate) can release the energy needed by the body, it must undergo a series of complex biochemical processes within

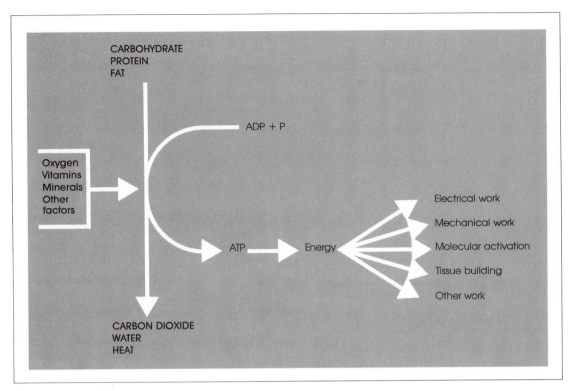

FIGURE 8-3. The role of ATP in body energy metabolism.

the cells. Three biological processes are involved: glycolysis, the citric acid cycle, and the respiratory chain.

Glucose comes from food and from internal production, which occurs mainly in the liver. Glycogen stored in the cells of the liver may be converted to glucose by the process of *glucogenolysis*. The synthesis of certain noncarbohydrate substances also produces glucose. These processes are briefly defined in Table 8-2.

Regulation of Blood Glucose

The balancing of blood glucose (or "blood sugar") levels is another important aspect of what happens to carbohydrates in the body. This subject is discussed below and also in Chapter 15 in relation to diabetes mellitus.

In a normal person, blood glucose levels fluctuate within narrow limits—between 70 and 100 mg/100 mL of blood. An appropriate level

TABLE 8-2. Definitions of Some Metabolic Terms

Term	Definition
Glycolysis	The breaking down of hexoses (six-carbon sugars), mainly glucose, into three-carbon substances (pyruvic or lactic acid). The process is sometimes termed the Embden-Meyerhof pathway.
Glycogenesis	The formation of glycogen from glucose.
Glycogenolysis	The breaking down of glycogen into glucose and its metabolites.
Gluconeogenesis	The synthesis of glucose (and thus glycogen) from noncarbohydrate sources, such as lactate, glycerol, and amino acids.
Citric acid cycle	Also termed Krebs cycle or tricarboxylic acid cycle. The process whereby carbohydrate, fat, and/or protein is completely oxidized to carbon dioxide, water, and energy. This is accomplished with the assistance of the respiratory chain.
Respiratory chain	The transport of hydrogen atoms from biological oxidation for acceptance by oxygen atoms to form water molecules.

is achieved by a balance between the supply and removal of blood glucose.

Hypoglycemia is characterized by subnormal blood glucose levels. These levels can be restored to normal by the provision of glucose from three sources: (1) additional dietary carbohydrates, (2) degradation of glycogen in liver and muscle, (3) the breakdown of protein and fat.

Hyperglycemia is characterized by elevated levels of blood glucose. Normally, the body spontaneously lowers these levels in one or more of the following ways: (1) More insulin is released to drive glucose into cells for oxidation; (2) more glycogen is formed (glycogenesis) in the liver and muscle; (3) more glucose is changed to fat in fat cells; (4) more glucose is excreted in the urine (glucosuria).

PROTEINS

There are three forms of dietary protein. The major portion is joined with other substances, a small fraction is associated with fat and carbohydrates, and only a very small part exists as free protein, such as that in egg white. All proteins must be broken down into amino acids to be used by the cells. The paths of protein digestion, absorption, and metabolism will be traced in the sections that follow.

Digestion

Protein digestion begins in the stomach (see Table 8-1), where acid activates the pepsinogen (an enzyme) to release pepsin (another enzyme). The pepsin divides the peptide linkages in the protein into polypeptides, each with two or more amino acids. In the small intestine, the protein molecules are formed into small polypeptides and dipeptides. These are further digested to form free amino acids, the only form that can be utilized by body tissues.

The nonpeptide linkage in protein molecules must be denatured (by heat or stomach acid) before they can be digested. Denaturation facilitates digestion by exposing protein molecules and providing more surface area for enzymatic action. However, excess heating or cooking can inhibit digestion by causing protein molecules to re-form other linkages.

Absorption

Normally, only amino acids are absorbed. In the small intestine all free amino acids, whether ingested or digested products, are absorbed via the mucosal cells into the hepatic portal vein. The L-amino acids are both more readily absorbed and more biologically active than the D-amino acids. While absorption occurs along the entire small intestine, with the slowest rate along the ileum, the stomach and colon may also absorb some amino acids. About 20 to 30 percent of ingested proteins are unabsorbed and are excreted in the stools.

Occasionally an allergic reaction to ingested protein occurs in infants who are unable to absorb undigested protein. Adults with a similar allergy are still probably capable of absorbing whole protein molecules.

The best utilization of amino acids seems to occur in accordance with the body's need for growth and function. Any excess absorbed is excreted rather than stored. Further, studies have shown that absorption and utilization of proteins are optimized when adults evenly distribute their protein intake throughout the day.

Erratic patterns of protein absorption may result from stomach irregularities rather than irregular protein ingestion. It is the stomach that regulates the emptying of protein into the small intestine. Loss of all or part of the stomach; the formation of excessive amounts of chemicals such as histamine, tyramine, and ammonia; and clinical disorders such as ulcerative colitis can have an undesirable effect on the absorption of protein.

Metabolism

The importance of protein to the body is indicated by its numerous functions and the complexity of its metabolism. Three major factors affect protein metabolism: (1) the quality and quantity of protein consumed, (2) the amount of calories ingested, and (3) the physiological and nutritional status of the body.

Because body tissues can utilize only amino acids, protein metabolism revolves around a body pool of amino acids that are continuously released by protein hydrolysis and resynthesized. Amino acids released by the liver are the same as those ingested; any amino acids filtered through the kidneys are reabsorbed. Individuals experiencing periods of growth, such as childhood, adolescence, or pregnancy, require a large pool of amino acids.

The major site of destruction of each amino acid is the liver, although protein is degraded to its individual amino acids in the muscle and other tissues. Under normal circumstances, the destruction (catabolism) of protein is balanced by its formation. However, during periods of stress such as disease, destruction can overcome synthesis.

When protein is degraded, amino acids are formed. Some amino acids circulate, some are oxidized, some converted to glucose, and some directed to other paths.

The process of linking different amino acids by groups (*peptide linkages*) to form a molecule of protein is known as *protein synthesis*. Amino acids in the right number, pattern, and sequence must be present to form a specific body structure, such as hair, saliva, tears, or hormones. The formation of each specific protein requires a highly specific genetic code.

FATS

A third set of chemical and biological pathways is followed by the digestion, absorption, transportation, and cellular metabolism of fats. They intersect the pathways of carbohydrates and proteins at several points. The following sections briefly describe the role of fats in the body. More details of fat metabolism are presented in Chapter 17.

Digestion, Absorption, and Transportation

The pancreas provides the most important *lipase,* or digestive enzyme, in the process of breaking down ingested fat (Table 8-1). Although the lipases in the saliva, stomach, and small intestine have a small effect on fat digestion, the major degradation occurs in the duodenum. When the exocrine gland of the pancreas is disabled, undigested and unabsorbed fat causes steatorrhea (bulky, clay-colored, fatty stools). The combined action of bile salts (from the gallbladder), fatty acids, and glycerides emulsifies fat and facilitates its digestion.

Free fatty acids and glycerols are formed in the small intestine from half of the ingested triglycerides. The rest are changed to monoglycerides and a small amount of diglycerides. The intestinal mucosa absorbs the monoglycerides, which are further hydrolyzed to glycerols and free fatty acids.

In the intestine, free fatty acids are absorbed in two ways: (1) by passing directly from the intestinal lumen, through mucosal cells, into the portal vein and thence to the liver (fatty acids with less than 10 to 12 carbon atoms); (2) by being absorbed into the mucosal cells, where they are regrouped with glycerols to form triglycerides (fatty acids with more than 10 to 21 carbon atoms).

Triglycerides attach themselves to very low density lipoproteins to form **chylomicrons,** which enter the bloodstream via the lymph and the thoracic duct. Chylomicrons are fat particles 1 μm in diameter visible under the microscope. Like the triglycerides, absorbed cholesterol becomes part of the chylomicrons that enter the bloodstream.

Blood plasma contains fat in the following forms: fatty acids, glycerol, glycerides, cholesterol, cholesterol esters, and phospholipids. The resulting *lipid-protein complexes* have varying densities. In general, *very low density lipoproteins* carry mainly triglycerides; *low density lipoproteins* carry mainly cholesterol; and A-*lipoproteins* carry phospholipids, albumin, and free fatty acids.

In a normal person, about 95 percent of ingested fat is absorbed, mainly in the duodenum and jejunum, with some absorption in the ileum. About 5 percent of fecal waste is fat, which comes from the diet, cell debris, and bacterial synthesis.

Fat is distributed to two main locations: *structural fats* in the membranes and other structural parts; *neutral fats* in fat cells. Neutral body fat contains mainly triglycerides, which are the main form of stored energy.

Metabolism

According to the body's need for energy, stored fat is degraded in two stages: (1) hydrolysis of glycerides and (2) oxidation of fatty acids. When glycerides are hydrolyzed, they form fatty acids and glycerols, which are released into the circulation and transported to the liver.

In the process of *beta-oxidation*, fatty acids are oxidized in the liver to form carbon dioxide, water, and energy. Unsaturated fatty acids generate less energy than the molecular equivalent of saturated fatty acids, because the former contains less hydrogen.

Fat synthesis occurs through the formation of either fatty acids or triglycerides. The body is able to synthesize unsaturated fatty acids from saturated ones by removing hydrogen. In the adipose tissues, fatty acids combine with glycerol to form triglycerides, or neutral fats.

Ketone Bodies

Ketone bodies are normal metabolic byproducts from protein and fat metabolism. Under normal circumstances, ketone bodies are metabolized as soon as they are formed. A person rarely excretes more than 1 mg of ketones each day, and blood levels are usually less than 1 mg/ 100 mL of blood.

However, ketones can accumulate under certain conditions, resulting in the disorder known as **ketosis.** This usually occurs when the body is metabolizing mainly fat and/or protein only. When the glucose supply to cells is reduced, ketosis may develop. Such a reduction may be related to diabetes mellitus or dietary alterations such as high fat/low carbohydrate intake or simple starvation. Chapter 15 explores this clinical condition in a diabetic patient.

Cholesterol Metabolism

Animal products such as fats, eggs, and organ meats provide most of our dietary cholesterol, which is absorbed via the lymphatic system. Cholesterol also can be synthesized by the body, mainly in the intestinal mucosa and liver. It is currently believed that the more cholesterol ingested the less cholesterol synthesized by the body.

The synthesis and degradation of cholesterol are ongoing processes that occur at the same time. Cholesterol is removed from the body via the liver and excretion in the bile; however, some cholesterol is reabsorbed. Other aspects of cholesterol metabolism are discussed in Chapters 3 and 20.

NUCLEIC ACIDS

Practically everything we eat contains nucleic acids, which occur in cell chromosomes. Nucleic acids are responsible for our heredity. During digestion, ingested nucleic acids are initially cleaved into nucleotides by pancreatic nucleases (see Table 8-1). Next, the small intestine secretes nucleotidase, which hydrolyzes nucleotides to form phosphoric acid and nucleosides. The latter are split by intestinal nucleosidases to form sugars, purine, and pyrimidine, all of which are absorbed by active transport. Undigested large molecules of nucleic acids are excreted in the stool.

Nucleic acids can also be resynthesized. In the body, purines, pyrimidines, and sugars are put together to form ribonucleic acid (RNA), deoxyribonucleic acid (DNA), nicotinamide adenine dinucleotide (NAD), and other related substances. However, the liver can also make pyrimidines and purines.

Within a cell, although DNA is stable throughout life, RNA is in constant equilibrium with a metabolic pool. Purines and pyrimidines may be excreted as such in the urine or be metabolized to uric acid (purines) or carbon dioxide and ammonia (pyrimidines).

Uric acid in the body comes from two sources: synthesis from glycine (amino acid) and degradation of purines. In humans, uric acid is excreted in the urine, although in most other mammals, it is converted to allantoin before excretion. The normal blood level of uric acid is 4 mg/100 mL. The kidney reabsorbs much of the filtered uric acid, but the body excretes about 1 g of uric acid in 24 hours. Consult a standard reference text for additional information on DNA, RNA, and molecular genetics.

WATER, VITAMINS, AND MINERALS

Most of us are aware that water is an essential nutrient. Although humans are known to survive for weeks and even months without food, they cannot live for long without water. The water within us is essential to a number of body processes and structures. One primary function of water is as a medium of transportation, carrying nutrients and wastes in and out of cells by both passive and active processes. Although the levels of fluid volume and electrolyte (mineral) concentration in a healthy person are subjected to a number of adjustments, they are always maintained at biological equilibrium. Similarly, the chemical conditions of acidity and alkalinity in a normal person are constantly maintained at a delicate balance despite the wide variety of foods and beverages consumed daily.

Functions, Distribution, and Balance of Body Water

Water makes up more than 60% of adult body weight. Water is an important substance with many major functions in the body. It transports nutrients to the cells and waste materials through the kidney for excre-

TABLE 8-3. Daily Water Balance in a Normal Adult

Factors Affecting Water Balance	Volume of Water Change (mL)
Sources of gain	
Food (meat, apples, etc.)	+500–1,000
Water, beverages, and liquid and semiliquid edible items (e.g., soups)	+1,100
Metabolic water (formed from chemical reaction, e.g., oxidation of food)*	+400
Total	+2,000–2,500
Sources of loss	
Urine	−1,000–1,300
Stools	−90–100
Perspiration, respiration	−410–500
Insensible loss	−500–600
Total	−2,000–2,500

*The oxidation of 1 g of fat, carbohydrate, and protein produces 1.1, 0.6, and 0.4 g of water, respectively.

tion. It is the main medium in which biological and chemical reactions take place. It serves as an important substrate and reactant in chemical and biological reactions. It regulates body temperature and lubricates joints. It maintains pressure and equilibrium for certain organs and structures, such as the eyeball and fetus. It provides an emergency fluid source.

Water exists both inside (intracellular) and outside (extracellular) the cells of the body. The extracellular water is distributed in the blood plasma, in the spaces between cells, in bone and connective tissue, and within the gastrointestinal tract, brain, and spinal column.

We take in water daily by actually drinking water and liquids and by eating foods. The liquids we ingest include coffee, tea, alcoholic beverages, sodas, and thin soups. Practically all foods contain some water. Also, in a healthy person, normal metabolic processes form water inside the body. On the other hand, we lose water daily in urine, bowel movements, perspiration, respiration, and the insensible loss—the constant but invisible evaporation of moisture from the skin surface. In a normal person daily losses and gains of water balance each other, as shown in Table 8-3.

Water balance in many clinical conditions deviates from those listed in Table 8-3. For example, a hospitalized patient may take in more water through a special tube or through an intravenous or rectal route. On the other hand, the same patient may lose water from the body through conditions such as abnormal gastrointestinal loss (stomach suction, vomiting, colitis, intestinal suction, presence of fistula, or diarrhea), exudates (burns, ulcers, bedsores, and wounds), respiratory diseases (bronchorrhea or acute laryngotracheobronchitis), injuries, edema of damaged tissues, massive urticaria, or swellings of the skin. Dehydration results when water loss exceeds gain; edema results when more water is ingested and retained than lost. Either kind of imbalance is dangerous to body functioning and can be fatal if severe.

To illustrate the principles of fluid-electrolyte imbalances in the body, Figure 8-4 shows how the body responds to a decrease in water intake or an increase in salt intake; Figure 8-5 illustrates fluid and electrolyte adjustments to compensate for perspiration; and Figure 8-6 shows varying fluid and electrolyte responses to an abnormally low protein intake, which is common in many undeveloped and developing countries (see Chapter 9).

From the stomach to the colon, water passes freely and reversibly between the intestinal lumen and body compartments, although less so in the stomach than elsewhere in the gastrointestinal tract. Water moves in or out of the intestinal lumen to assure osmotic equilibrium on the two sides. In general, the osmolality of the contents of the small intestine resembles that of the plasma. After nutrients in the intestine have been absorbed, the excess water in the lumen is passed out with fecal waste to maintain osmotic equilibrium. Sodium moves freely according to the concentration gradient on the two sides of the mucosal cells. In the colon, sodium moves from body to lumen in accordance with the osmotic gradient; that is, from areas of lower concentration to higher.

All water-soluble vitamins are absorbed along the small intestine. Except for vitamin B_{12}, a healthy person can absorb these vitamins rapidly. All fat-soluble vitamins require the presence of pancreatic enzymes, bile salts, glycerides, and fatty acids for absorption, as does fat itself. Chapter 6 discusses in detail the absorption and metabolism of each vitamin.

In a healthy person, all essential minerals are absorbed easily by the body, although the extent varies with individual minerals. Chapter 7 provides a detailed discussion of the absorption and metabolism of each mineral.

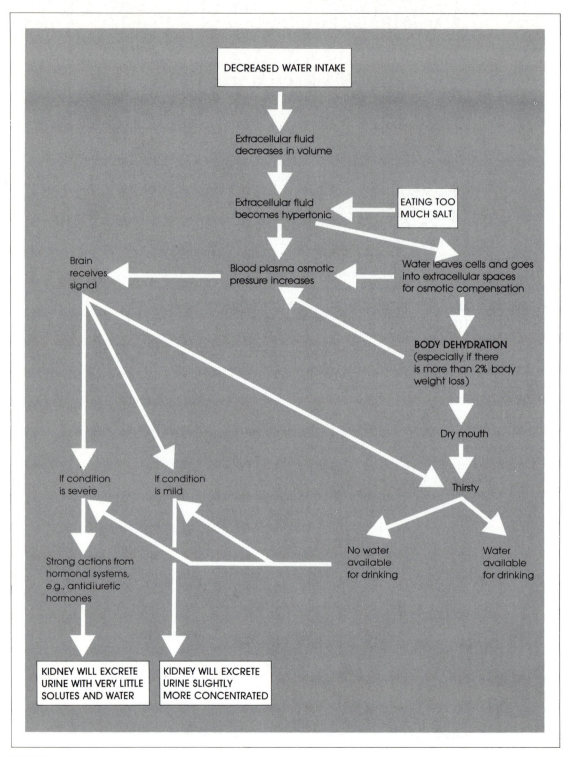

FIGURE 8-4. Body fluid and electrolyte adjustment caused by decreased water intake or excessive salt intake.

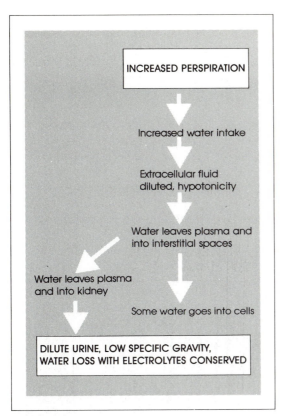

FIGURE 8-5. Body fluid and electrolyte adjustment caused by perspiration.

STUDY QUESTIONS

1. Describe the digestive system.
2. What is the role of enzymes? Of coenzymes?
3. To what form are all carbohydrates eventually reduced in the digestive process?
4. Discuss one way in which energy is released or stored in relation to carbohydrate metabolism.
5. How is blood sugar level usually maintained within a narrow range?
6. What is the end product of protein digestion? In what areas do protein digestion, absorption, catabolism, and synthesis take place?
7. What pancreatic enzyme is important in fat digestion? What disor-

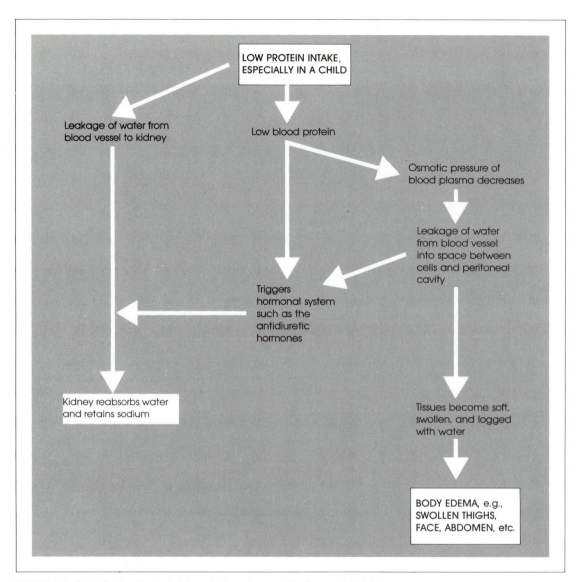

FIGURE 8-6. Body fluid and electrolyte adjustment caused by low protein intake.

der arises when the pancreas is unable to provide enough of this enzyme?

8. What forms of fat can be absorbed and are therefore found in blood plasma? To what are they bound?
9. Define ketosis.
10. Define osmosis. Give three clinical conditions in which osmotic equilibrium is not maintained in the body.

REFERENCES

Berdanier, C. D., ed. 1976. *Carbohydrate metabolism: regulation and physiological role.* New York: Halsted Press.

Danowski, T. S., et al. 1975. Hypoglycemia. *World Rev. Nutr. Dietet.* 22:288.

Edholm, O. H., and Weiner, J. S. 1981. *The principles and practice of human physiology.* New York: Academic Press.

Guyton, A. G. 1981. *Textbook of medical physiology.* 6th ed. Philadelphia: Saunders.

Hui, Y. H. 1983. *Human nutrition and diet therapy.* Monterey, Calif.: Wadsworth Health Sciences Division.

Lit, A. K. C., et al. 1980. *Fluid, electrolytes, acid-base and nutrition.* New York: Academic Press.

Meneely, G. R., and Battarbee, H. D. 1976. Sodium and potassium. *Nutr. Rev.* 14:225.

Munro, H. N. 1976. Regulation of body protein metabolism. *Proc. Nutr. Soc.* 35:297.

Robinson, J. 1970. Water, the indispensable nutrient. *Nutr. Today* 5:16.

Weldy, N. J. 1980. *Body fluids and electrolytes: a programmed presentation.* 3rd ed. St. Louis: C. V. Mosby.

Part Two

NUTRITION DURING THE LIFE CYCLE

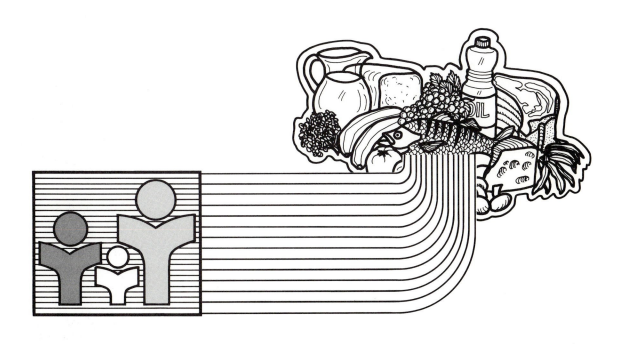

9 UNDERNUTRITION

The diets of many people throughout the world are extremely inadequate (see Chapter 10). Hunger, starvation, and *undernutrition* are terms that refer to a lack of essential nutrients in the human body caused by *insufficient food intake. Malnutrition*, on the other hand, means "bad" nutrition that may or may not be caused by inadequate intake.

Undernutrition is a serious problem in developing countries such as India, the Philippines, West Africa, Ethiopia, Ghana, Guatemala, and Brazil. In the United States, undernutrition is less extensive and severe. Malnutrition, by contrast, is widespread owing to such factors as alcoholism, drug abuse, overeating, unbalanced meals, and social isolation.

The focus of this chapter is on undernutrition: its prevalence, symptoms, and treatment as well as the attempts currently being made to alleviate the suffering caused by world hunger.

UNDERNUTRITION IN THE UNITED STATES

Most cases of undernourishment in the United States involve newborn infants, children, adolescents, college students, and the elderly.

The major cause of underweight in newborns is the mother's improper nourishment before and during pregnancy. Lack of protein foods and inadequate prenatal care can cause growth retardation in the fetus.

Children who live in poverty are more likely to be substandard in both weight and height. Lack of food, unsanitary living conditions, poor housing, unsafe drinking water, unemployment, and lack of education are among the factors contributing to undernourishment.

TABLE 9-1. A 3,000-kcal Menu Plan

Breakfast	Lunch	Dinner
6 oz unsweetened grapefruit juice	Salad:	1 c tomato soup
¾ c oatmeal, cooked with raisins	¼ head lettuce wedge	½ peach (canned)
1 sl bacon	1 sliced tomato	¼ c cottage cheese
½ English muffin, toasted	1 sliced hard-boiled egg	3 oz roast beef, chuck
1 t margarine	¼ c tuna, oil pack	1 medium baked potato
1 t jam	1 T thousand island dressing	1 t butter
¼ c whole milk	1 large hard roll	½ c cooked carrots
Coffee or tea	1 t butter	½ c tapioca pudding
	8 oz sweetened fruit yogurt	Coffee or tea
Snack	1 c whole milk	
1 medium orange	Coffee or tea	**Snack**
		2 fresh apricots
	Snack	1 c whole milk
	1 sl pecan pie	
	1 c whole milk	

TABLE 9-2. A 2,000-kcal Menu Plan

Breakfast	Lunch	Dinner
½ c oatmeal	Sandwich	1 chicken drumstick, fried
1 t sugar	1 T peanut butter	10 pieces french fried potatoes
2 T raisins	1 T jelly	½ c cooked mustard greens
1 sl whole wheat toast	2 sl white bread	1 dinner roll
1 T butter	Raw carrot sticks	1 T butter
1 T jelly	1 medium orange	1 c whole milk
1 c whole milk	1 iced brownie	
	½ c whole milk	
Snack		
1 banana	**Snack**	
	1 c apple juice	
	2 oatmeal cookies	

Note: This menu plan is acceptable for a 5- or 6-year-old who needs to gain weight.

Occasionally, high school and college students as well as the elderly show signs of undernutrition. Causes of their inadequate nutrition vary. For example, an adolescent may deliberately avoid food to lose weight. A college student may adopt a vegetarian diet that is nutritionally unsound, or an elderly person may not want to cook and eat alone.

For those individuals who need to gain weight, a high-calorie, high-protein diet is recommended. Tables 9-1 and 9-2 provide 3,000-kcal and 2,000-kcal sample menus for an adult and a child, respectively.

UNDERNUTRITION IN DEVELOPING COUNTRIES

Pronounced undernutrition is widespread in countries with only minimal resources. The children of these countries are the most likely to show the general symptoms that characterize undernutrition. After reviewing these symptoms, we will examine two of the most common syndromes of gross undernutrition: marasmus and kwashiorkor.

General Symptoms

In prolonged food deprivation, the functioning and regeneration of organ tissues slow down, and the body's demand for nutrients declines. The body becomes emaciated from loss of fat and muscle. Physical activity is reduced in an effort to conserve energy, and the victim becomes quiet and withdrawn.

Specific Symptoms

Other specific changes that may occur include:

- **Hair**—becomes dry and falls out easily.
- **Skin**—develops brown, gray, or red patches; becomes pale, dry, and loose.
- **Body weight**—gradual loss of water, fat, muscle, and skin can cause victim's weight to dwindle by half.
- **Edema**—sometimes experienced as result of fluid retention.
- **Cardiovascular system**—blood pressure and heartbeat slow down, and the heart shrinks.
- **Respiratory system**—rate, depth, and efficiency of respirations decrease.
- **Basal metabolic rate**—body metabolism slows down.
- **Endocrine system**—growth hormone decreases; adrenal and thyroid secretions remain normal.
- **Nervous system**—behavioral changes, such as apathy, irritability, and inability to concentrate, are common.
- **Gastrointestinal system**—in addition to the problems of malabsorption and diarrhea, digestive difficulties may occur because the stomach does not make enough hydrochloric acid. Also, the small intestine secretes fewer and less active enzymes.
- **Anemia**—some patients develop anemia.
- **Activities**—the adult victim has difficulty moving around because of the lack of energy and muscle, reduced capacity of the cardiovascular system, and anemia.

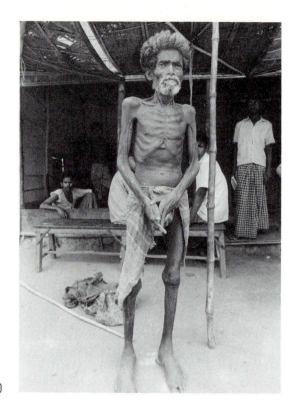

FIGURE 9-1. Undernutrition in an adult in Bangladesh. (Courtesy of the Agency for International Development)

Forms of Undernutrition

The victims of gross undernutrition are deficient in energy and in protein, vitamins, minerals, and other essential nutrients. One name given to classic undernutrition is *protein-calorie malnutrition,* or PCM.

The range of nutritional deficiency diseases included in the term PCM includes nutritional marasmus at one extreme and kwashiorkor at the other, with many variations in between. **Marasmus** is caused by a deficiency of calories and nearly all other essential nutrients, as in simple starvation. **Kwashiorkor** is the result of a severe lack of quantity and quality of protein, but an adequate or even excessive calorie intake and only a moderate lack of other essential nutrients.

Figure 9-1 shows an adult suffering from PCM. Table 9-3 compares marasmus and kwashiorkor symptoms in children. Figure 9-2(a) shows drawings comparing a marasmic child with a kwashiorkor child. In the following sections marasmus, kwashiorkor, and the infections that complicate these conditions will be described in more detail.

TABLE 9-3. Comparison of Marasmus and Kwashiorkor Symptoms in Children

Criterion	Marasmus	Kwashiorkor
Clinical symptom		
Subcutaneous fat	Little	Some
Lean body mass	Wasted	Wasted
Edema	No	Yes
Potbelly	No	Yes
Hair	Changes common	Changes very common and severe
Skin	Occasional minor changes	Characteristic dermatosis
Liver	Frequently enlarged	Very frequently enlarged
Anemia	Usually mild	Varies from mild to severe
Symptoms from vitamin deficiencies	Yes	No
Mental status	Usually normal	Apathetic
Age of occurrence	Under 1 year old	After 1 year old
Prognosis	Fair	Good
Permanent damage		
Liver	No	No
Neurological	Yes	No
Body organs and tissues	Major	Somewhat
Some chemical and biochemical analyses		
Body potassium depletion	Mild	Severe
Fatty liver	No	Yes

Marasmus

Nutritional marasmus refers to emaciation, or wasting, related to a lack of food. The symptoms of marasmus, such as weight loss, failure to thrive, irritability, and loss of appetite, are usually most apparent in children under 1 year old.

The marasmic child has the face of a little old man (see Figure 9-2a,c). Growth is retarded, with a significant loss of fat and muscle. There is no edema, and changes in the skin, hair, mucous membranes, and liver are less noticeable than in kwashiorkor. Watery diarrhea is common and may lead to dehydration.

Because caloric insufficiency rarely occurs without other clinical problems, respiratory and intestinal infections, tuberculosis, and parasitic infection often accompany marasmus. Vitamin deficiencies also can be severe.

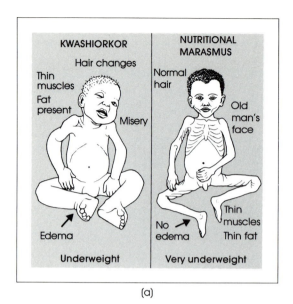

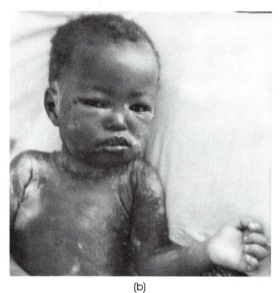

(a)

(b)

FIGURE 9-2. Children with marasmus and kwashiorkor: (a) Comparison of marasmus and kwashiorkor. (From D. B. Jelliffe, *Clinical Nutrition in Developing Countries*, 1968, U.S. Department of Health, Education and Welfare, Public Health Service) (b) A child in Chad with kwashiorkor. (UNICEF photo by Diabate) (c) A marasmic child in Uganda. (UNICEF photo by Arild Vollan)

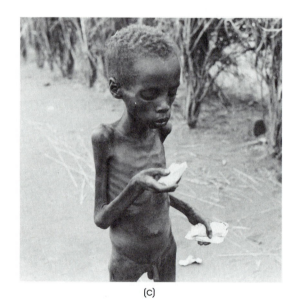

(c)

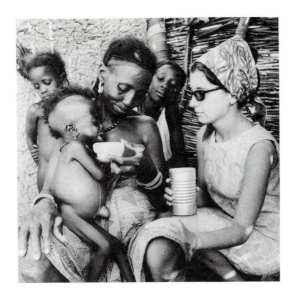

FIGURE 9-3. Edema in a kwashiorkor child. (Courtesy of the Agency for International Development)

Kwashiorkor

A kwashiorkor child, usually over 1 year old, shows some weight loss and is apathetic and irritable. Diarrhea, lack of appetite, and edema are all present. There is muscle wasting, but some body fat remains. More details on each symptom are given below.

- **Edema**—a characteristic symptom, particularly of the lower part of the body. Figure 9-3 shows a kwashiorkor child with edema; note the characteristic potbelly. Also see the swollen face of a kwashiorkor child in Figure 9-2(b).
- **Hair**—thin, soft, and "flagged" with alternating bands of gray, blonde, or red color. See Figure 9-4.
- **Liver**—the child shows a fatty liver that is often enlarged.
- **Skin**—cracks, flakes off, and sometimes develops infection that can be fatal. See Figures 9-2(b) and 9-5.
- **Anemia**—victim may develop practically any type of anemia.
- **Mucous membranes**—oral inflammation, lesions, and cracking at the corners of the mouth, tongue atrophy, and ulcers around the anal membranes.

Infection

Marasmus and kwashiorkor are often associated with infection of many kinds, because in such cases of malnutrition the lack of calories and protein impairs the body's ability to ward off illness. Infection can com-

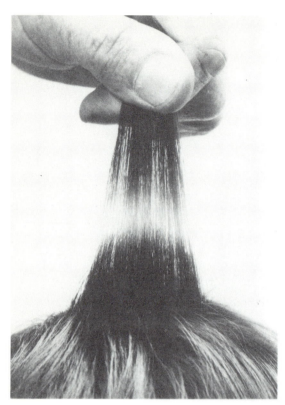

FIGURE 9-4. The flag sign in the hair of a child with kwashiorkor. (From N. S. Scrimshaw and M. Behar, *Science*, vol. 133, pp. 2039–2047, June 30, 1961. Copyright 1961 by the American Association for the Advancement of Science.)

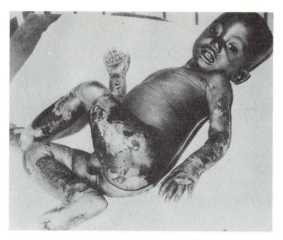

FIGURE 9-5. Skin lesions in a kwashiorkor child. (From A. J. Radford and A. J. H. Stephens, *The Lancet*, December 7, 1974, p. 1391)

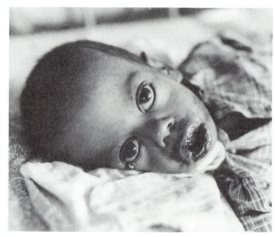

FIGURE 9-6. Oral infection in a malnourished child (Courtesy of the Agency for International Development).

pound the problems of the child already suffering from malnutrition. First, infection further depletes the body's protein, increasing the loss of muscle tissue. As a result, still more vitamins and minerals that the child can ill afford to lose are excreted. Second, malnutrition and infection combine to retard body growth and produce a subnormal weight: height ratio. Third, infection can severely reduce appetite, causing the child to refuse to eat and thereby magnifying the undernutrition problem. Fourth, the treatment of infection with antibiotics can further reduce the victim's immune response and interfere with the absorption of nutrients.

It is estimated that half the world's malnourished children may also be suffering from infection. Figure 9-6 shows a malnourished child with an oral infection.

MANAGEMENT OF PROTEIN-CALORIE MALNUTRITION

The nutritional and dietary care of a child suffering PCM requires special considerations and is conducted in two stages: immediate treatment and long-term rehabilitation.

Immediate Treatment

A child hospitalized for severe malnutrition and/or infection receives immediate treatment to restore fluid and electrolyte balance. Antibiotic therapy and blood transfusion also are important. Diet therapy is the next step.

At first the child is fed small amounts of milk to provide protein and calorie needs. Most undernourished children also need vitamin and mineral supplements. The child is fed progressively, beginning with the milk and gradually working up to a mixture of milk and cereal, mashed potato or banana, or any other combination of locally available nutrient-dense foods. Modern commercial nutrient supplements, though good sources of calorie and protein, are expensive and difficult to obtain in remote areas of the world.

In addition to medical treatment and diet therapy, tender care is an important part of the child's recovery. A comfortably warm environment and plenty of touching, holding, and emotional support are essential.

Signs of the child's improved well-being, good appetite, subsiding edema, and normal reactions to the environment indicate recovery from the emergency stage, sometimes as soon as one month after treatment begins. Figure 9-7 shows mothers feeding their emaciated children at the Kaabong emergency center in drought-stricken Karamoja Province.

Long-term Rehabilitation

The problem of long-term rehabilitation is a difficult one, because food is not abundant in most poverty-stricken countries. Increasing the food supply is complicated by such interrelated issues as population, poverty, culture, food preference, and politics.

There are many causes of malnutrition. Primary causes include natu-

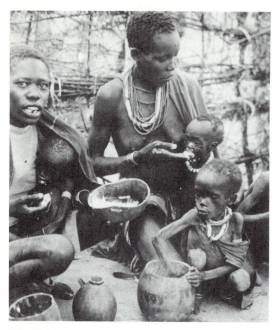

FIGURE 9-7. Emergency feeding of malnourished children. (UNICEF photo by H. Dalrymple)

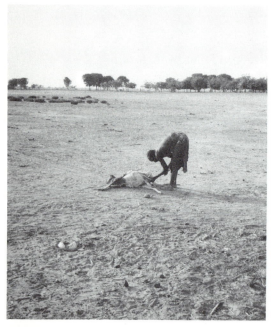

FIGURE 9-8. Drought in Mauritania. (UNICEF photo by Davico)

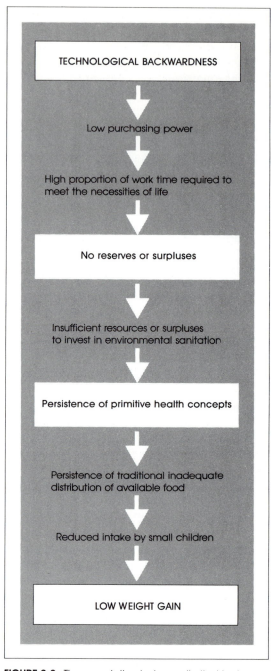

FIGURE 9-9. The association between limited technology and childhood undernutrition in a poor country. (Adapted from "Malnutrition and early childhood," J. Cravioto and E. R. Delicardie, *Food Nutrition* 2:2, 1976)

ral and man-made disasters (accidents, sickness, drought, war, and floods), poverty and unequal distribution of wealth, lack of natural resources, culturally ingrained food habits, unsanitary living conditions, malabsorption from all causes, lack of prenatal care, infection, and ignorance and lack of education. In the great Sahelian drought in Mauritania in 1968 through 1973, for example, thousands of people died of starvation when parched grazing grounds no longer could support livestock as shown in Figure 9-8.

Factors such as limited technology, resources, education, health knowledge, and large families contribute to childhood undernutrition, especially in developing countries. Figure 9-9, one of a series of flow diagrams constructed by Doctors J. Cravioto and E. R. Delicardie of the United Nations, illustrates the relationship between limited resources and childhood undernutrition in a poor country.

Because of the complex nature of world hunger, solutions are difficult. Undernutrition in underdeveloped countries will continue. There are, however, three simple and economical ways in which malnourished children have been successfully helped.

Use of Local Foods

One way of combating persistent malnutrition is to promote the use of local foods that are inexpensive but nutrient rich. This method has been successful in ending moderate undernutrition among the children of Nepal (M. R. Bomgaars, *Journal of the American Medical Association* 1976, *236*:2513).

In Nepal, many parents believed their young Nepalese children had been cast under a spell because of their miserable behavior, such as whining and refusing to eat. These children subsequently were diagnosed by members of a nearby modern health project as being underfed. By utilizing their knowledge of local food availability and dietary practices, the health personnel showed residents how to prepare a high-protein, high-calorie mixture of roasted corn, soybeans, and wheat called *sarbottam pitho* (or "super flour"). The children ate it, and their nutrition improved. Their behavior also returned to normal. It is important to note that the disturbance of native beliefs was kept to a minimum.

Promotion of Relactation

A second method of combating PCM involves the promotion of relactation in some women (R. E. Brown, *Clinical Pediatrics* 1978, *17*:333). Relactation simply means the stimulation of milk production in women either who have never breast-fed or who have stopped breast-feeding for a time.

Breast-feeding by Female Relatives. In many developing countries, when a mother dies from childbirth, it is the custom to entrust the care of the surviving infant to a female relative or friend. The baby is allowed to suckle on her as often as possible, and she is given herbs and medicine. Many babies are able to induce a flow of milk after only a brief interval. Emotional support and encouragement play an important role in the success of this effort.

Interrupted Breast-feeding by the Mother. A second form of relactation is the renewal of breast milk in the baby's own mother. Certain unique circumstances have provided ample evidence that mothers' breasts can easily be induced to produce a normal flow of milk by letting the baby suckle as often as possible. Again, the encouragement of friends and relatives enhances the success of this relactation effort. Government officials in Bangladesh and India recognize the convenience and economy of feeding the mothers well instead of buying medicine and formula milk for the infants.

Wet-nursing Orphans. Hiring women to wet-nurse orphaned babies is the basis of a third form of relactation. At the end of the Vietnam war, large-scale employment of nearby women to wet-nurse orphaned babies was initiated. Sincere interest, effort, and support enabled most "substitute mothers" to achieve a normal milk flow. Both the women and the babies benefited.

The practice of relactation has been shown to be cheap, convenient, and practical. The extent to which it can be applied to a world full of hungry children remains to be seen.

Nutrition Rehabilitation Units

During the past 30 years, the use of local nutrition units to rehabilitate malnourished children has become a common and successful practice in many impoverished countries (*British Medical Journal* 1975, *2*:246). These units, established according to the limitations and needs of the local people, have three major functions: (1) to provide low-cost nutrition and dietary care to everyone; (2) to rehabilitate malnourished children; (3) to teach natives about proper dietary practices.

A number of significant health benefits have resulted from such units. Natives are more willing to follow health guidelines because they are no longer threatened by the hospital atmosphere. Satisfied recipients of health care and training spread the news so that more people are willing to come. The community is brought closer together by such units and becomes exposed to some elements of medical care, education, agriculture, and community development.

TABLE 9-4. Special High-protein Products Used by Different Countries to Combat Protein-Calorie Malnutrition*

Country or Area	Product	Major Ingredients
Algeria	Superamine	Dried skim milk, chick-peas, legumes, wheat
Brazil	Incaparina	Soya, maize
Chile	Lache alim	Soya, fish protein concentrate, dried skim milk
Colombia	Duryea	Soya, dried skim milk, maize
Central America	Incaparina	Cottonseed, maize
Egypt	Weaning food	Dried skim milk, chick-peas, broad beans, wheat
Ethiopia	Faffa	Soya, dried skim milk
India	Bal-Amul	Soya, dried skim milk, legumes, wheat
Kenya	Simba	Dried skim milk, maize
Madagascar	Weaning food	Soya, dried skim milk, rice
Mexico	Conasupo products	Soya, kidney bean
Mozambique	Super Maeu	Soya, dried skim milk, maize, malt
Nigeria	Arlac	Groundnut, dried skim milk
Peru	Peruvita	Cottonseed, dried skim milk, quinoa
Senegal	Ladylac	Groundnut, dried skim milk, millet
South Africa	Pronutro	Soya, groundnut, dried skim milk, maize, yeast, wheat germ
Taiwan	Weaning food	Soya, dried skim milk, rice
Thailand	Noodles	Soya, wheat
Turkey	Weaning food	Soya, dried skim milk, chick-peas, wheat
Uganda	Soya porridge	Soya, dried skim milk, maize
United States	WSB (wheat and soy blend)	Soya, wheat
Venezuela	Incaparina	Soya, cottonseed, maize
Zambia	Milk biscuit	Soya, casein, wheat

*Though some products have existed for many years, others change constantly. Current references should be used to supplement this list.

HIGH-PROTEIN FOODS

Many efforts have been made to increase the availability of high-protein foods in underdeveloped countries. One effort, called the "green revolution," is a highly technological approach to intensified food production. Perhaps a more successful approach is supplying children with special cheap and semisynthetic high-protein foods from locally available sources. Many governments are issuing products that contain all the essential amino acids as well as other essential nutrients. Table 9-4 presents a partial list of those products and their major ingredients.

Figure 9-10 shows a severely malnourished child in the Provincial Hospital in Kuito, Angola, drinking K-Mix II (a high-protein food mixture developed by UNICEF). Figure 9-11 shows children in Dacca (Bangladesh) sharing a bowl of CSM (Corn-Soya-Milk plus sugar, a high-protein food supplied by UNICEF).

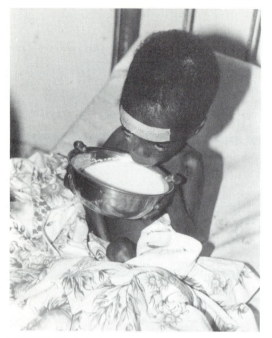

FIGURE 9-10. Rehabilitating an Angolan child. (UNICEF photo by Horst Ulax Cerni)

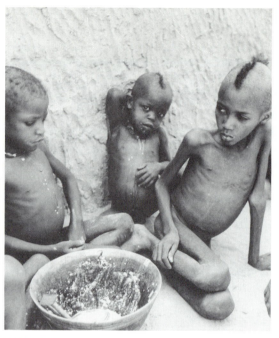

FIGURE 9-11. Rehabilitating children in Bangladesh. (UNICEF photo by Jacques Danois)

The effort to cure and prevent worldwide malnutrition is dependent upon concerned individuals all over the world.

STUDY QUESTIONS

1. Distinguish between the terms *undernutrition* and *malnutrition*.
2. In the United States which age groups are most likely to be undernourished? Why?
3. Describe the general symptoms of gross undernutrition.
4. What is protein-calorie malnutrition? In what way is this term misleading?
5. What is the theoretical difference between kwashiorkor and marasmus? Describe some characteristic symptoms of each condition.
6. Discuss three successful approaches to rehabilitating young victims of malnutrition in some underdeveloped countries.

7. What is being done at the national and international levels to increase the supply of high-protein foods in countries in danger of widespread malnutrition?

REFERENCES

Ashworth, A. 1980. Practical aspects of dietary management during rehabilitation from severe protein-energy malnutrition. *J. Human Nutr.* 34:360.

Austin, J. E. 1981. *Nutrition programs in the third world.* Cambridge, Mass.: Oelgeschlager, Gunn, and Hain.

Cameron, M., and Hofvander, Y. 1971. *Manual on feeding infants and young children.* Protein Advisory Group, United Nations.

Golden, M. H. N., and Jackson, A. A. 1984. Chronic severe undernutrition. In *Present knowledge in nutrition,* 5th ed. Washington, D. C.: The Nutrition Foundation.

Hensley, E. S. 1981. Basic concepts of world nutrition. Springfield, Ill.: C. C. Thomas.

Morley, D., and Woodland, M. 1980. *See how they grow: monitoring child growth for appropriate health care in developing countries.* New York: Oxford University Press.

Olson, R. E., ed. 1975. *Protein-calorie malnutrition.* New York: Academic Press.

Presidential Commission on World Hunger. 1979. *Overcoming world hunger: the challenge ahead, presidential commission on world hunger, final report.* Washington, D. C.: Government Printing Office.

10 AN ADEQUATE DIET

Understanding the importance of various nutrients to our health is the first step in planning daily diets with adequate amounts of all these nutrients. However, careful meal planning is not an easy task. Certain guidelines have been devised by nutritionists to facilitate the process, including: food composition tables, Recommended Dietary Allowances (RDAs), nutrient labeling, and the four food groups. Daily food guides based on the four food groups provide a way to ensure that diets are adequate.

In addition to examining these guidelines, we shall consider other factors involved in meal planning such as: the frequency and timing of meals, the effects of cooking on nutrient loss, and ways to keep food costs down without sacrificing essential nutrients.

FOOD COMPOSITION TABLES

Food composition tables provide important information about nutrients. Some of the major American food composition tables are:

- *Composition of Foods—Raw, Processed, and Prepared.* USDA Agricultural Handbook No. 8. The 1963 edition, continuously revised, now has many volumes (see below).
- *Nutritive Value of American Foods in Common Units.* USDA Agricultural Handbook No. 456, 1980.
- "Nutritive Value of Foods." USDA Home and Garden Bulletin No. 72, 1981.

TABLE 10-1. Revised Sections of USDA Handbook No. 8 as of 1984

Section No.	Food Group	Year Issued	No. of Items
8-1	Dairy and egg products	1976	144
8-2	Spices and herbs	1977	43
8-3	Baby foods	1978	217
8-4	Fats and oils	1979	128
8-5	Poultry products	1979	304
8-6	Soups, sauces, and gravies	1980	214
8-7	Sausages and luncheon meats	1980	80
8-8	Breakfast cereals	1982	142
8-9	Fruits and fruit juices	1982	263
8-10	Pork products	1983	186

- *Food Values of Portions Commonly Used*, 13th edition. J. A. T. Pennington and H. N. Church, Lippincott, 1985.
- "Amino Acid Contents of Foods." USDA Home Economics Research Report No. 4, 1968.
- "Vitamin B-6, Pantothenic Acid, and Vitamin B-12." USDA Home Economics Research Report No. 36, 1969.

A major revision of USDA Handbook No. 8 is currently in progress. When completed, it will provide information on 61 nutrients in about 4,000 foods. Table 10-1 lists sections of the revised edition released as of 1980.

Food composition tables are convenient, cheap, and widely used, but they have some limitations. For example, factors such as soil and climate, harvesting and storage, and preparation and serving methods can cause different food composition tables to give different data. Some uncommon or ethnic foods may not be listed.

RECOMMENDED DIETARY ALLOWANCES (RDAs)

In addition to learning the nutrient content of foods, we must know how much of each nutrient we need to consume every day. Some standard guidelines for determining a number of nutrients for people in different age and sex categories have been developed by the National Research Council of the National Academy of Sciences. These are the well-known Recommended Dietary Allowances (RDAs). The latest RDAs, which were released in 1980, indicate the recommended daily amounts of kilocalories, protein, vitamins A, D, E, B_1, B_2, B_6, B_{12}, and C, niacin, folacin, calcium, phosphorus, magnesium, zinc, iodine, and iron, as well as ranges of estimated safe and adequate daily dietary intakes (recommended) of vitamin K, biotin, pantothenic acid, molybdenum, selenium, chromium, copper, manganese, fluoride, and the electrolytes sodium, potassium, and chloride. The complete RDAs are reproduced in Table 1 of the appendix.

The RDAs are designed to provide a nutrient intake guide for normal, healthy people. They are not appropriate for people with clinical conditions such as hereditary diseases, acute or chronic illness, or trauma. A combination of methods to evaluate a person's nutritional status is the safest and includes: (1) an analysis of nutrient intake; (2) physical examination; (3) clinical evaluation; and (4) blood, urine, and other laboratory studies.

DAILY FOOD GUIDES: THE FOUR FOOD GROUPS

Because there is no "perfect" food that can supply all the RDAs, we must eat a variety of foods to meet our nutritional needs. Nutritionists have translated the RDA guidelines into daily meal plans, known as *daily food guides*, to provide an easy way to make good food choices.

The daily food guides recommend a large number of nutritious foods, grouped into four broad categories. These *four food groups* are: (1) milk and milk products, (2) meat or meat equivalents, (3) fruits and vegetables, and (4) breads and cereals. Each group contributes a substantial amount of the major nutrients needed for health.

In addition to sorting "nutrient-dense" foods into four basic groups, the USDA has suggested an appropriate number of servings from each group to be consumed daily (Table 10-2). However, both the food guides and the RDAs should be used as suggestions for sound nutrition rather than ironclad rules.

Recently, the USDA introduced a fifth food group: fats, sweets, and alcohol. Because this new group has not yet been widely adopted, this book will adhere to the four food groups previously mentioned and consider fats, sweets, and some other items as *supplementary foods* (see below). However, these may be considered the fifth food group if preferred.

In the following sections the foods commonly chosen in the United States—in other words, the "standard American diet"—and the nutrients these foods provide will be examined.

Milk and Milk Products

Each of us should consume at least a minimal amount of milk each day. Some common varieties of milk and milk products follow:

TABLE 10-2. Recommended Numbers of Servings from the Four Food Groups

Food Group	Serving Size	No. of Daily Servings
Milk and milk products		
Fluid milk	1 c, 8 oz, ½ pt, ¼ qt	Children under 9: 2–3 Children 9–12: ≥3 Teenagers: ≥4 Adults: ≥2 Pregnant women: ≥3 Nursing mothers: ≥4
Calcium equivalent	1 c milk 2 c cottage cheese 1 c pudding 1¾ c ice cream 1½ oz cheddar cheese	
Meat and meat equivalents	2–3 oz cooked lean meat without bone 3–4 oz raw meat without bone 2 oz luncheon meat (e.g., bologna) ¾ c canned baked beans 1 c cooked dry beans, peas, lentils 2 eggs 2 oz cheddar cheese ½ c cottage cheese 4 T peanut butter	≥2
Fruits and vegetables	Varies by item: ½ c cooked spinach 1 potato 1 orange ½ grapefruit	≥4, including 1 of citrus fruit and another fruit or vegetable that is a good source of vitamin C and 2 of a fair source 1, at least every other day, of a dark green or deep yellow vegetable for vitamin C ≥2 or more of other vegetables and fruits, including potatoes
Bread and cereals	1 slice of bread, 1 oz ready-to-eat cereal ½ to ¾ c cooked cereal, corn-meal, grits, macaroni, noodles, rice, or spaghetti	≥4

- **Fluid milk:** whole, low-fat, skim, fat-free
- **Dry milk:** whole, low-fat, skim, fat-free
- **Other milk:** evaporated, condensed
- **Milk products:** yogurt, cheese, cottage cheese
- **Milk alternates:** soy milk, powdered soy milk, soy cheese

The recommendations range from 2 or more cups of fluid whole milk for adults and children, to 4 or more cups for teenagers and nursing mothers.

Milk's major contributions are calcium, protein, and vitamin B_2. Milk also is a source of vitamins B_1, B_6, B_{12}, A and D, niacin, and magnesium. Milk protein is cheap, easily digested, and of high quality; lactalbumin and casein make up about 80 percent of the protein in milk.

For those people who cannot digest fluid whole milk, fermented milk products such as cheese, yogurt, or buttermilk may be substituted. Cottage cheese and low-fat, skim, or nonfat milk also are good sources of protein. Such products do not contain the same nutrients as fluid whole milk, however. For example, if low-fat, skim, or nonfat milk are used, the intake of vitamins A and D and essential fatty acids may be low. Some of the water-soluble vitamins are lost in the preparation of cheese. Cottage cheese prepared by acid coagulation is low in calcium and has reduced water-soluble vitamins.

In general, cheeses tend to have higher fat and calorie content and lower levels of protein, calcium, and vitamin B_{12} than fluid whole milk. Otherwise, the nutrient content is similar to that of milk.

Ice cream, although made from milk, milk solids, and cream, also contains additives, flavorings, and sweeteners. It is higher in calories than milk. Most commercial yogurt is low in fat and high (20 percent) in galactose. More than half the weight of some yogurts consists of added sugar and fruit.

One milk product may be replaced with another to get equivalent amounts of nutrients. Table 10-3 shows the amounts of milk products that provide the same amount of protein and calcium as 1 cup of fluid whole milk.

Meats and Equivalents

According to the daily food guides (Table 10-2), we should eat two or more servings from the meat and meat-equivalent groups every day. These two servings of meat provide approximately 50 percent of the protein, 25 to 50 percent of the iron, 25 to 30 percent of vitamins B_1 and B_2, and 30 percent of the niacin in the RDAs. Meat is not a good source of vitamins C and A or calcium. Common foods in the meat group are:

- **Lean meat:**   Beef, veal, lamb, pork (fresh or cured), liver
- **Variety meat:**   Heart, brain, tongue, kidney

TABLE 10-3. Milk Products That Contribute As Much Protein and Calcium As 1 Cup of Fluid Whole Milk

Milk Product	Amount of Product Containing Given Amount of Nutrient	
	9 g Protein	280 g Calcium
Nonfat milk	1 c	1 c
Cheddar cheese	1⅓ oz	1⅓ oz
Cottage cheese	1⅓ c	⅓ c
Ice cream	1½ c	1½ c
Cream cheese	30 T	9 T

- **Wild meat:** Squirrel, rabbit, bear, deer, buffalo
- **Fish:** Shellfish, fresh and saltwater varieties (fresh, dried, frozen, canned)
- **Poultry:** All fowl (e.g., chicken, turkey, guinea hen, duck, goose) and their giblets
- **Game birds:** Pheasant, wild duck, grouse
- **Miscellaneous:** "Turkey ham" (made from turkey meat but treated and smoked to look and taste like ham), "hot dogs" (made from a variety of meats including organ meats)
- **Dry legumes:** Navy beans, lima beans, lentils, peanuts, others
- **Nuts:** Nuts, nut butters
- **Peas:** All split, dried peas; pinto beans, chick-peas, pigeon peas
- **Meat analogues:** Textured vegetable proteins (TVPs), largely soy, which may be processed to simulate meat products such as sausage and bacon in shape and flavor
- **Meat equivalents:** Eggs, cheese

Muscle meats and organ meats are high sources of iron. By contrast, chicken and fish have relatively low iron content. In addition to iron, muscle meats contribute zinc and phosphorus.

A major source of protein, meats have varying levels of the nutrient. For example, pork contains about 13 percent protein, whereas fish may contain as much as 30 percent. Eggs, cheese, beans, peas, and peanut butter contain less protein, but are nevertheless good inexpensive sources. Dried beans and peas are 30 percent protein; nuts are 15 percent protein.

The fat content of meat may vary from 1 to 40 percent, with prime beef containing 25 percent, standard beef 16 percent, and utility beef less than 15 percent. By contrast, fish has only 1 to 7 percent fat.

Fruits and Vegetables

Four or more servings of fruits and vegetables each day are recommended by the daily food guides. This food group is the major source of iron and vitamins A and C. Fruits and vegetables are also good sources of calcium, magnesium, and folic acid. Fruits stimulate appetite and aid the absorption of iron and calcium.

Most fruits and vegetables are nutrient-dense, low in calories, low in fat, and high in cellulose. A good intestinal environment is provided by the bulk and roughage in fruits and vegetables. Some of them—such as celery, apples, and carrots—even help clean our teeth.

Although this group as a whole is a major source of vitamin A, very few vegetables and fruits contain ample amounts of this vitamin. Fruits and vegetables that are high in vitamin A include dark green leafy vegetables, orange-colored vegetables, and orange-fleshed fruits (see Table 10-4).

This food group is our main source of vitamin C. Citrus fruits are particularly high in vitamin C: a 4-oz serving of citrus fruit juice provides 30 mg of the vitamin. Fruits such as strawberries, cherries, and cantaloupe are also good sources. Vegetables such as spinach, broccoli, and cabbage are rich in vitamin C, especially when eaten raw. Since vitamin C can be destroyed by heat, air, and light, food should be prepared in ways that minimize its loss.

About one quarter of our daily iron need and a small amount of calcium are derived from fruits and vegetables. Certain vegetables, such as beans and peas, are good sources of protein, while tuber vegetables such as potatoes provide some protein. Both groups are high in carbohydrate calories.

Cereals and Cereal Products

The daily food guides recommend four or more servings of grain products each day. Major nutrients contributed by these foods are calories, iron, niacin, and vitamins B_1 and B_2.

Cereals and cereal products include all grains served in whole grain, enriched, or fortified forms: for example, wheat, corn, oats, buckwheat, rice, and rye. Some common items in this food group are as follows:

- **Breads:** Yeast breads, rolls, quick breads, biscuits, buns, muffins, pancakes, waffles, crackers, others
- **Breakfast cereals:** Ready–to–eat types, including flaked, rolled, and puffed forms; cooked types including whole grain, and rolled forms

TABLE 10-4. Foods in the Fruit and Vegetable Group

Varieties Rich in Vitamin A and Carotene

Dark green leafy vegetables: beet greens, broccoli, chard, collard, watercress, kale, mustard greens, spinach, turnip tops, wild greens (dandelion and others)

Orange-colored vegetables: carrots, pumpkins, sweet potatoes, winter squash, yams

Orange-fleshed fruits: apricots, muskmelon, mangoes

Varieties Rich in Vitamin C

Citrus fruits: grapefruit, oranges, lemons, tangerines; juices of these fruits

Other good and excellent sources: muskmelon, strawberries, broccoli, several tropical fruits (including guavas), raw sweet green and red peppers

Significant sources: tomatoes, tomato juice, white potatoes, dark green leafy vegetables, other raw vegetables and fruits

Other Fruits and Vegetables

Vegetables: asparagus, lima beans, green beans, beets, cabbage, cauliflower, celery, corn, cucumber, eggplant, kohlrabi, lettuce, okra, onions, green peas, plantain, rutabaga, sauerkraut, summer squash, and turnips

Fruits: apples, avocados, bananas, berries, cherries, dates, figs, grapes, nectarines, peaches, pears, pineapple, plums, prunes, raisins, rhubarb, watermelon; juices and nectars of many fruits

---

- **Other grain foods:** Macaroni, spaghetti, noodles, flour, rice, cornmeal
- **Whole grain products:** Whole wheat flour and its products, bulgur, dark rye flour, brown rice, whole ground cornmeal

The protein in grains is incomplete. Grains can be used to provide complete proteins, however, as discussed in Chapters 5 and 9, by combining several different cereals. Combining grains with protein-rich foods—for instance, macaroni and cheese, rice with chicken, and milk on cereal—increases our amino acid intake.

Grains provide a fair amount of nutrients at low cost. Also, adding milk to grain products adds not only protein but also calcium and other nutrients. The enrichment and fortification of grain products is an important health protection measure.

TABLE 10-5. A Daily Foundation Diet for an Adult Using the Basic Foods

Food Group	No. of Servings
Milk	2 c fluid milk
Meat	3½ oz broiled round steak
	1 medium egg
Fruits and vegetables	½ c cooked asparagus
	1 medium baked potato
	½ c cooked summer squash
	6 oz orange juice
	1 pear
Bread and cereals	3 slices enriched bread
	⅔ c corn flakes

THE FOUNDATION DIET AND SUPPLEMENTARY FOODS

Foundation Diet

A foundation diet consists of only the recommended numbers of servings from the four food groups. An example of such a diet is shown in Table 10-5. A foundation diet provides more than 90 percent of most essential nutrients and over 75 percent of the calories in the RDAs, as shown in Table 10-6.

Supplementary Foods

Most of us eat more than a foundation diet, however, both through extra servings and by adding foods not included in the four food groups. Such items are called *supplementary foods*. They include spices, butter, margarine, and other fats. Many snacks and soft drinks, sweets, and fabricated foods such as breakfast bars also can be included in this group.

Some common supplemental foods are: beverages (coffee, tea, soft drinks, alcoholic beverages); fats (butter, cream, margarine, mayonnaise, oils); sweets (sugar, jam, sweet desserts, candy, pastries, syrups); snack items (cookies, potato chips); spices and seasonings (flavorings, seasonings, all herbs and spices, sauces).

Fats, though classified as supplemental foods, are essential to health (see Chapter 3). Vegetable oil should be included among the fats used. Common sources of fats are butter, margarine, shortening, cooking and salad oils, cream, most cheeses, mayonnaise, salad dressings, nuts, and bacon. Meats, whole milk, eggs, and chocolate contain some fat naturally.

TABLE 10-6. Nutrient Contribution by the Foundation Diet

Nutrient*	Amount of Nutrient Contributed†	RDA for a 25-year-old	
		Male	Female
Kilocalories	1,200–1,300	2,700	2,000
Protein	60–70 g	56	44
Vitamin A	1,100–1,400 μg RE	1,000	800
Vitamin E	1–5 mg	10	8
Vitamin C	125–135 mg	60	60
Thiamin	0.8–1.2 mg	1.4	1.0
Riboflavin	1.5–1.8 mg	1.6	1.2
Niacin	13.0–13.5 mg	18	13
Vitamin B_6	1 mg	2.2	2.0
Folacin	200–250 μg	400	400
Vitamin B_{12}	2–4 μg	3	3
Calcium	700–800 mg	800	800
Phosphorus	900–1,000 mg	800	800
Iron	10 mg	10	18
Zinc	5–8 mg	15	15

*Vitamin D and iodine are not included. All units used comply with the RDA system. Check Table 1 in the appendix for more details.

†Because of the variation in the nutrient content of foods, only a range or an approximation is given.

Although supplementary foods round out meals and make them more tasty, these foods tend to be low in nutrients. Each of the four food groups provides at least 25 percent of three or more nutrients. By contrast, the nutrient contribution of supplementary foods is relatively insignificant except for calories and fats. For example, supplementary foods provide 20 percent of the total caloric intake, 30 to 35 percent of the total fat intake, and 10 percent of the vitamin A need. The approximate nutrient contributions of the different food groups to the American diet are shown in Table 10-7. The more calories one eats from the basic four food groups, the greater the likelihood of obtaining the RDAs. A low-calorie diet, therefore, should emphasize the basic food groups rather than the supplementary foods.

Meal Planning

Normal, healthy people may eat any food they like so long as they know how to combine foods to provide a good diet. Familiarity with the basic food groups allows us to plan balanced and nutritious meals. Table 10-8 suggests a meal plan for an adult, while Table 10-9 presents a sample menu of 2,400 kcal and 95 g of protein.

TABLE 10-7. Approximate Nutrient Contributions of the Different Food Groups

Food Group	Major Nutrient Contributed	Proportional Contribution to the American Diet
Milk	Protein	1/3
	Calcium	2/3
	Riboflavin	1/2
Meat	Protein	1/2
	Thiamine	1/4
	Iron	>1/3
	Niacin	>1/3
Fruits and vegetables	Vitamin C	practically all
	Vitamin A and carotene	3/4
	Iron	1/4
Bread and cereals	Iron, thiamine, niacin, other B vitamins, fiber	>1/4
Supplementary foods		
Fats, oils	Calories, fat-soluble vitamins	varies
Sweet products	Fluids, calories, small amount of nutrients	varies
Spices and seasonings	Iodine	varies
Alcohol	Calories	insignificant to 1/3

TABLE 10-8. Suggested Meal Plan

Breakfast	Lunch	Dinner
Fruit/juice, ½ c/1 serving	Soup, ½ c	Soup, ½ c
Cereal: hot/6 oz; dry/1 oz	Meat (regular/substitute), 2–3 oz	Meat (regular/substitute), 3–4 oz
Egg (regular or substitute), 1 serving	Vegetable (cooked/salad), ½ c	Fruit/juice, ½ c/1 serving
Meat: 2 strips bacon; 2 sausages; or 1 oz regular meat	Potato (regular/substitute), ½ c	Vegetable (cooked/salad), ½ c
	Salad dressing, 1 T	Potato (regular/substitute), ½ c
Bread, 1–2 slices	Bread/roll, 1–2 servings	Salad dressing, 1–2 t
Butter/margarine, 1–3 t	Butter/margarine, 1–3 t	Bread/roll, 1–2 servings
Jelly/jam/preserves, 1–3 t	Dessert, 1 serving	Butter/margarine, 1–3 t
Milk, 1 c	Milk, 1 c	Dessert, 1 serving
Hot beverage (coffee/tea), 1–2 c	Hot beverage (coffee/tea), 1–2 c	Milk, 1 c
Cream (regular/substitute), 1–3 t	Cream (regular/substitute), 1–3 t	Hot beverage (coffee/tea), 1–2 c
Sugar, 1–3 t	Sugar, 1–3 t	Cream (regular/substitute), 1–3 t
Salt, pepper	Salt, pepper	Sugar, 1–3 t
		Salt, pepper

TABLE 10-9. Menu Plan Providing 2,400 kcal and 95 g of Protein

Breakfast	Lunch	Dinner
Orange juice, ½ c	Pea soup, ½ c	Chicken broth, ½ c
Oatmeal, 6 oz	Crackers, 2	Fried chicken, 3 oz
Egg, 1	Ham, 2 oz	Spinach, ½ c
Bread, 2 slices	Lettuce/tomato salad, ½ c	Rice, ½ c
Margarine, 2 t	Noodles, ½ c	Bread, 1 slice
Jelly, 1 t	Toast, 1 slice	Margarine, 1 t
Milk, 1 c	Margarine, 1 t	Milk, 1 c
Coffee, 1 c	Milk, 1 c	Coffee, 1 c
Cream, 1 t	Ice cream, 1 c	Cream substitute, 1 t
Sugar, 2 t	Coffee, 1 c	Sugar, 1 t
Salt, pepper	Sugar, 1 t	Salt, pepper
	Salt, pepper	

COOKING METHODS AND NUTRIENT LOSS

Minimizing nutrient losses caused by home cooking and commercial food preparation is a second concern. Even food storage has an effect on nutrient retention. For example, the cool moist temperatures provided by refrigeration not only help keep vegetables and other foods fresh but also help retain nutrients.

Methods of preparing foods, such as chopping, slicing, crushing, and shredding, increase nutrient loss. Trimming vegetables or removing coarse outer leaves often results in a loss of vitamins A and C and calcium.

The high temperatures used in dry heat cooking—frying, roasting, baking, grilling, and broiling—may destroy any heat-sensitive nutrient. Vitamin C, thiamine, folic acid, pyridoxine, and pantothenic acid are readily destroyed at high temperatures. Prolonged use of dry heat changes the quality of protein and destroys polyunsaturated fatty acids.

Moist cooking methods such as stewing or simmering are less likely to destroy nutrients. If a small amount of liquid is used, nutrient loss is minimized. Minerals and water-soluble vitamins may be saved if cooking liquid is reused as a soup or base.

FOOD BUDGETING

There are a number of ways to keep the food budget under control without sacrificing nutrients. Some of these are:

- **Planning ahead:** Making a grocery list can save time, money, and frustration.

- **Sales, specials, and coupons:** To be cost effective, sales and coupons are useful only if the advertised items are needed and purchasing them does not require going to many different stores.
- **Low-cost brands:** Savings of 5 to 10 percent may be realized by buying store brands and nonbrand items.
- **Inexpensive to moderate-cost items:** Less expensive foods can provide as many nutrients as costlier foods.
- **Produce in season:** Vegetables, fruits, and other foods are usually less expensive when they are plentiful.
- **Wholesale or quantity purchases:** Purchasing a large quantity of food can save money, if freezer or storage space is available.
- **Pricing by units:** Unit pricing—by the pound, ounce, or cup, for example—makes it easier to compare the cost of goods.
- **Cooperatives:** Because cooperatives are nonprofit, most of their products are cheaper than those in other stores.
- **Less-frequent shopping:** Less money is spent when major shopping is reduced to once or twice a month.
- **Fewer fast and convenience foods:** Preparing a dish at home instead of relying on fast and convenience foods usually saves money.

STUDY QUESTIONS

1. What is the purpose of food composition tables? What are their drawbacks?
2. What do the RDAs represent? Which agency or organization established them? How can the RDAs be used in conjunction with other criteria to determine a person's nutritional status?
3. What are the Five Food Groups? How many servings of each are recommended by the daily food guides? What are the major nutritional contributions of each group?
4. What is a foundation diet? Discuss the role of supplementary foods.
5. How does food processing or preparation cause a loss of nutrients? How can these losses be minimized?
6. List at least seven ways of keeping food costs down without scrimping on nutritional needs.
7. Plan a 3-day menu for a family of four.

REFERENCES

Harper, A. E. 1978. Meeting recommended dietary allowances. *J. Florida Med. Assoc.* 66:419.

King, J. C., et al. 1978. Evaluation and modification of the basic four food guide. *J. Nutr. Edu.* 10:27.

National Academy of Sciences, National Research Council, Food and Nutrition Board, 1980. *Recommended dietary allowances.*

Peckham, G. C., and Freeland-Graves, J. H. 1979. *Foundations of food preparation.* 4th ed. New York: Macmillan.

Rezabek, K. 1979. *Nutritive value of convenience foods.* Hines, Ill.: West Suburban Dietetic Association.

Shannon, B. M., and Parks, S. C. 1980. Fast foods: a perspective on their nutritional impact. *J. Amer. Dietet. Assoc.* 76:242.

U. S. Department of Agriculture, Science and Education Administration. 1979. *Family food budgeting for good meals and good nutrition.* Home & Garden Bulletin, no. 94, revised.

U. S. Department of Agriculture. 1982. *Your money's worth in foods.* Home & Garden Bulletin, no. 183.

White, A., and the Society for Nutrition Education. 1980. *The family health cookbook.* New York: McKay.

11 NUTRITION DURING PREGNANCY AND LACTATION

NUTRITION AND PREGNANCY

Every culture since time began has had its own ideas about pregnancy and diet. What a woman should or should not eat is a matter of great interest. The Chinese, for example, believe that pregnant women should eat sweet and sour pigs' feet because of the variety of nutrients contained. Dietary recommendations during pregnancy are, however, often more folklore than fact.

The most significant nutritional fact about pregnancy is that the fetus is, from the instant of conception, completely dependent upon the mother for nourishment. At the beginning of pregnancy the fetus receives nutrients through the placenta; eventually the amniotic fluid provides additional nourishment.

Because the baby's need for nourishment is added to that of the mother, her nutritional status both at conception and during pregnancy is vital. For the woman who breast-feeds her baby, the need for extra nutrients continues until the child is weaned.

Maternal Nutrition and Pregnancy

Few statistics on the nutritional status of American women entering pregnancy are available. It is known, however, that a significant number of women are: (1) not at ideal weight; (2) deficient in iron, folic acid, and vitamin B_{12}; (3) below the minimum dietary allowance (RDA) of vitamins A and C, calcium, and iodine.

A well-nourished woman is obviously more likely to successfully complete nine months of pregnancy than a malnourished one. She is most likely to deliver a healthy baby who is nutritionally sound with few complications. The child is expected to show normal growth and development the first year. The mother probably will be able to nurse her baby successfully.

Studies indicate that a poorly nourished mother is a higher risk to herself and to her infant. She may have many problems, including: (1) miscarriage or infant death; (2) an incompetent placenta; (3) complications during pregnancy, labor, and delivery; (4) high-risk infant. Such infants may be premature or suffer from clinical disorders including birth defects. They also have a higher mortality rate than normal infants.

Nutritional Risk Factors in Pregnancy

The dangers of malnutrition to both the mother and the fetus should be discussed when counseling pregnant women. Factors such as physical appearance, body development, weight, and oral hygiene help the clinician evaluate her nutritional status.

Physical Characteristics

Certain women are at particular risk of being malnourished. Teenage mothers, for example, must consider their own development as well as that of the fetus. Body weight significantly above or below normal ranges and height under 5 feet can cause problems. The presence of irregular eating habits or clinical disorders such as high blood pressure can also lead to complications. Other factors contributing to high risk during pregnancy include the use of cigarettes, alcohol, and drugs as well as emotional upsets.

Reproductive History

An unsatisfactory reproductive history that includes complications in pregnancy, labor, or delivery tends to identify a high-risk patient. Other indicators are long-term breast-feeding, multiple births, short intervals between pregnancies, and use of oral contraceptives within 6 months of conception.

Clinical Progress of Pregnancy

If the mother shows unusually low or high weight gain, and if such complications as poor circulation or abnormal hormone changes are present, she may be at high risk. Other factors are unsatisfactory fetal growth and/or unusual retention of fluids.

TABLE 11-1. Distribution of Weight Gain During Pregnancy

Component	Approximate Weight (lb)
Fetus	7½ (5–10)
Placenta	1½
Amniotic fluid	2
Uterus	2
Mother's tissue fluid	3
Blood volume	4
Breasts*	½
Fat and other reserve†	3½
Total	24

*The increase is much bigger in some women and is considered as reserve.

†In some women, fat reserve may be as high as 8 lb.

Weight Changes

One of the most important criteria of a healthy pregnancy is a normal weight gain. Body tissue storage accounts for most of the mother's increased weight during early pregnancy. By midpregnancy she begins to store reserves of fat for energy, especially during lactation. The last two months, when the weight of the fetus doubles, are the most crucial for adequate nutritional intake.

The National Academy of Sciences, the American College of Obstetrics and Gynecology, and experts in the field of nutrition agree on certain aspects of weight gain during pregnancy. A discussion follows.

Normal Weight Gain

Weight gain during pregnancy should be smooth and steady. Most American women gain between 27 and 29 lb, with the ideal gain about 25 lb. Table 11-1 indicates the approximate distribution of the weight gained during pregnancy. An adequate fat reserve reduces health risk to both mother and child.

Excessive Weight Gain

Numerous problems may be encountered by a woman of ideal weight who gains more than 28 to 30 lb during pregnancy or one who is already 20 percent or more overweight at conception. These include: (1) in-

Chapter 11
NUTRITION
DURING
PREGNANCY
AND LACTATION

187

creased risk of toxemia or occurrence of a number of pathological conditions identified only in pregnant women; (2) difficult labor and delivery; (3) higher health risks for both mother and baby.

A daily food plan that is nutritionally sound and satisfying and helps the patient maintain a slow and steady weight gain is recommended. Water retention may account for excess weight gain and is more undesirable and dangerous than fat storage.

Weight reduction during pregnancy should be discouraged. There is no evidence to support the myth that weight loss during pregnancy results in a smaller baby and an easier labor and delivery. A common-sense approach to nutrition during pregnancy is advisable—adequate calories, well-balanced and nourishing meals, and vitamin/mineral supplements when indicated.

Inadequate Weight Gain

Problems encountered by women who gain less than 10 to 12 lb during gestation include: (1) increased risk of toxemia, (2) premature separation of the placenta, and (3) higher health risks for both mother and baby. The baby is likely to be smaller and more fragile at birth.

Nutritional Needs During Pregnancy

Pregnant and nursing women have increased needs for many specific nutrients. Table 11-2 describes the RDAs for women at three physiological stages. The following sections discuss a pregnant woman's increased needs for protein, calories, iron, calcium, sodium, iodine, and folic acid.

Protein

Women eating an adequate amount of protein are more likely to experience a satisfactory pregnancy. Protein intake should be increased by about 30 g per day (see Table 14-2). Inadequate protein intake may result in smaller babies with more complications and a higher risk of mortality. Some may suffer brain damage. Adequate protein intake, on the other hand, may increase the infant's resistance to disease.

Calories

A pregnant woman needs approximately 300 additional calories per day, or about 2,300 total. Less than 1,800 calories will result in a negative nitrogen balance (see Chapter 5), causing the fetus to grow at the mother's expense. Ideal caloric intake must, of course, be balanced with the mother's physical activity.

TABLE 11-2. 1980 RDAs for a 25-year-old Woman at Three Physiological Stages

Nutrient	Daily Amount Needed	Additional Daily Amount Needed	
		Pregnancy	Lactation
Energy (kcal)	2,000	300	500
Protein (g)	44	30	20
Vitamin A (μg)	800	200	400
Vitamin D (IU)	200	200	200
Vitamin E (mg)	8	2	3
Vitamin C (mg)	60	20	40
Vitamin B_1 (mg)	1.0	0.4	0.5
Vitamin B_2 (mg)	1.2	0.3	0.5
Niacin (mg)	13	2	5
Vitamin B_6 (mg)	2.0	0.6	0.5
Folic acid (μg)	400	400	100
Vitamin B_{12} (μg)	3.0	1	1
Calcium (mg)	800	400	400
Phosphorus (mg)	800	400	400
Magnesium (mg)	300	150	150
Iron (mg)	18	>18*	>18*
Zinc (mg)	15	5	10
Iodine (mg)	150	25	50

*The excess need cannot be supplied by a regular diet. Supplementation is needed.

Iron

Pregnancy requires a considerable increase in iron—about 1 mg per day over the RDA of 18 mg/day. Blood loss during delivery and increased oxygen demands account for most of the increase. In addition, a woman's blood volume increases 20 to 30 percent during the second to eighth months of pregnancy.

Two facts help offset the need for iron—the lack of menstruation during gestation and the body's increased ability to absorb iron. During pregnancy, iron absorption increases 25 to 30 percent from a normal of 10 percent. This increase occurs during the second half of pregnancy, when the placenta permits iron transfer to the fetus.

Iron deficiency during pregnancy may occur for a number of reasons. Many women enter pregnancy already anemic. Repeated pregnancy without replenishing iron levels is another cause. A diet low in meat and animal products may lead to iron deficiency. Women who eat 25 percent or more of their calories from animal sources are less likely to become iron deficient. The best practice is to eat an adequate amount of iron before pregnancy so that there is a large reserve.

Chapter 11
NUTRITION
DURING
PREGNANCY
AND LACTATION

189

Even though iron intake may be adequate, poor absorption may still result in iron deficiency. Iron from animal sources is readily absorbed, for example, whereas the iron contained in cereals is not.

If iron deficiency occurs during pregnancy, both the mother and the newborn may become anemic. The baby is able to store very little iron when the mother is deficient. During the first 1 to 3 months after birth, the child must depend on stored iron, since milk has relatively little.

Two forms of anemia may occur during pregnancy. The first and by far the most common is *iron deficiency anemia*, which occurs in 15 to 20 percent of pregnant women. About 90 to 95 percent of pregnant women who become anemic are deficient in iron. Anemia is a dangerous condition that may be life-threatening to both mother and child.

The second type of anemia, called *megaloblastic anemia*, is caused by a lack of folic acid. Since one form of anemia may lead to the other, iron and folic acid supplements are usually prescribed together.

To build body storage and satisfy the needs of the fetus, iron supplements should be prescribed beginning sometime during the second trimester of pregnancy and continuing through lactation. From 30 to 60 mg per day for the last 6 months of pregnancy are recommended.

Calcium

If the mother takes in an adequate amount of vitamin D and calcium, her blood calcium is maintained at the proper level and supplementation is unnecessary. A low intake of vitamin D, however, must be balanced by a higher intake of calcium. Studies show that the absorption rate of calcium is doubled and its excretion decreased during the last few months of pregnancy.

As the pregnancy advances, the amount of calcium deposited in the fetus steadily increases. About 24 g is deposited in the fetus during the last 3 months of gestation, which accounts for two thirds of the total calcium in its body.

Calcium deficiency results in newborn rickets and may also cause serious damage to deciduous and permanent teeth. Appropriate amounts of calcium and phosphorus during the last months of gestation and the first year of infancy are also necessary to proper formation of the jaws. Poor dental conditions among children in underdeveloped countries must be attributed in part to calcium and phosphorus deficiencies.

Lack of calcium may also be responsible for leg cramps during pregnancy, especially if phosphorus intake is high (from milk, eggs, and meat). Other complications resulting from inadequate calcium include restlessness, muscle twitching, insomnia, thigh and back pain, and a hyperactive fetus. Although evidence is not conclusive, a lack of calcium may also lead to complications of labor.

Sodium

All pregnant women retain fluids to some degree; therefore, a certain amount of edema is to be expected. Recent studies indicate, however, that a reduced salt intake during gestation can be harmful to both mother and baby. Diuretics usually are not recommended, particularly in combination with salt restriction.

Iodine

One reason that iodine deficiency occurs in pregnant mothers, especially teenage ones, and in newborn infants is that iodine is excreted more readily during pregnancy. If the mother lacks iodine, the baby's risk of iodine deficiency is increased.

A high iodine intake, on the other hand, can cause the mother's thyroid gland to enlarge and can also increase the risk to the fetus. Excessive use of substances such as cough medicine and sea salt should be avoided.

Folic Acid

It is recommended that a pregnant woman increase folic acid intake to 800 μg per day. Folic acid deficiency results in megaloblastic anemia and is characterized by such symptoms as lethargy, depression, nausea, and loss of appetite. Vomiting, diarrhea, and gum disorders may also be present. Although anemia due to folic acid deficiency occurs in only 2 to 3 percent of pregnant women in the United States, its incidence is as high as 50 percent in developing countries such as India.

Women who eat plenty of meat, eggs, fish, and green leafy vegetables with an adequate caloric intake are not usually deficient in folic acid. If there is evidence of anemia or other serious conditions, however, a folic acid supplement may be prescribed about the third month and continue through lactation. The amount prescribed is usually 5 to 10 mg per day.

Megaloblastic anemia during pregnancy is not often life-threatening unless accompanied by toxemia or infection. In extreme cases that do not respond to conservative treatment, blood transfusion may be necessary.

Diet

A pregnant woman needs a well-balanced and nutritious diet. Table 11-3 compares the recommended daily servings from the four food groups for a woman in three physiological conditions: nonpregnant, pregnant, and lactating. Table 11-4 describes a sample meal plan, and Table 11-5 a sample menu for a pregnant woman. Note that Table 11-4 includes

Chapter 11
NUTRITION
DURING
PREGNANCY
AND LACTATION

191

TABLE 11-3. Protective Foods for Women

Protective Food*	Recommended No. of Daily Servings		
	Nonpregnant, nonlactating	Pregnant	Lactating
Milk and milk products	3	4	5
Protein products	3	4	4
Grain products	3	3	3
Vegetables and fruits			
Rich in vitamin C	1	1	1
Green leafy vegetables	2	2	2
Others	1	1	1

*The grouping follows the basic four food groups (also see Chapter 10).

TABLE 11-4. Sample Meal Plan for a Pregnant Woman

Breakfast	Lunch	Dinner
Milk or milk products, 1 serving	Milk or milk products, 1 serving	Milk or milk products, 1 serving
Fruits or vegetables rich in vitamin C, 1 serving	Other fruits and vegetables, 1 serving	Green leafy vegetables, 2 servings
Grain products	Protein products, 1 serving	Protein products, 2 servings
	Grain products, 2 servings	

Snack*		**Snack***
Milk or milk products, ½ serving		Milk or milk products, ½ serving
Protein products, 1 serving		

*The snacks may be consumed at any time of the day.

mainly foods from the basic food guides, while Table 11-5 includes protective and supplemental foods.

Although a diet slightly higher in calories and greatly increased in other nutrients is recommended, most pregnant women find it difficult to fulfill these requirements. Many physicians prescribe nutrient supplements—usually iron, folic acid, and calcium—but their use must be carefully monitored. Large doses of vitamins A and D, for example, may harm the mother and child.

TABLE 11-5. Sample Menu for a Pregnant Woman Including Protective (Basic) and Supplemental Foods

Breakfast	Lunch	Dinner
Orange juice, 4 oz	Sandwich	Roast beef, 6 oz
Oatmeal, ½ c	Whole wheat bread,	Egg noodles, ½ c, with
Brown sugar, 1–2 t	2 slices	sauteed poppy seeds
Milk, 8 oz	Tuna fish, ½ c	Cut asparagus, ¾ c
Coffee or tea	Diced celery with onion	Salad
	Mayonnaise	Torn spinach, 1 c
	Lettuce	Sliced mushrooms
	Banana, 1 small	Radishes
	Milk, 8 oz	Oil
	Coffee or tea	Vinegar
		Milk, 8 oz
		Coffee or tea
Snack	**Snack**	
Salted peanuts, ½ c	Oatmeal raisin cookies, 2	
Milk, 4 oz	Milk, 4 oz	

Clinical Complications

Some of the minor clinical problems encountered by pregnant women will be discussed in the following sections.

Digestive Problems

Changes in food preferences and in appetite are not uncommon in pregnant women. Although their appetite must be satisfied, they should develop good eating habits and avoid extremes. Small, frequent meals reduce the effects of morning sickness and the discomfort of an overfull stomach. A pregnant woman may also develop strong likes and dislikes of specific foods. The reason for this is not yet known.

Morning sickness, though rarely serious, is a common complaint during the early months of pregnancy. Nausea and vomiting begin at about six weeks and usually disappear by the fourth or fifth month.

The cause of morning sickness is unknown. Some physicians suggest that it is the result of a poor psychological adjustment to motherhood. Certain clinical disorders, such as hernias and ulcers, may also account for the symptoms of nausea and vomiting. Dry foods given at frequent intervals often make the patient feel better. The restriction of fats, spicy dishes, and strong-smelling foods may also help. A rare complication

Chapter 11
NUTRITION
DURING
PREGNANCY
AND LACTATION

193

known as *hyperemesis gravidarum*, characterized by persistent and severe vomiting, requires hospitalization and extreme precautions.

Many pregnant women suffer discomfort from heartburn. This condition is caused by regurgitation of stomach contents and the reduction of stomach secretion and activity. As the pregnancy advances, the expanding uterus can displace the stomach and further aggravate the heartburn. When severe heartburn occurs during late pregnancy as the result of hiatus hernia (in about 15 percent of pregnancy patients), it leads to nausea and vomiting. Conservative treatment for heartburn is recommended, such as hard candy, hot tea, and postural changes.

Constipation in pregnancy may result from bowel sluggishness or from fetal pressure upon portions of the intestine. A large intake of roughage and fluid, plus a program of regular exercise, helps restore regularity. Strong laxatives are not recommended.

Abdominal pain may be caused by pressure or by gas. As the uterus becomes heavier, it presses on the abdominal wall, sometimes causing pain. Changes in position, frequent rest periods, and a maternity girdle offer some relief. Excess gas and bloating can result in constipation and other intestinal discomforts. The avoidance of poorly tolerated foods and frequent small meals instead of large, heavy ones usually reduce the symptoms.

Oral Hygiene

Pregnant women are more likely to experience dental decay and gum infection. Bleeding gums, in fact, afflict from 50 to 70 percent of pregnant women. Such disorders result from reduced oral hygiene, an increase in sugary foods, and hormonal imbalance. Most symptoms subside within two months of delivery with proper dental care.

Other Related Conditions

Faintness during early pregnancy may occur either because the brain's blood supply is temporarily reduced by postural changes or because of hypoglycemia before meals. Stimulants such as coffee or tea, frequent but slow changes of position, and small meals close together usually help.

Frequency and urgency of urination, especially in late pregnancy, result from pressure of the fetus on the bladder. Sedatives are effective when urinary tract infections appear. The patient should avoid possible irritants such as coffee, tea, spices, and alcohol.

Cramping of the calves, thighs, or buttocks occurs in some women with the stretching of leg and foot muscles. Possible causes include high phosphorus or low calcium level, fatigue, and slow blood circulation.

Balanced calcium and phosphorus levels as well as adequate rest and exercise can alleviate cramping.

About two out of three women develop mild edema of the lower extremities late in pregnancy. This kind of edema results from sodium and water retention and is unrelated to toxemia. Possible reasons include: (1) varicose veins, (2) increased levels of steroid hormones, and (3) sitting or standing for too long. Some common preventive measures are sleeping with the feet elevated, avoiding tight clothing, and mildly restricting salt (preferably with medical supervision).

NUTRITION AND LACTATION

The current trend in the United States seems to be toward breast-feeding, although no one knows the exact incidence. Studies done as recently as 1975 indicate a correlation between the mother's education and her decision to breast-feed—the more educated she is, the more likely she is to breast-feed her baby. The decision of whether to breast-feed and the special dietary considerations that are a part of that decision are discussed in the following sections.

The Decision to Breast-feed

Expectant mothers may elect to nurse their babies because of the physiological advantages to the infant or because of the intimacy and security nursing provides. The production and secretion of breast milk are influenced by many factors, including: (1) a strong desire to breast-feed, (2) emotional support from physician and family, (3) satisfactory nutritional status, (4) a basic knowledge of the process of milk production, (5) adequate fluid intake, and (6) a nutritious and balanced diet.

In general, a woman will make more milk if she has a large body or breast size. Frequent nursing unsupplemented by formula increases the volume of milk produced.

Nutritional Needs

It is obvious that a woman who is breast-feeding should eat a nutritious diet. Experts agree that most nutrients in milk can be derived from the mother's storage, including vitamins, minerals, calories, and protein. A nursing mother whose nutritional status is borderline, therefore, and who fails to eat adequately is running a risk of nutrient deficiency.

The nursing mother needs more protein, vitamins, minerals, and especially calories to produce wholesome milk without depleting her own body's nutrient storage. The sections below discuss the nursing mother's need for additional nutrients.

Chapter 11
NUTRITION
DURING
PREGNANCY
AND LACTATION

195

Calories

A nursing mother should eat about 500 kcal more per day. These extra calories and the fat reserve in her body combine to provide the 700 to 900 kcal needed for nursing.

Despite the additional calories, many women find that nursing helps them lose weight. If the food supply is adequate, mothers who choose to breast-feed can develop sound eating habits and maintain a trim figure even after several pregnancies.

Fat

Although the amount of the mother's fat intake does not affect the fat level of her milk, the type of fat makes a difference. Increased poly-unsaturated fats in the diet, for example, will most likely result in a similar increase in the milk.

Iron

An adequate diet plus an iron supplement is recommended during the first few months of nursing to replenish the woman's depleted storage of iron. After three to four months, she should eat a nutritious diet for her iron need without a supplement.

The woman's intake of iron does not generally influence the iron content of her milk. For the first three months after birth, the baby should have good reserves of iron, and the intake from breast milk will be adequate.

Calcium and Phosphorus

The calcium need of a woman increases during nursing, partly for the milk and partly for her body storage. Calcium level in breast milk varies and is not directly related to the woman's intake. The secretion of calcium in breast milk is a continuous drain on the woman's calcium reserve. Dietary compensation must be made if a negative balance of calcium and phosphorus is to be avoided.

Vitamins

Within limits, the levels of vitamin C, B_1, B_2, B_6, and B_{12} in the breast milk reflect the mother's dietary intake. Her RDAs for vitamins, therefore, are about 150 percent those of a nonpregnant woman. The intake of folic acid also requires careful monitoring.

TABLE 11-6. Sample Meal Plan for a Lactating Woman

Breakfast	Lunch	Dinner
Milk or milk products, 1 serving	Milk or milk products, 1 serving	Milk or milk products, 1 serving
Fruits or vegetables rich in vitamin C, 1 serving	Other fruits or vegetables, 1 serving	Green leafy vegetables, 2 servings
Grain products, 1 serving	Protein products, 1 serving	Protein products, 2 servings
	Grain products, 2 servings	

Snack*	Snack*
Milk or milk products, 1 serving	Milk or milk products, 1 serving
Protein products, 1 serving	

*The snacks may be consumed at any time of the day.

TABLE 11-7. Sample Menu for a Lactating Woman Including Protective (Basic) and Supplemental Foods

Breakfast	Lunch	Dinner
Orange juice, 4 oz	Sandwich	Roast beef, 6 oz
Oatmeal, ½ c	Whole wheat bread, 2 slices	Egg noodles, ½ c, with sauteed poppy seeds
Brown sugar, 1–2 t	Tuna fish, ½ c	Cut asparagus, ¾ c
Milk, 8 oz	Diced celery	Salad
Coffee or tea	Onion	Torn spinach, 1 c
	Mayonnaise	Sliced mushrooms
	Lettuce	Radishes
	Banana, 1 small	Oil
	Milk, 8 oz	Vinegar
		Milk, 8 oz
		Coffee or tea

Snack	Snack
Salted peanuts, ½ c	Oatmeal raisin cookies, 2
Milk, 8 oz	Milk, 8 oz

Diet

What should a nursing mother eat? Table 11-3 gives recommended amounts of protective foods for a lactating woman. Table 11-6 gives a sample meal plan, and Table 11-7 gives a sample menu. If a woman eats according to these regimens, she will receive adequate nutrients.

Chapter 11
NUTRITION
DURING
PREGNANCY
AND LACTATION

197

STUDY QUESTIONS

1. What nutritional deficiencies are common among women entering pregnancy? What health risks are greater among malnourished pregnant women than among well-nourished pregnant women?
2. Describe the currently recommended pattern and extent of weight gain during pregnancy. Why is a fat reserve important?
3. When is weight loss in an overweight woman preferable: before, during, or after pregnancy? Why?
4. What are the risks of being underweight when entering pregnancy? What advice should such women be given?
5. What nutrient needs are increased during pregnancy? What can be said about the intakes of calcium, sodium, iodine, and vitamins A, D, C, and K during pregnancy?
6. What general dietary advice should be given to a pregnant woman? Plan one week's menus for a 25–year–old pregnant woman.
7. Name at least six minor health problems in a pregnant woman that may be related to nutrition. What dietary or related advice may be helpful in each case?
8. How does the recommended diet for a nursing mother differ from that for a pregnant woman?

REFERENCES

Aebi, H., and Whitehead, R. 1980. *Maternal nutrition during pregnancy and lactation.* Bern, Switzerland: Hans Huber.

Dobbing, J., ed. 1981. *Maternal nutrition in pregnancy.* New York: Academic Press.

Duhring, J. L. 1984. Nutrition in pregnancy. In *Present knowledge in nutrition,* 5th ed. Washington, D. C.: The Nutrition Foundation.

Filer, L. J. 1975. Maternal nutrition in lactation. *Clin. Perinatol.* 2:353.

Larson, B. L., ed. 1978. In *Lactation: a comprehensive treatise,* vol. 4. The mammary gland, human lactation, milk synthesis. New York: Academic Press.

Luke, B. 1979. *Maternal nutrition.* Boston: Little, Brown.

National Academy of Sciences, National Research Council, Committee on Maternal Nutrition, Food and Nutrition Board. 1970. *Maternal nutrition and the course of pregnancy.* Washington, D. C.

Rush, D., et al. 1980. *Diet in pregnancy.* New York: Alan R. Liss.

Shanplin, D. R., and Hodin, J. 1979. *Maternal nutrition and child health.* Chicago: C. C. Thomas.

Chapter 11
NUTRITION
DURING
PREGNANCY
AND LACTATION

199

12 NUTRITION AND THE GROWING YEARS

Because the need for nutrients is high during the growing years, the diets of infants, children, and adolescents are important concerns. Deficiencies at this time can create health problems that persist in later life. In infancy, breast- versus bottle-feeding and the introduction of solid foods are the issues in question. During childhood and adolescence, feeding problems, snacking, obesity, food allergies, and nutrient deficiencies are the major concerns. From infancy through adolescence, sound nutritional education is crucial for both parents and children to help them make wise food choices.

NUTRITION AND INFANTS

All infants need an adequate amount of essential nutrients for the proper development of body organs, cells, and tissues. One major index of health for an infant is its growth rate. Table 12-1 shows the weight gain from birth to age 1 year.

The normal development of the child's brain in structure, size, and function is especially important. Experiments have shown that a newborn's mental development and learning potential can be adversely affected by undernourishment, though the permanence of such effects is not known.

The health and nutrition of the mother during pregnancy contribute to the newborn's nutritional status. If a child is born with nutritional problems because of a malnourished mother, however, there is a good

TABLE 12-1. Weight Gain from Birth to 1 Year Old

	Average Weight Values	
Age (mo)	Weight (lb)	Weight gain rate (lb/mo)
0	7½	1
4–6	15	2
10–12	22–23	3

Note: Consult the appendix for the standard growth grid.

chance of complete recovery if the child receives adequate nutritional care after birth.

Facts About Breast-feeding

The issue of whether to bottle-feed or breast-feed a baby has been a controversial one since World War II. In the following sections, the advantages, disadvantages, and techniques of breast-feeding will be discussed.

Nutritional Benefits

Several nutritional benefits are associated with breast-feeding. First, the higher level of lactose in breast milk creates a better intestinal environment and enhances bowel activity. The child becomes hungry and eats more frequently. Lactose also increases the absorption of amino acids and magnesium as well as promoting formation of myelin, a fatty material that coats nerve endings.

Second, breast milk contains a special enzyme that promotes protein digestion. Third, digestion and utilization of fat are facilitated by the high level of polyunsaturated fatty acids in breast milk. Fourth, breast milk usually contains more vitamin C and B_1 than unfortified cow's milk, since pasteurization destroys these vitamins. Finally, even malnourished mothers secrete milk of acceptable quality and quantity.

Fewer Allergies

Breast-fed infants tend to develop fewer allergies. Because the intestinal system of an infant allows the absorption of large protein molecules, a baby receiving cow's milk may absorb "foreign protein," sometimes resulting in allergic reactions and/or a tendency to lifelong allergies.

Protection Against Infection

In some way not yet understood, breast milk protects the infant from infection, especially intestinal infection due to *Escherichia coli* (*E. coli*).

Bottle-fed infants, therefore, are more likely to develop diarrhea; in fact, diarrhea in a bottle-fed baby can be stopped by switching to breast milk. In the United States, greater morbidity and mortality rates from diarrhea among bottle-fed infants have been documented for years. Breast-fed babies also have fewer constipation problems, possibly because of the higher level of lactose in breast milk.

One possible source of immunity to infection in infancy is **colostrum,** the yellowish fluid that is secreted before white milk. Certain particles contained in colostrum may reduce the number of intestinal bacteria or may digest bacteria and viruses. Colostrum may contain lactoferrin, which is believed to inhibit bacterial growth.

Breast milk contains immunoglobulin A (IgA), which is active against *E. coli*. Like colostrum, breast milk may contain lactoferrin, suspected of inhibiting the growth of bacteria. Milk may contain lysozymes, which have an antiinfective property. The presence of *Lactobacillus bifidus* (a bacteria) in breast milk stops the multiplication of some undesirable organisms and crowds out others, such as *E. coli* or viruses. Nonintestinal infections such as respiratory infections also seem to be less prevalent among breast-fed babies.

Psychological Factors

Many women feel that breast milk provides the best food for their babies because it was designed for them. They are, furthermore, able to establish an important bond with the child by breast-feeding. Direct and immediate contact between mother and the newborn in the delivery room seems to promote successful breast-feeding.

Oral Muscles and Speech Development

An infant must work harder to suck milk from the breast than from a bottle. It is suggested that this effort improves the development of oral muscles, jaws, teeth, and tongue. The result may be stronger oral tissues and the absence of overcrowded teeth.

Breast-feeding may also have a beneficial effect on the speech development of the child. The natural act of sucking, for example, can accelerate development of the neuromuscular system involved in speech. On the other hand, the tongue thrusting that the child is forced to use to arrest the rapid flow of milk from a bottle may have an adverse effect on the child's later speech movement.

Uterus Size

Breast-feeding causes vigorous contraction of the uterus, which returns to its normal size in a shorter time than in a woman who elects to bottle-feed her baby. Bleeding of the uterus is also reduced.

Miscellaneous Benefits

Other benefits from breast-feeding include contraception, weight reduction, and the reduced risk of breast engorgement and trauma. In most mothers who successfully breast-feed, ovulation is postponed until at least the tenth week after childbirth, and sometimes longer for those who maintain full breast-feeding without any formula supplementation. Breast-feeding as a means of contraception is not reliable, however, since some nursing mothers do become pregnant. On the other hand, the hormones in some oral contraceptives may be passed through the mother's milk and pose a risk to the infant. For reasons not yet clear, devices such as the IUD can increase lactation.

Some nursing mothers find that breast-feeding is effective in reducing weight. Breast-feeding is also a natural protection against engorgement of the breast tissues from milk. Women who choose to bottle-feed their babies find their breasts initially painful and tender from engorgement, possibly increasing their susceptibility to breast trauma and cancer.

Problems of Breast-Feeding

Some women who wish to breast-feed are unable to produce enough milk. The reasons for an inadequate supply of milk include: (1) insufficient fluid intake; (2) inadequate caloric intake; (3) negative attitude, confusion, or poor emotional status; (4) fatigue; and (5) excessive use of supplemental bottle-feeding. A relaxed atmosphere in which the mother can learn those techniques that work best for herself and her baby is most conducive to successful breast-feeding.

A second disadvantage to breast-feeding is the woman's fear that her physical appearance may be impaired, either by overlarge or sagging breasts. Some mothers also may feel that nursing will prevent them from returning to their normal weight.

Breast-feeding can restrict a woman's freedom of movement. For women who work outside the home full time, nursing is especially difficult. Recreational pursuits also must be planned around the nursing needs of the child.

Certain chemicals in drugs of any kind, including prescriptions, cigarettes, and alcohol, may appear in the milk, causing varying degrees of risk to the child.

TABLE 12-2. Growth Rates and Body Size of Infants by Method of Feeding

Type of Feeding	Growth Rate (mo)		Body Size at 2 Years
	0–5	5–24	
Breast	Faster	Slower	Same
Bottle	Slower	Faster	Same

A newborn infant occasionally has sucking difficulties for the first two to three days owing to the mother's sedation or difficult labor. These problems do not normally persist.

Finally, some women are afraid that nursing may increase the risk of breast infection. Still another concern is that breast milk is lower than cow's milk in a number of nutrients.

Facts About Formula Feeding

Although breast milk is nature's food for human infants, 50 years of clinical observations have confirmed that bottle-fed babies grow equally well, as shown in Table 12-2. As Table 12-3 illustrates, whole cow's milk is higher in certain nutrients and lower in others than breast milk. Cow's milk can be modified in various ways to make it similar to breast milk, as indicated below.

The protein and some minerals in cow's milk must be reduced in quantity. This is usually accomplished by diluting the milk with water. The resulting loss of calories is compensated for by adding a carbohydrate such as sucrose, dextromaltose, or lactose to either commercial or home-prepared formulas. An additive is also used to give the milk a soft texture for easier digestion. To approximate the content of sodium in breast milk, this mineral is partially removed from cow's milk. The high content of saturated fat in cow's milk is reduced by replacing part of it with vegetable oil such as corn oil, which is high in polyunsaturated fats. Vitamin E also may be added to prevent oxidation.

Disadvantages of Bottle-feeding

Lack of sanitation in preparing the formula can result in infection. This problem is especially common among families of low socioeconomic status and in developing countries.

Not enough attention to preparation instructions can result in a formula that is underdiluted. This can overload the infant with too much

TABLE 12-3. Approximate Nutritional Content of Colostrum, Breast Milk, and Whole Cow's Milk*

Nutrient Per 100 mL	Colostrum	Breast Milk	Cow's Milk
Water (mL)	87	87	87
Kcal	59	75	68
Protein (g)	2.8	1.2	3.5
Lactose (g)	5.5	6.9	4.9
Fat (g)	2.8	4.4	3.7
Calcium (mg)	30	34	120
Phosphorus (mg)	15	14	94
Sodium (mg)	45	160	505
Potassium (mg)	75	407	1,360
Iron (mg)	0.1	0.13	0.1
Vitamin A (IU)	200	210	150
Vitamin D (IU)	No information	0.5	2.0
Vitamin E (mg)	1.0	0.6	0.06
Vitamin K (μg)	No information	1.4	5.8
Vitamin C (mg)	5.0	4.3	1.81
Vitamin B_1 (mg)	13	16	41
Vitamin B_2 (μg)	25	40	160
Vitamin B_6 (μg)	No information	10	50
Vitamin B_{12} (μg)	No information	0.03	0.4
Folic acid (μg)	0.05	5	5
Pantothenic acid (μg)	180	190	340
Niacin (μg)	70	170	90

*Information obtained from a number of investigators' reports. All values are averages.

protein and sodium while depriving it of adequate liquid. An over-diluted formula, on the other hand, fails to provide the baby with adequate nourishment. Changing formulas frequently is also not recommended, since it varies the child's caloric intake and interferes with its hunger/satiety rhythm.

Certain conditions are more likely to occur among formula-fed than breast-fed babies. These include allergy and constipation, diarrhea, and infections of the respiratory and gastrointestinal tracts. The tendency for a formula-fed baby to overfeed is also high.

Because the fat content of some formula milk is high, an infant fed such milk may accumulate lipids in its blood. Exposure to sweeteners added to formula, juice, vitamin C supplement, or plain water may condition the bottle-fed baby to prefer sweet things. A higher incidence of cavities may result, especially if the child is allowed to have a bottle for a prolonged period.

Babies who fall asleep with a bottle of sugary liquid in their mouth may develop "nursing bottle syndrome" in which the teeth and gums

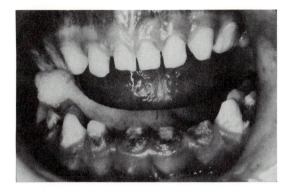

FIGURE 12-1. Rampant decay in primary dentition of 4-year-old boy with continuous history of bottle-feeding prior to sleeping. Lower anterior teeth are not carious because of protection from tongue during sucking and swallowing. (From T. E. Cone, Jr., *Journal of the American Medical Association* 245 [1981]: 2334. Copyright 1981, American Medical Association.)

show excess rotting. The sugar solution soaks the mouth for hours and causes the decay. See Figure 12-1.

Advantages of Bottle-feeding

There are many advantages to bottle-feeding. First, it affords mothers more freedom of movement. Second, the supply and cost of formula is dependable and not necessarily more expensive than breast milk, depending on the formula used and the diet of the mother. Third, bottle-feeding is preferable for women who drink and smoke excessively, use drugs or medication, or are exposed to chemicals. Fourth, some babies do not thrive on breast milk. Bottle-feeding is advised for these infants.

Skim, nonfat, or low-fat milk is not recommended for feeding infants, because these products are not nutritionally adequate as an only food. Deficiencies of linoleic acid and vitamins A and D may result.

The low fat content of skim milk can lead to diarrhea as well as a failure to gain weight in some babies. Lack of fat also decreases the absorption of vitamins A and D and interferes with the proper formation of myelin.

Although skim milk has a high content of both nitrogen and sodium, it has relatively low levels of iron and copper. The value of using low-fat milk to decrease cholesterol intake and avoid obesity has not been determined. Because condensed milk contains too much sugar and can result in an overweight baby, its use is not advised.

NUTRITION AND CHILDREN

There are many questions about the nutritional and dietary intake of children in the United States. We will discuss their nutritional status, feeding problems, and sound family menus during the childhood years.

Nutritional Status

The nutritional status of children under 6 years of age has been reported in several national surveys, including the Preschool Nutritional Survey (1968–1970) (G. Owen, *Pediatrics* 1974, *53*:11 [supplement]), the Ten-State Nutrition Survey (1968–1970) (Department of Health, Education and Welfare publication no. [HSM] 72-8132), and the Health and Nutrition Examination Survey (1971–1974) (Department of Health, Education and Welfare publication no. [HRA] 74-1219-1).

From these surveys, it appears that the nutritional status of most children in the United States is satisfactory. Deficiencies are most common among children from poor families, although iron deficiency appears in 7 to 12 percent of all children studied. From one quarter to one half of preschool children receive vitamin supplements. Some black and Hispanic children, however, are deficient in vitamin A, and about 10 to 15 percent of children have a low intake of vitamin C. From 10 to 30 percent of children, especially blacks, do not eat an adequate amount of calcium. About 5 to 10 percent of children are overweight, a more common problem among families with moderate to high incomes. Protein intake is in general higher than the RDA.

Feeding Problems

Feeding children sometimes becomes a problem. Professionals recommend a number of pointers to avoid or manage eating problems.

One important factor is to consider the child's food preferences. Table 12-4 summarizes general attitudes of children toward foods. Another consideration is the mealtime environment. An attractive setting and relaxed surroundings help establish mealtimes as pleasant experiences.

Refusing to eat is a way for a child to attract attention. A child's food obsessions also may cause concern. Parents' overreaction may prolong rather than correct such behaviors.

Children should be encouraged to eat only until they are satisfied. The "clean plate policy" of early childhood years—the requirement that everything on the plate must be eaten before leaving the table—may help account for adult overeating and obesity.

Meal Plans

What is a nutritious meal for a child? Tables 12-5, 12-6, and 12-7 provide meal plans and sample menus for children aged 1 to 2, 3 to 6, and

TABLE 12-4. Criteria for the Acceptance of Foods by Children

Food Characteristics	Preferred by Children	Disliked by Children
Texture	Soft; e.g., thin soup or puddings, tender beef, moist ground meat, soft mashed potatoes, soft bread	Thick, tough, stringy, dry; e.g., stringy beans, dry toast, coarse bread, thick soup, dry fish
Temperature of foods	Lukewarm; e.g., milk that is out of the refrigerator for a while, slightly melted ice cream	Very cold or hot; e.g., hot soup, cold rice, and meat
Flavor	Normal, unspoiled flavor	Any off flavors; e.g., slightly colored (e.g., very light yellow) or scorched milk, strong cabbage or onion flavor unless they are creamed to modify the flavor
Color	Colorful meal setting including the food, plate, table, and room decoration	Strange color such as blue or purple foods
Serving portion	Small portions and small utensils	Large portions and large utensils
Food shapes	Forms that they can manipulate with their hands rather than with utensils; e.g., strips of vegetables or meats	Shapes and forms that they cannot manipulate with their utensils and hands

7 to 12 years old, respectively. The meal plans in these tables are based on the four food groups (see Chapter 10). They must, of course, be adjusted to the individual needs of the child.

NUTRITION AND ADOLESCENCE

The period of pubescence and adolescence spans the years from 12 to 18 and is characterized by major body compositional and developmental changes. Adolescence places a greater nutritional demand on the body than any other phase, with the exception of pregnancy and lactation.

TABLE 12-5. Suggested Meal Plan and Sample Menu for 1- and 2-year-olds*

Meal Plan	Sample Menu
Breakfast	**Breakfast**
Juice or fruit	Orange juice
Cereal (hot or dry) with milk	Hot oatmeal with milk
Toast or egg (soft-boiled)	Whole wheat toast
Butter or margarine	Butter
Milk	Milk
Snack	**Snack**
Milk or juice	Apple juice
Lunch	**Lunch**
Meat, cheese, egg, or alternate	Grilled cheese sandwich
Potato, bread, crackers, or alternate	Peas
Vegetable	Milk
Butter or margarine	Ice cream
Milk	
Dessert	**Snack**
	Rice pudding
Snack	
Milk, juice, pudding, or crackers with cheese or alternate	**Dinner**
	Meat loaf
	Spinach or carrots
	Roll
Dinner	Butter
Meat, cheese, poultry, or alternate	Applesauce
Vegetable or salad	Milk
Potato, bread, roll, or alternate	
Butter or margarine	
Dessert	
Milk	

*Serving size varies with the child. Other nutritious items not shown may be used; e.g., jams, oatmeal, cookies, peanut butter. Their inclusion must be integrated into the child's overall daily intake of calories and nutrients.

TABLE 12-6. Suggested Meal Plan and Sample Menu for 3 Through 6-year-olds*

Meal Plan	Sample Menu
Breakfast	**Breakfast**
Juice or fruit	Apple
Cereal (hot or dry)	Bran flakes with milk
Egg, meat, or toast	Egg (soft-boiled) with whole wheat toast
Milk	Milk
Snack	**Snack**
Dry fruits or nutritious cookies	Dates
Lunch	**Lunch**
Meat, egg, or alternate	Peanut butter and jelly sandwich
Potato, bread, or alternate	Vegetable soup with rice
Vegetable	Margarine
Butter or margarine	Milk
Milk	Custard pudding
Dessert	
	Snack
Snack	Orange juice
Milk or juice	Apple wedges with peanut butter
Crackers, pudding, or dried fruits	
	Dinner
Dinner	Fish sticks
Meat, cheese, poultry, or alternate	Sweet corn
Vegetable or salad	Baked potato
Potato, bread, roll, or alternate	Butter
Butter or margarine	Fruit pudding
Dessert	Milk
Milk	

*Serving size varies with the child. Other nutritious items not shown may be used; e.g., jams, oatmeal, cookies, peanut butter. Their inclusion must be integrated into the child's overall daily intake of calories and nutrients.

TABLE 12-7. Suggested Meal Plan and Sample Menu for 7 Through 12-year-olds*

Meal Plan	Sample Menu
Breakfast	**Breakfast**
Juice or fruit	Pear(s)
Cereal (hot or dry) with milk	Farina with milk
Toast	Toast
Egg, meat, or alternate	Egg or sausages
Butter or margarine	Margarine
Milk	Milk
Lunch	**Lunch**
Meat, cheese, or alternate	Macaroni and cheese
Potato, bread, or alternate	Coleslaw
Vegetable	Milk
Butter or margarine	Fresh peaches
Milk	
Dessert	**Snack**
	Molasses cookies
Snack	Apple juice
Dried fruits or nutritious cookies	
Milk or juice	**Dinner**
	Hamburger
Dinner	Carrots and peas
Meat, cheese, or alternate	Shredded raw cabbage salad
Vegetable	Baked potato
Salad	Bread
Potato or alternate	Butter
Bread or alternate	Ice cream
Butter or margarine	Milk
Dessert	
Milk	

*Serving size varies with the child. Other nutritious items not shown may be used; e.g., jams, oatmeal, cookies, peanut butter. Their inclusion must be integrated into the child's overall daily intake of calories and nutrients.

Eating Habits

Teenagers whose health and family relationships play an important role are more apt to develop good eating habits than those who seek social acceptance by peers. The latter group likes to eat outside the home and share meals with peers. Their nutritional intake is frequently poor.

Adolescents may have a number of bad food habits: the omission of meals, especially breakfast; irregular meals; dislike for nutritious foods such as milk; frequent consumption of unbalanced meals outside the home; and concern for appearance at the risk of good health.

Eating a nutritious meal in the morning is particularly important, since breakfast ideally contributes about 500 kcal and provides significant amounts of vitamins C and B_2 and calcium. Furthermore, eating a good breakfast helps maintain normal to high levels of blood glucose and reduces the appetite for snacks.

Snacking and Obesity

As indicated earlier, snacks that contribute needed nutrients without reducing the appetite for regular meals are not undesirable. Whether or not snacking is good or bad for a person depends on his or her dietary intake.

Making nutritious snacks available at such strategic places as home refrigerators, vending machines, and school lunch counters is one remedy for the problem of improving the nutritional status of teenagers. A second suggestion is to fortify popular snack foods with nutrients that are likely to be lacking, such as calcium and iron. Nutrition education is, however, the most important step.

In addition to inadequate nutrition, a common teenage problem is overweight. It is estimated that approximately 20 to 30 percent of adolescents may be considered obese. A young adult should be advised to learn to stop eating when full and to engage in a program of regular exercise.

American teenagers desperately need nutrition education. Implementing nutritional knowledge is as important as acquiring it. In addition to learning about good dietary intake, teenagers should be exposed to behavioral modification to change old eating habits to positive new eating behaviors.

STUDY QUESTIONS

1. Discuss some nutritional benefits of breast milk. What are some other advantages of breast-feeding? What are the potential disadvantages?

2. What are some differences between the modified milk in most common infant formulas and regular cow's milk?
3. Discuss some advantages and disadvantages of bottle-feeding.
4. What are some nutrition problems revealed by national surveys of American children?
5. What is the current thinking among nutritionists about the "clean–your–plate" rule often laid down by parents?
6. Using an appropriate reference source, compile a list of foods to which children are commonly allergic.
7. Why is it important that teenagers learn not to skip breakfast?

REFERENCES

Acheinin, A. 1984. The role of dietary carbohydrates in plaque formation and oral disease. In *Present knowledge in nutrition*, 5th ed. Washington, D. C.: The Nutrition Foundation.

American Academy of Pediatrics. 1979. *Pediatric nutrition handbook*. Evanston, Ill.

American Academy of Pediatrics, Committee on Drugs. 1981. Breast-feeding and contraception. *Pediatrics* 68:138.

Beal, V. A. 1980. *Nutrition in the life span*. New York: Wiley.

Dairy Council Digest. 1981. Nutritional concerns during adolescence. 52:7.

Dunnig, J. M. 1976. *Dental care for everyone: problems and proposals*. Cambridge, Mass.: Harvard University Press.

Endres, J. B., and Rockwell, R. E. 1980. *Food, nutrition, and the young child*. St. Louis: C. U. Mosby.

Foman, S. 1980. *Infant nutrition*. Philadelphia: Saunders.

Goldfarb, J., and Tibbetts, E. 1980. *Breastfeeding handbook: a practical reference for physicians, nurses, and other health professionals*. Hillside, N. J.: Enslow Publishers.

MacLean, W. C., Jr. 1984. Nutrition in infancy. In *Present knowledge in nutrition*, 5th ed. Washington, D. C.: The Nutrition Foundation.

13 NUTRITION AND THE ELDERLY

During the twentieth century, life expectancy has increased from only about 50 years in the early 1900s to 65 to 70 for males and 70 to 75 years for females in the 1970s. This older population is now the fastest-growing minority group in the United States. In the early 1900s only about 3 million people were over 65 years; in 1976, there were more than 25 million.

Today, because of the larger number of older people, many of their problems such as housing, income, diet, and health are being given more recognition. The first focus of this chapter is on one of the most significant considerations of the elderly—their health status.

HEALTH PROBLEMS OF SENIOR CITIZENS

Among people over 65, about 60 to 75 percent have at least one chronic illness, and 30 to 50 percent are chronically disabled. Economic status and the degree of independence can influence health status.

A variety of physical factors also can affect the health of an older person. These include heredity; the quality of the air and water; the presence of harmful substances such as pesticides; tobacco, alcohol, and drug use; and nutritional intake, both short- and long-term.

Older people are more concerned with health, since illness frequently accompanies old age. They are susceptible to quick cures and unsubstantiated medical claims.

PERSONAL FACTORS AFFECTING NUTRITIONAL STATUS

In addition to disturbing body changes, certain personal factors may limit the adequacy of an elderly individual's diet. Some of these factors are food habits, financial problems, limited resources, physical handicaps, and psychological problems. An outline of these factors follows:

Food Habits

Unwholesome eating patterns should be modified as age advances. Even those elderly people with a lifetime of good eating habits may require a new nutritional pattern because of unavoidable changes in later years, such as limited income, loneliness, and physical handicaps.

Financial Problems

Food selection and eating out are severely limited by the fixed income of many seniors and constantly rising food prices. An already meager income may be further depleted by the purchase of such "miraculous" special foods as yeast and seaweed.

Scarcity of Food-related Resources

The eating patterns of many older people are affected by the lack of cooking utensils, refrigerators, adequate housing, storage, and kitchen facilities. Inaccessibility of markets also may be a problem. The wide variety of foods in a supermarket can be confusing, especially when shopping for the right foods on a limited income.

Physical Handicaps

The frailty of some elderly people poses numerous problems in food shopping, cooking, and eating. Decayed or missing teeth are a major problem. "Old age" conditions of the esophagus (see Chapter 18) such as hiatus hernia, spasm, and diverticular diseases can affect eating and drinking. Some may be unable to feed themselves because of paralysis resulting from stroke.

Psychological Problems

Nutritional and dietary intakes are greatly influenced by the emotional and psychological climate of older people. Some significant factors include: death of a spouse or close friend, lack of meaningful work and/or close relationships, poor adjustment to changes in self-esteem, loss of vitality and deterioration of health, social isolation, and constant fear of death.

Psychological problems can make an older person susceptible to depression, which may lead to either disinterest in food or overeating. Also, boredom, inconvenience, and unwillingness to shop, cook, and eat alone can create undesirable eating habits and patterns.

NUTRITIONAL NEEDS

An adequate intake of nutrients and food is essential for an elderly person. There is, however, no single "right" or "special" food for someone who is growing old.

Information about the exact nutrient requirements of the elderly is very limited. Most experts agree that the RDAs of an older person are about the same as those of a 25–year–old, with the exception of calories. A brief analysis is provided below.

Calories

There are no fixed daily caloric recommendations for ages above 50; caloric intake should be determined on an individual basis according to the person's age, physical activity, and body condition. For example, a man between 60 and 70 uses about 75 to 90 percent of the calories of a 25–year–old. Reasons for the decline in caloric need include a decrease in the basal metabolic rate, atrophy of the lean body mass, and decreased activity.

Protein

The latest RDA suggests protein intake of about 0.8 g per kilogram body weight for adults. Most seniors in this country consume about 40 to 50 g of protein a day, less than is usually recommended. Low protein consumption usually means that the intake of many essential nutrients contained in protein-rich foods is also inadequate.

Among the many reasons for insufficient protein intake in older people are: (1) the high cost of protein foods, (2) adverse intestinal reactions to certain high-protein foods such as milk, and (3) dental problems such as loss of teeth and ill-fitting dentures. In addition, protein absorption and utilization and nitrogen retention may all be affected by the chronic illnesses of old age. Reduced physical activity and emotional instability also may contribute to nitrogen loss.

Carbohydrate

An older person's daily caloric intake should include about 50 to 55 percent carbohydrate. A balance between carbohydrate and protein intakes should be maintained.

Ideally, starch makes up about 40 to 45 percent of carbohydrate consumption, with sugar intake limited to about 5 to 10 percent. Too much sugar can increase dental problems and inhibit the intake of essential nutrients. Persons over 40 also are susceptible to the development of diabetes.

Fat

The current recommendation concerning fat intake is that it should make up about 30 percent or less of the total caloric intake of people over 50. Many questions about the relationship between dietary fat and the cause and outcome of heart disease have yet to be answered.

Vitamins and Minerals

Although the elderly are said to have the same vitamin requirements as 25–year–olds, their actual vitamin need is suspected of being higher. Vitamin and mineral deficiencies in old people are common. A brief analysis of the vitamin needs of senior citizens is provided below.

Vitamin C is the vitamin most likely to be low in the diet and blood of older people. Low intake and retention problems can reduce the levels of vitamin C in tissues, blood, and cerebrospinal fluid. Less efficient utilization can increase the need for the vitamin, and drug use can interfere with its absorption and retention.

Thiamine, or vitamin B_1, deficiency in old age can be brought about in several ways. Old age itself increases the need and decreases the utilization of the vitamin. Substances such as diuretics and alcohol can distort proper metabolism of the vitamin. Decreased hydrochloric acid secretion can inactivate thiamine in the stomach. Further, certain clinical circumstances, such as fever, can lead to deficiency of the vitamin. Finally, a low-cost, starchy diet can lead to thiamine deficiency, since the metabolism of carbohydrate requires a large amount of the vitamin.

Riboflavin, or vitamin B_2, may be required in larger amounts with age. Certain clinical conditions also may increase the requirement. The types and quantity of intestinal bacteria may adversely affect the utilization, synthesis, and secretion of the vitamin.

Pyridoxine, or vitamin B_6, may be required in greater quantity in old age. Deficiency of the vitamin B_6 may be precipitated by use of drugs such as penicillamine, adverse effects of intestinal bacteria, decreased secretion of the vitamin, and urinary tract infections.

Folic acid deficiency is common in old people. Reasons for the deficiency include increased body need; the effects of drugs; insufficient intake; destruction during cooking; decreased absorption, utilization, and secretion; and reduced intestinal synthesis.

Vitamin B$_{12}$ and its relationship to folic acid is discussed in Chapter 6. For example, it is well known that a decreased iron intake will decrease the absorption of these two vitamins. The nutritional anemia that occurs in some older Americans results from insufficient iron, vitamin B$_{12}$, and folic acid. Deficiency of B$_{12}$ may reflect decreased absorption, gastric atrophy with a decrease in intrinsic factor (see Chapter 6), or abnormal bacterial growth in the small intestine.

Fat-soluble vitamin deficiency is caused by decreased absorption. A low fat intake, insufficient secretion of bile, pancreatic failure, and prolonged use of antibiotics and laxatives are all factors contributing to malabsorption. The conversion of provitamin A to the vitamin may be affected by old age. Vitamin D deficiency may result from low milk consumption and little exposure to sunlight, contributing to osteoporosis. The requirement for vitamin E may increase with age. Vitamin K deficiency most often results from certain clinical conditions, such as gallbladder disease, rather than from insufficient intake.

According to the 1980 RDAs, an older person requires the same essential minerals as a 25–year–old, including calcium, phosphorus, iodine, iron, magnesium, and zinc. Older people may have a special need for fluoride. Adequate amounts of iron, calcium, and possibly fluoride are especially important because of the incidence of nutritional anemia and osteoporosis among the elderly.

Calcium deficiency can contribute to the development of osteoporosis. Low calcium intake may be due to consuming too few dairy products. Iron deficiency is common in older people, especially among elderly women, and can lead to anemia. The water and fiber requirements of the elderly are important in preventing constipation. Consult Chapters 2, 14, and 18 for more information on the importance of fiber in the diet.

PLANNING A GOOD DIET

Nutritional assistance to the elderly is effective only when the entire environment in which they live is taken into consideration, including the social, economic, psychological, environmental, and clinical factors involved. Because each person has specific habits and unique problems, he or she must be nutritionally evaluated on an individual basis. Such factors as present nutritional status and eating patterns, age, lifelong eating habits, income, social status, education, activity, illnesses, handicaps, psychological problems, and degree of independence all play an important part in the individual's general well-being.

Although the total calories of an older person should be reduced, all other essential nutrients must be provided in adequate quantities. Consult Chapter 10 for basic information about planning a balanced diet. The four basic food groups should be considered in supplying a foundation diet of about 1,100 to 1,200 kcal a day, which may be provided by serving the following:

Food Groups	Sample Serving
Milk and equivalents; e.g., yogurt, ice cream	2 to 8 oz milk
Meat and equivalents; e.g., eggs, legumes, peas, peanut butter	2 to 4 oz cooked lean meat 1 egg
Vegetable and fruit group	½ c yellow or deep green vegetable ½ c other vegetable 1 medium cooked (baked) potato 6 oz tomato, orange, or grapefruit juice (citrus juices) 1 serving other fruit or juice, such as apple, banana
Cereal and equivalents; e.g., bread, macaroni	3 sl bread ⅔ c cereal

The above diet meets the RDAs for older people in all nutrients except calories. This diet may be used as a foundation in meal planning, with flavor (and calories) added by the use of sweeteners, sauces, gravies, and butter or margarine.

Protein-rich foods such as cheese, poultry, meat, and fish are an important part of the foundation diet for older people. Such foods often are lacking, however, because of their cost and because the elderly may be unaware of protein values and requirements. Also, dental problems can make meat difficult to chew. Milk, although a good source of protein, can create problems for the elderly because it is costly, can cause diarrhea or constipation, and is sometimes inadvisable because of its high saturated fat and cholesterol content. If milk is excluded from the diet, other similar high-protein food such as yogurt may be substituted to promote an adequate intake of calcium and vitamin B_2 as well as protein.

Body weight is important in determining how many calories should be added to the foundation diet to meet a particular older person's needs. It is assumed that a person 60 years old should weigh the same as when he or she was 25. Someone of average weight who gets a fair amount of light activity daily should consume 1,600 to 1,900 kcal for a male and about 1,500 to 1,700 kcal for a female. The caloric intake may be adjusted to achieve and maintain optimal weight.

TABLE 13-1. A Week's Sample Menus for Older People

Snacks: Some suggested items are fresh fruit; soft, dried prunes; whole wheat crackers with cheese; cheese sticks; peanut butter on toast; and yogurt. Snacks may be served in mid-morning, mid-afternoon, and/or before bedtime.

Breakfast	Lunch	Dinner
Monday		
½ c orange juice	1 c creamed tuna on noodles	1 c chicken, rice, and pea casserole
Poached eggs	Celery or carrot sticks	½ c buttered spinach
Whole wheat toast	1 c skim milk	Fresh fruit; banana, melon
2 slices bacon	1 orange	Decaffeinated coffee
Tuesday		
½ c grapefruit juice	Cottage cheese with pineapple	3 oz broiled fish
½ c cooked oatmeal, sugar, and	salad	½ c mashed potato
milk	Banana	½ c creamed peas
1 fruit or 2 sausages	Toasted raisin bread with butter	Celery sticks
	Tea or decaffeinated coffee	Gingerbread, 1 square
		Decaffeinated coffee
Wednesday		
Sliced banana and milk	1 c split pea soup	1 c beef and vegetable stew
2 bran muffins	Tomato and shredded lettuce salad	½ c cabbage coleslaw
1 baked egg with cheese	Crackers and cheese	½ c rice pudding
1 orange	Skim milk	Decaffeinated coffee
	1 pear	
Thursday		
3 stewed prunes	1 c minestrone soup	3 oz hamburger steak
2 French toast slices with butter and	Cottage cheese and peach salad	½ c mashed potatoes
syrup	2 crackers	½ c buttered broccoli
8 oz skim milk	Skim milk	1 sliced tomato with dressing
	Decaffeinated coffee	2 oatmeal cookies
		½ c gelatin
Friday		
Sliced orange	Tomato and rice soup	1 c tuna noodle casserole
1 c puffed rice with milk and sugar	⅔ c potato salad	½ c mixed vegetables
Sliced cheese	Celery or green pepper sticks	½ c lettuce salad
Hot tea	½ c strawberries	1 slice angel food cake
	Skim milk	Decaffeinated coffee
Saturday		
Melon or fresh fruit	1 c creamed chicken and	1 c spaghetti and meatballs in
3 hotcakes	mushrooms on toast	tomato sauce
2 sausages	½ c carrot and raisin salad	½ c string beans
8 oz skim milk	Fresh fruit	½ c fruit gelatin
	Skim milk	Decaffeinated coffee

TABLE 13-1. (continued)

Snacks: Some suggested items are fresh fruit; soft, dried prunes; whole wheat crackers with cheese; cheese sticks; peanut butter on toast; and yogurt. Snacks may be served in mid-morning, mid-afternoon, and/or before bedtime.

Breakfast	Lunch	Dinner
Sunday		
3 stewed figs	2-egg cheese omelet	1 baked pork chop with applesauce
½ c hot cream of wheat	½ c steamed rice	½ c buttered peas
Milk	½ c asparagus	1 baked potato
2 slices crisp bacon	Celery or carrot sticks	Lettuce wedge
8 oz hot chocolate made with skim milk	8 oz skim milk	½ c custard
		Decaffeinated coffee

Older people should eat the foods they enjoy most, with as few restrictions as possible. A reasonable arrangement is to use a combination of the foundation foods and a fair amount of those other items that the person likes. Attention should be given to food preparation and the size of serving portions. Table 13-1 gives sample menus for 7 days for an elderly person.

STUDY QUESTIONS

1. Use a reference source to summarize the health problems of the elderly population.
2. Describe the personal factors affecting the nutritional status of an old person.
3. Analyze the vitamin needs of senior citizens.
4. Prepare one week's menus for an old person with specific caloric needs. Make sure that they are different from the ones provided by the book.
5. Do some library research and summarize different government programs that aim at improving the nutritional and dietary needs of senior citizens.

REFERENCES

Gupta, C. P. 1980. Nutrition in geriatrics. *J. Indian. Med. Assoc.* 74:91.

Holmes, M. B., and Holmes, D. 1979. *Handbook of human services for older persons.* New York: Human Sciences Press.

Morrison, S. D. 1984. Nutrition and longevity. In *Present knowledge in nutrition*, 5th ed. Washington, D. C.: The Nutrition Foundation.

Natow, A. B., and Heslin, J. 1980. *Geriatric nutrition*. Boston: CBI Publishing.

Posner, B. M. 1979. *Nutrition and the elderly*. Lexington, Mass.: Lexington Books.

Rockstein, M., and Sussman, M. L., eds. 1976. *Nutrition, longevity and aging*. New York: Academic Press.

Somers, A. R., and Fabian, D. R., eds. 1981. *The geriatric imperative: an introduction to gerontology and clinical geriatrics*. New York: Appleton-Century-Crofts.

Winick, M., ed. 1976. *Nutrition and aging*. New York: Wiley.

Part Three

BASICS OF DIET THERAPY AND PATIENT CARE

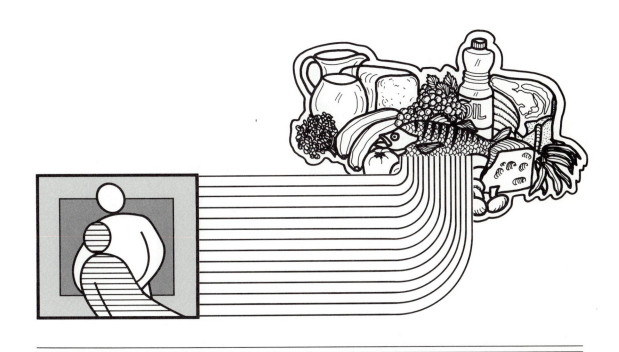

14 DIET AND THE HOSPITALIZED PATIENT

Applying basic nutritional and dietary principles in the treatment and prevention of human diseases is an important part of the practice of **dietetics.** According to the American Dietetic Association (*Journal of the American Dietetic Association, 54*:92, 1969), dietetics is "a profession concerned with the science and art of human nutrition care, an essential component of the health sciences. It includes the extending and imparting of knowledge concerning foods which will provide nutrients sufficient for health and during disease throughout the life cycle and the management of group feeding for these purposes."

Diet therapy for a particular disorder may be described in terms of the disorder, as in ulcer diet, kidney diet, or diabetic diet. Diet therapy may also be described in terms of nutrient contents, as in low-calorie diet, low-protein diet, or high-fat diet.

There are six categories of hospital feedings, including: (1) regular diets; (2) diets with texture and blandness modifications; (3) diets with nutritional modifications; (4) diets with miscellaneous modifications; (5) artificial feeding methods; (6) special test diets for diagnoses. Table 14-1 provides examples for each of these categories. Categories 1, 2, and 5 are discussed in this chapter. Category 3 is discussed in the remaining chapters. Information concerning categories 4 and 6 may be located in the references for this chapter.

TABLE 14-1. Examples of Different Types of Hospital Diets

Category of Diet	Examples of Diets or Descriptions of Usage
1. Regular diets	Regular foods with simple adjustments
2. Diets with texture and blandness modifications	Fluid-regulated diet Liquid diet Soft diet Fiber-regulated diet Diet for dental problems Bland diet
3. Diets with nutritional modifications	Calorie-controlled diet Protein-controlled diet Fat-controlled diet Carbohydrate-controlled diet Mineral-controlled diet (electrolyte-controlled diet)
4. Diets with miscellaneous modifications	Tyramine-controlled diet Uric-acid-controlled diet Purine-controlled diet Coal tar regimen
5. Artificial feeding methods (semi-synthetic, synthetic, and regular foods may all be used)	Enteral feedings Parenteral feedings
6. Special test diets for clinical diagnosis, confirmation, and assessment of a disorder	The diet may be a test for: Fat excretion Metabolic studies X-ray studies Stool blood Glucose tolerance Ketogenic hypoglycemia Hyperaldosteronemia Pheochromocytoma Carcinoid tumors Collagen degradation Urinary creatinine excretion

BASIC CONCEPTS OF DIET THERAPY

Diet and nutrition may be related to disease in two ways:

1. **Therapy**—Special dietary and nutritional care and perhaps even cure for people with certain forms of illness. Therapeutic nutrition can affect the course of illness. For example, diet therapy can reduce or control the symptoms of diabetes. Also, how burn patients eat affects their recovery. Many aspects of the scope of diet therapy have yet to be explored.
2. **Prevention**—The use of the knowledge that certain dietary practices or substances may produce or worsen specific clinical disorders. For example, eating too much salt may cause high blood pressure. Conversely, avoiding excess intake of salt may help prevent high blood pressure. Lifelong dietary habits can influence disease prevention.

The two approaches—therapy and prevention—may be used together to meet the patient's needs and particular disease. A well-nourished patient with a good appetite is fed a regular diet to maintain nutritional status and promote a speedy recovery. Other patients need special diets to control a disease, to correct nutrient deficiencies, and to provide life support.

THE HEALTH TEAM

Usually, three care providers interact to implement diet therapy: the doctor, the dietitian, and the nurse. Each of these professionals has clearly defined responsibilities to the patient under ideal circumstances. For example, if a patient needs a special diet, the doctor prescribes a diet order. The dietitian devises the meal plan to be prepared by the food service staff. The nurse serves the meals and monitors the amount and kind of food consumed by the patient. However, the current practice in many hospitals is less clear-cut.

The Doctor

Only the doctor is authorized to diagnose illness and decide whether special nutritional or dietary care will benefit the patient. On the basis of that decision, the doctor may recommend a prescription for the patient's nutritional and dietary needs.

The Dietitian

Following the doctor's prescription, the dietitian usually develops the specific dietary plan.

According to the American Dietetic Association, a registered dietitian (R.D.) is "a specialist educated for a profession responsible for the nutrition care of individuals and groups. This care includes the application of the science and art of human nutrition in helping people select and obtain food for the primary purposes of nourishing their bodies in health or disease throughout the life cycle. This participation may be in single or combined functions; in food service systems management; in extending knowledge of food and nutrition principles; in teaching these principles for application according to particular situations; or in dietary counseling." (Copyright The American Dietetic Association. Reprinted by permission from *Journal of the American Dietetic Association,* 77:62, 1981.)

Dietitians are the best-trained personnel to administer nutritional and dietary care to patients. However, institutions vary in the degree of responsibility they give to dietitians. Figure 14-1 indicates the ideal relationship among the doctor, dietitian, and nurse.

The Nurse

Nurses play an extremely important role in clinical dietetics: They coordinate the activities of doctors, dietitians, and patients, including diet prescription, food service, meal serving, and patient response.

Arranging food trays, helping patients eat, and answering questions are among the nurse's duties. In addition, the nurse observes patients directly and records the amounts of fluids, foods, and nutrient supplements consumed. Measuring the amount of urine voided and evaluating patient response to the dietary regimen are related duties of the nurse.

Enteral and parenteral feeding practices are defined and discussed in detail later in this chapter. These feedings are administered and monitored by the nurse. In the case of intravenous fluids and electrolytes, the doctor's prescription is carried out only by the nurse, who also checks the patient's response. The dietitian or nutritionist is helped in planning other aspects of the patient's nutritional and dietary needs by the nurse's observations and the patient's health history.

Drugs profoundly affect a person's nutritional status. A nurse must know firsthand what drugs the patient is taking, what the dosages are, and when they are taken. If drugs cause nausea or drowsiness, the patient may not eat enough.

The nurse frequently is the patient's only source of nutritional and dietary information and advice. In any case, the nurse has the best opportunity to teach the patient principles of nutrition in the course of the

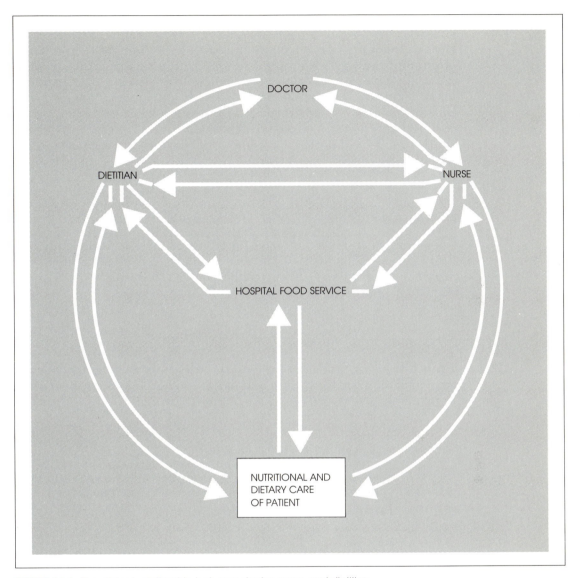

FIGURE 14-1. The clinical relationship between doctor, nurse, and dietitian.

day-to-day care. After the patient is discharged, the nurse may be the only health professional in contact with the patient.

It is not uncommon for a nurse to assume the roles of nutritionist and dietitian as well as nurse. Some nurses even assume certain aspects of the physician's role. Because of the nurse's importance in the nutritional and dietary care of the patient, nurses may need a stronger background in nutrition and dietetics.

NUTRITIONAL MAINTENANCE

Hospital malnutrition is a continuing problem. In the last few years, a large number of cases of hospital undernutrition have been documented, especially protein and calorie deficiencies. The reasons for inadequate nutritional care include: the patient's poor nutritional status; adverse effects from medical and drug treatment; pain, nausea, and vomiting; inadequate care resulting from poor communication between patient and care givers; lack of nutritional knowledge; and/or the patient's inability to follow the dietary prescription.

Knowing the Patient

One of the most important ways for a hospital and health team to prevent malnourishment is to know the patient and monitor his or her progress, especially regarding nutrition. The following factors are of particular importance:

Personal History

The health history and interviews of patient, family members, and health personnel may reveal relevant details such as health and special feeding problems.

Lifelong Eating Habits and Nutritional Status

Information should include number of meals eaten daily, time and location of each meal, sizes and servings, types and quantities of food, food habits, and eating difficulties.

Body Weight History

Especially important in disorders such as diabetes and renal diseases, body weight information should include: degree of overweight or underweight, body weight history since childhood, family weight history, weight at hospital admission, and ideal body weight.

Drug Use History

A thorough knowledge of the patient's drug use history is vitally important because of the relationship between drugs and nutritional status.

Ideal Body Weight and Caloric Intake

Standard tables and sex/frame/height rules of thumb help establish a patient's ideal body weight. RDAs and other methods may be used to determine caloric intake. More information is presented in Chapter 4.

Eating Pattern During the Hospital Stay

The importance of monitoring the patient's food consumption cannot be overemphasized. Indications are that from 5 to 40 percent of some items, such as bread, meat, vegetables, and salad, are not eaten. For patients with fevers, infections, and conditions of stress, overall monitoring is even more important. If protein and calorie consumption fall below certain levels, drastic measures such as **enteral feeding** (via the gastrointestinal tract) or **parenteral feeding** (via the veins) may be indicated.

Health History

The patient's records should include nutritional status; results of blood and urine analyses; medications administered; and a complete description of hospital feeding, such as diets ordered, nutrient intake, and use of enteral and parenteral feeding.

Consultation with Other Medical Personnel

The best patient care results from close communication among the doctor, nurse, and dietitian. Coordination with other professionals—pharmacists, oral surgeons, and physical therapists, for example—also may be required in certain disorders such as cancer, burns, and chronic illness.

HELPING THE PATIENT COMPLY

A lack of well-funded nutritional support programs is not the only reason for malnourishment among hospital patients. Another problem is a patient's unwillingness or inability to eat what is provided.

To some degree all sick people experience physical and psychological trauma. Hospitalization can increase anxiety and confusion. The sterile environment and the presence of so many health personnel add to the discomfort for most patients. Physical interferences, psychological factors, personal preferences, and gaps in health team communication all contribute to possible trouble in eating, as discussed below.

Other major considerations in patient compliance include: conditions on admission, diet prescription, the patient's level of knowledge, and adjustments for specific problems.

Basic eating patterns are largely determined by socioeconomic, ethnic, cultural, family, and religious factors. These eating patterns and the patient's conditions on admission provide important clues to appropriate dietary care. The more restricted the prescribed diet, the more difficult it is to prepare appetizing meals that the patient will eat. Diet prescriptions are more readily followed if they are explained to the patient. Certain problems may require modification of the original treatment plan to help a patient accept the diet and eat what is provided. For example, if pain is interfering with eating, a medication can be used to relieve the pain.

Some hospitalized patients have one or more feeding problems mentioned in this chapter. However, many patients are cooperative, eat well, adhere to the prescribed diet, and achieve a speedy recovery. These patients are given a regular diet, which acts as a frame of reference for developing more specialized diets for patients who require them.

REGULAR DIETS

The regular hospital diet contains all the essential nutrients, such as calories, protein, fat, carbohydrate, minerals, and vitamins, in adequate amounts to satisfy the RDAs. Such a diet is based on the basic four food groups and the formulation of a foundation diet, the details of which are presented in Chapter 10. Table 14-2 shows a meal plan for a regular diet for a healthy adult male that contributes 2,600 to 2,900 kcal, 95 to 105 g of protein, 95 to 125 g of fat, and 300 to 320 g of carbohydrate.

As indicated in Chapter 10, the patient's age, sex, and activity level must be considered in adjusting a diet to individual needs. In planning any regular or therapeutic diet, the major objective is nutritional adequacy. If the diet is modified to treat a patient with a disease, the nutrient contents must still comply with the RDAs.

A regular diet sometimes requires only slight adjustment for a hospitalized patient. For example, a patient recovering from minor surgery needs foods high in protein and calories in addition to the regular diet. Such foods as cheese, meat, bread, fat, ice cream, and milkshakes help to rebuild body muscle. Table 14-3 provides an example of 3,500-kcal, 150-g-protein menu. Three large meals may be divided into a number of small feedings (perhaps five to seven) or three medium-sized meals with two to four snacks.

TABLE 14-2. Sample Meal Plan for a Regular Diet

Breakfast	Lunch	Dinner
Fruit or juice, ½ c	Soup, ½ c	Soup, ½ c
Cereal: hot, 6 oz; or dry, 1 oz	Meat or alternate, 2–3 oz	Meat or alternate, 3–4 oz
Egg or substitute, 1	Potato or alternate, ½ c	Potato or alternate, ½ c
Meat: regular meat, 1 oz; or bacon, 2 strips	Vegetable (cooked or in a salad), ½ c	Vegetable (cooked or in a salad), ½ c
Bread, 1–2 sl	Salad dressing, 1 T	Salad dressing, 1–2 t
Butter or margarine, 1–3 t	Bread or roll, 1	Bread or roll, 1
Jelly, jam, or preserves, 1–3 t	Butter or margarine, 1–2 t	Dessert
Milk, 1 c	Dessert	Milk, 1 c
Hot beverage, 1–2 c	Beverage (cold or hot)	Butter or margarine, 1–2 t
Cream (regular or substitute), 1 t	Cream (regular or substitute), 1 t	Hot beverage, 1–2 c
Sugar, 1–3 t	Sugar, 1–3 t	Sugar, 1–3 t
Salt, pepper	Salt, pepper	Cream (regular or substitute), 1–2 t
		Salt, pepper

TABLE 14-3. Sample Menu for a 3,500-kcal, 150-g-Protein Diet

Breakfast	Lunch	Dinner
Orange juice, ½ c	Split pea soup, 1 c	Chicken, broiled, 6 oz
Eggs, scrambled with milk, 2	Corn muffins, 2	Sweet potato, baked, 1
Ham, 3 oz	Butter, 2 pats	Broccoli, steamed, 1 stalk
Waffle, 1	Jam, 2 T	Bread, whole wheat, 1 sl
Syrup, 2 T	Cheddar cheese, 1 oz	Butter, 1–2 pats
Margarine, 1 T	Salad:	Pear poached in wine and sugar:
Banana, sliced, 1	Tomato, medium, 1	Pear, 1
Yogurt, 1 c	Raw spinach, 1 c	Wine, white, 3½ oz
Cocoa, 1 c	Celery, 1 stalk	Sugar, 1 T
Salt, pepper	Almonds, ¼ c	Milk, 1 c
	Olive oil and vinegar dressing, 2 T	Tea, 2 c
	Applesauce, sweetened, 1 c	Honey, 1 T
	Brownies, 2	Salt, pepper
	Coffee, 1 c	
	Sugar, 1 t	
	Salt, pepper	

Note: If meals are too large, they can be divided into five to seven feedings or three medium-sized meals with two to four snacks.

DIETS WITH TEXTURE AND BLANDNESS MODIFICATIONS

Some patients who have no need for a special modified diet are nevertheless not ready for a regular diet because of their physical condition or food tolerances. Although the types of diets for this group of patients vary from hospital to hospital, they usually include the following: a clear-liquid diet, a full-liquid diet, a pureed diet, a mechanical soft diet, and a soft diet. The following sections describe each of these types.

Clear-Liquid Diet

A clear-liquid diet consists of fluids that are liquid at body temperature, with mono- and disaccharides as the major caloric sources. Such a diet is beneficial in the following clinical conditions: (1) before and after an operation, (2) during acute stages of a number of clinical disorders, (3) during a fever, or (4) under circumstances that require very little residue or fecal waste in the bowel (for example, when certain tests are scheduled).

The clear-liquid diet prevents dehydration until a full-liquid diet or solid food can be tolerated. About 600 to 1,000 kcal and 50 to 150 g of carbohydrate are provided. This diet is inadequate in all essential nutrients and in some cases may not provide enough fluid; therefore it should not be used for more than 14 hours without supplementation. The use of commercial nutritional supplements should be encouraged.

The list below describes those foods and beverages permitted in a clear-liquid diet.

- **Soups:** Clear broth, bouillon, consommé
- **Desserts:** Plain or clear-flavored gelatin, Popsicles, fruit-flavored ices without pieces of fruit or milk, water ices without pieces of fruit or milk
- **Sweets:** Honey, jelly, syrup, sugar; plain sugar candy; sugar substitutes
- **Fruits:** All strained or clear fruit juices; apple and citrus juices only if tolerated
- **Vegetables:** Vegetable broth
- **Beverages:** Clear tea and regular coffee, decaffeinated coffee, water, strained lemonade and limeade, strained fruit punches, fruit-flavored drinks, cereal beverages, carbonated beverages and certain commercial beverages such as Gatorade and Kool-aid
- **Miscellaneous:** Salt

Table 14-4 provides a sample menu plan for a clear-liquid diet.

TABLE 14-4. Sample Menu for a Clear-Liquid Diet

Breakfast	Lunch	Dinner
Juice, ⅔ c	Juice, ⅔ c	Juice, ⅔ c
Coffee or tea	Broth (chicken, beef, or	Broth (chicken, beef, or
Sugar	vegetable), ⅔ c	vegetable), ⅔ c
	Flavored gelatin, ½ c	Fruit ice or flavored
Snack	Coffee or tea	gelatin, ½ c
Juice, ⅔ c; or broth,	Sugar	Coffee or tea
clear, ½ c		Sugar
	Snack	
	Flavored ice, ½ c	**Snack**
		Carbonated beverage

Full-Liquid Diet

The full-liquid diet includes certain foods and beverages that are liquid at body temperature. This diet is beneficial under the following conditions: (1) swallowing and chewing difficulty, (2) any condition that prevents the patient from eating semisolid or solid foods, (3) postsurgical recovery, and (4) acute infections.

Because the full-liquid diet is inadequate in most nutrients, it would be used for a minimal period only. Whenever the patient tolerates them, commercial nutrient solutions should be given. This diet provides approximately 1,500 to 2,000 kcal, 50 to 70 g of protein, and 180 to 250 g of carbohydrate. The foods and beverages permitted in a full-liquid diet are listed below.

- **Milk and milk products:** Whole milk, skim milk, chocolate, buttermilk, smooth or plain yogurt, whey, milkshakes, cocoa
- **Cheeses:** Cheese soup
- **Eggs:** Eggnog from pasteurized mix or other egg forms prepared in a beverage; scrambled or soft-cooked eggs if tolerated
- **Cereals:** Cream of Rice, Cream of Wheat; cooked, refined cereals such as farina, grits, cornmeal, strained thin oatmeal and granulated rice, gruels
- **Meats, fish, poultry, legumes, and nuts:** Strained and pureed forms added to broth and cream soup
- **Potatoes:** Pureed form added to soup
- **Soups:** Any pureed or strained soup; cream soup, broth, bouillon
- **Fruits:** All juices, including nectars
- **Vegetables:** All juices and pureed forms used in preparing soups
- **Beverages:** Coffee (regular, decaffeinated, or substitute), tea, carbonated types, lemonade, commercial types such as Kool-aid, other tolerated varieties

TABLE 14-5. Sample Meal Plan for a Full-Liquid Diet

Breakfast	Lunch	Dinner
Juice, ½ c	Juice, ½ c	Juice, ½ c
Cereal, ½ c	Soup, ⅔ c	Soup, ⅔ c
Milk, ½ c	Milk, ½ c	Milk, 1 c
Beverage, 1–2 c	Dessert, ½ c	Dessert, ½ c
Cream	Beverage, 1–2 c	Beverage, 1–2 c
Sugar	Cream	Cream
Salt	Sugar	Sugar
	Salt	Salt
Snack		
Eggnog (from pasteurized mix), 1 c	**Snack**	**Snack**
	Custard, ½ c	Milkshake, 1 c

TABLE 14-6. Sample Menu for a Full-Liquid Diet

Breakfast	Lunch	Dinner
Orange juice, ½ c	Pineapple juice, ½ c	Grapefruit juice, ½ c
Cream of Rice, ½ c	Cream soup, strained, ⅔ c	Vegetable soup, strained or pureed, ⅔ c
Milk, ½ c	Milk, ½ c	Milk, 1 c
Coffee or tea, 1–2 c	Gelatin, strawberry flavored, ½ c	Pudding, ½ c
Cream	Coffee or tea, 1–2 c	Coffee or tea, 1–2 c
Sugar	Cream	Cream
Salt	Sugar	Sugar
	Salt	Salt
Snack		
Apple juice, 1 c	**Snack**	**Snack**
	Ice cream, 1 c	Custard, ½ c; or nutritional supplement

- **Desserts:** Custards, plain or flavored (no fruits) gelatin, smooth ice cream, plain water ices, ice milk, puddings, sherbets, Popsicles
- **Sweets:** Honey, molasses, sugar, syrup, hard candy, jellies
- **Fats:** Margarine, butter, cream, oils
- **Miscellaneous:** Nutritious protein supplements (homemade or commercial); Instant Breakfast; salt; any finely ground herbs, spices, or flavorings tolerated by the patient

Table 14-5 shows a sample meal plan for the full-liquid diet, and Table 14-6 shows a sample menu.

High-Nutrient or Modified Full-Liquid Diet

As already stated, a full-liquid diet is nutritionally inadequate. For long-term home and hospital use, a high-nutrient or modified full-liquid diet that is nutritionally adequate has been developed. It consists of nutritionally rich liquids and semisolid foods that are appropriate for patients with broken or wired jaws, oral or throat injuries, or other clinical disorders that require prolonged liquid feedings.

The diet provides about 2,300 to 2,800 kcal, 120 to 150 g of protein, 90 to 100 g of fat, and 250 to 300 g of carbohydrate and is high in cholesterol, saturated fats, and fat-soluble vitamins. Additional foods can be given as tolerated. Those foods and beverages permitted in a high-nutrient or modified full-liquid diet are as follows:

- **Beverages:** All types including coffee (regular or decaffeinated), milk, milk beverages, high-protein solutions, cocoa
- **Cereals:** Cream of Wheat, Cream of Rice; cooked refined cereals diluted with milk, such as farina, grits, granulated rice; certain strainable cereals; for example, oatmeal
- **Cheeses:** Finely grated cheese in soup; blended cottage cheese; melted cheese if tolerated
- **Meats** (beef, pork, poultry, fish): Strained or baby food meats (thinned with gravy, broth, or milk)
- **Eggs:** Cooked, preferably incorporated into beverages such as eggnog; soft or scrambled eggs if tolerated
- **Fruits:** All nectars and juices; strained or baby food fruits diluted with fruit juice
- **Vegetables:** Baby food or strained vegetables (thinned with strained vegetable juice, cream, or milk); juices
- **Potatoes:** Mashed potatoes, thinned with gravy or milk
- **Soups:** Strained, pureed, or cream soups without solids
- **Sweets:** Syrup, sugar, jelly, honey, molasses
- **Desserts:** Melted, smooth sherbet and ice cream; thin, strained puddings; thin Jello; custard sauce; thin yogurt
- **Fats:** Butter, margarine, cream, or plain gravy used in food preparation
- **Miscellaneous:** Salt; all finely chopped or ground herbs and spices; commercial nutrient supplement solutions

Table 14-7 provides a sample meal plan for the modified full-liquid diet and Table 14-8 presents a sample menu.

Pureed Diet

The pureed diet is appropriate for patients who cannot chew or swallow well. Its food items are easy to digest and of a consistency between liquid and soft. All meats and vegetables are pureed. Additional foods that

TABLE 14-7. Sample Meal Plan for a Modified Full-Liquid or High-Nutrient Liquid Diet

Breakfast	Lunch	Dinner
Fruit juice, ½ c	Soup or broth, ½ c	Meat or broth, ½ c
Cereal, ½ c	Meat or broth, ½ c	Potato or gravy, ½ c
Milk, 1 c	Vegetable, ¼ c	Vegetable, ½ c
Butter or margarine	Fruit, ¼ c	Fruit, ¼ c
Beverage	Milk, 1 c	Milk, 1 c
Cream	Butter or margarine	Butter or margarine
Sugar	Beverage	Beverage
Salt	Sugar	Cream
	Cream	Sugar
Snack	Salt	Salt
Nutritional		
supplement*	**Snack**	**Snack**
	Nutritional	Nutritional
	supplement*	supplement*

Note: The portion sizes refer to undiluted items; the appropriate amount of fluid at the correct temperature is added to permit drinking or sucking through a straw.

*Any commercial liquid or high-nutrient diet supplement, milkshake, malted milk, or eggnog.

TABLE 14-8. Sample Menu for a Modified Full-Liquid or High-Nutrient Liquid Diet

Breakfast	Lunch	Dinner
Orange juice, strained, ½ c	Vegetable soup, strained, ½ c	Chicken, strained, thinned with broth, ½ c
Farina, cooked, refined, thinned with milk, ½ c	Beef, baby food, thinned with broth, ½ c	Potatoes, mashed, thinned with milk and gravy, ½ c
Milk, 1 c	Spinach, strained, thinned with spinach juice, ¼ c	Carrots, strained, thinned with carrot juice, ¼ c
Margarine or butter, 1 t	Peach, strained, thinned with peach juice, ¼ c	Apricots, strained, thinned with apricot juice, ¼ c
Sugar	Milk, 1 c	Milk, 1 c
Cream	Butter or margarine	Margarine or butter, 1 t
Salt	Coffee or tea	Coffee or tea
	Sugar	Sugar
Snack	Cream	Cream
Milk shake, 8 oz	Salt	Salt
	Snack	**Snack**
	Meritene liquid, 1 c	Sustacal liquid, 1 c

are tolerated may be given. The diet is nutritionally adequate and provides about 1,800 to 2,500 kcal, 60 to 70 g of protein, 180 to 220 g of carbohydrate, and 60 to 80 g of fat. A list of those foods and beverages permitted in a pureed diet follows. To increase nutritional content, pureed regular foods such as casseroles may be served rather than commercial pureed products.

- **Dairy products:** All types of fluid milk, including whole, skim, and chocolate and buttermilk; milkshakes, cocoa, yogurt, eggnog; cottage cheese, cream, and mild cheese sauces; other tolerated melted cheeses
- **Eggs:** Poached, soft, scrambled
- **Meats, fish, poultry:** All strained or pureed products
- **Cereals:** Cooked cereals, Cream of Wheat, Cream of Rice, grits, oatmeal (thinned); white bread and toast if tolerated
- **Soups:** Strained cream soups, broth, and pureed soups from permitted foods; broth, bouillon, consommé
- **Potatoes:** Mashed, whipped, and creamed potatoes (white and sweet)
- **Beverages:** All types including coffee (regular or decaffeinated), tea, carbonated beverages, lemonade; other commercial beverages such as Kool-aid
- **Fruits:** Mashed, strained, and pureed fruits and juices
- **Vegetables:** Mashed, strained, and pureed vegetables and juices
- **Sweets:** Sugar, honey, jelly, syrup
- **Desserts:** Plain custard, ice cream, gelatin, sherbet, ices, puddings, fruit whip, plain or smooth desserts without any fruit
- **Fats:** Margarine, oils, sour cream, cream, butter, mayonnaise, cream cheese
- **Miscellaneous:** Salt; other flavorings such as pepper, herbs, and spices if tolerated (in moderation); cream sauces and gravies

Table 14-9 provides a sample meal plan for the pureed diet, and Table 14-10 gives a sample menu.

Mechanical Soft Diet

The mechanical soft diet is a sample modification of the regular diet and is made up of foods and beverages that require little chewing. It is appropriate for patients with few or no teeth, poor teeth, or ill-fitting dentures. It provides about 2,200 to 2,600 kcal, 85 to 95 g of protein, 100 to 110 g of fat, and 295 to 315 g of carbohydrate.

Pureed, ground, chopped, and mashed foods are served according to individual desires and needs. A diet should be based on both the patient's chewing ability and food preferences as well as nutritional adequacy.

The foods permitted in a mechanical soft diet are as follows:

TABLE 14-9. Sample Meal Plan for a Pureed Diet

Breakfast	Lunch	Dinner
Fruit or juice, ½ c	Meat, poultry, or fish, 2 oz	Meat, fish, or poultry, 3–4 oz
Cereal, ½ c	Vegetable, ½ c	Potato, ½ c
Egg, 1	Cereal, ½ c; or mashed potatoes	Vegetable, ½ c
Butter or margarine, 1 t	Dessert, ½ c	Butter or margarine, 1 t
Milk, 1 c	Butter or margarine, 1 t	Dessert, ½ c
Hot beverage, 1–2 c	Milk, ½ c	Hot beverage, 1–2 c
Sugar	Hot beverage, 1–2 c	Cream
Cream	Cream	Sugar
Salt	Sugar	Salt
	Salt	

TABLE 14-10. Sample Menu for a Pureed Diet

Breakfast	Lunch	Dinner
Orange juice, ½ c	Chicken, pureed, 2 oz	Beef, pureed, with gravy, 3–4 oz
Oatmeal, ½ c	Beets, pureed, ½ c	Potatoes, mashed, ½ c
Egg, scrambled, soft, 1	Applesauce, ½ c	Asparagus, pureed, ½ c
Butter or margarine, 1 t	Sweet potato, mashed, ½ c	Butter or margarine, 1 t
Coffee or tea, 1–2 c	Margarine or butter, 1 t	Pudding, butterscotch, ½ c
Milk, 1 c	Coffee or tea, 1–2 c	Coffee or tea, 1–2 c
Sugar	Cream	Cream
Cream	Sugar	Sugar
Salt	Salt	Salt

- **Milk:** All forms
- **Cheeses:** All forms
- **Eggs:** Any cooked form
- **Breads:** White, rye without seeds, refined whole wheat; cornbread; any cracker not made with whole grains; French toast made from permitted breads; spoon bread; pancakes; plain soft rolls
- **Cereals:** All cooked, soft varieties; puffed flakes and noncoarse ready-to-eat varieties
- **Flour:** All forms
- **Meats, fish, poultry:** Small cubed and finely ground or minced forms; as ingredients in creamed dishes, soups, casseroles, and stews

- **Seafoods:** Any variety of fish without bone (canned, fresh, or frozen; packaged prepared forms in cream sauces); minced, shredded, ground, and finely chopped shellfish
- **Legumes, nuts:** Fine, smooth, creamy peanut butter; legumes (if tolerated) cooked tender, finely chopped, mashed, or minced
- **Potatoes:** White potatoes: mashed, boiled, baked, creamed, scalloped, cakes, au gratin; sweet potatoes: boiled, baked, mashed
- **Soups:** All varieties, preferably without hard solids such as nuts and seeds
- **Fruits:** Raw: avocado, banana; cooked and canned: fruit cocktail, cherries, apples, apricots, peaches, pears, sections of mandarin oranges, grapefruits or oranges without membranes; all juices and nectars
- **Vegetables:** All juices; all vegetables cooked tender, chopped, mashed, canned, or pureed; canned, pureed, or paste forms of tomato
- **Sweets:** Marshmallow and chocolate sauces; preserves, marmalade, jelly, jam; candy: hard, chocolate, caramels, jellybeans, marshmallows, candy corn, butterscotch, gumdrops, plain fudge, lollipops, fondant mints; syrup: sorghum, maple, corn; sugar: granulated, brown, maple, confectioner's; honey; molasses
- **Desserts:** All plain or certain flavored varieties (permitted flavorings include liquids, such as juice; finely chopped or pureed fruits without solid pieces of fruit, seeds, nuts, etc.); gelatins, puddings; ice cream, ice milk, sherbet; water ices; cakes, cookies, cake icing; cobblers
- **Fats:** Butter, margarine, cream (or substitutes), oils and vegetable shortenings, and bacon fat; salad dressings, tartar sauce, sour cream
- **Seasonings:** Salt, pepper, soy sauce, vinegar, catsup; all other herbs, especially finely chopped or ground, that can be tolerated

Table 14-11 gives a sample meal plan for the mechanical soft diet, and Table 14-12 presents a sample menu.

Soft Diet

Although there is no solid scientific basis for use of the soft diet, many patients experience abdominal discomfort and flatulence if their diet includes fried foods, raw fruits and vegetables, very hard or coarse breads or cereals, and highly seasoned foods. Hospitals traditionally have used a soft diet during the transition from liquid to regular foods, especially when patients are convalescing (for example, after surgery). The consistency of the diet is easy to chew and can be adjusted to suit individual needs, preferences, and intolerances.

TABLE 14-11. Sample Meal Plan for a Mechanical Soft Diet

Breakfast	Lunch	Dinner
Fruit or juice, ½ c	Soup, ½ c	Soup, ½ c
Cereal, ½ c	Meat, fish, or poultry,	Meat, fish, or poultry,
Egg, 1	2–3 oz	3–4 oz
Bread or toast, 1 sl	Potato, ½ c	Potato, ½ c
Butter or margarine, 1 t	Bread or toast, 1 sl	Vegetable, ½ c
Milk, 1 c	Vegetable, ½ c	Bread or toast, 1 sl
Hot beverage, 1–2 c	Butter or margarine, 1 t	Butter or margarine, 1 t
Cream	Dessert, 1 serving	Dessert, 1 serving
Sugar	Milk, 1 c	Milk, 1 c
Salt, pepper	Hot beverage, 1–2 c	Hot beverage, 1–2 c
	Cream	Cream
	Sugar	Sugar
	Salt, pepper	Salt, pepper
		Snack
		Beverage, fruit, or
		dessert

TABLE 14-12. Sample Menu for a Mechanical Soft Diet

Breakfast	Lunch	Dinner
Orange juice, ½ c	Clam soup, ½ c	Cream soup, ½ c
Oatmeal, ½ c	Chicken, minced and	Roast beef, chopped,
Egg, scrambled, soft, 1	creamed, ½ c	with gravy, 3–4 oz
Toast, 1 sl	Potato, baked, ½ c	Potato, mashed, ½ c
Butter or margarine, 1 t	Toast, 1 sl	Spinach, ½ c
Milk, 1 c	Beets, diced, ½ c	Toast, 1 sl
Coffee or tea	Butter or margarine, 1 t	Butter or margarine, 1 t
Cream, 1 T	Custard, plain, ½ c	Ice cream, ½ c
Sugar, 1–2 t	Milk, 1 c	Milk, 1 c
Salt, pepper	Coffee or tea	Coffee or tea
	Cream, 1 T	Cream, 1 T
	Sugar, 1–2 t	Sugar, 1–2 t
	Salt, pepper	Salt, pepper
		Snack
		Cookies, plain, 3

The soft diet provides about 2,200 to 2,600 kcal, 90 to 100 g of protein, 90 to 110 g of fat, and 250 to 300 g of carbohydrate. Table 14-13 describes the foods permitted and prohibited in a soft diet; Table 14-14 shows a sample meal plan for the diet; and Table 14-15 gives a sample menu.

Special Dietary Foods

Special diet foods are used by some hospitals to satisfy the particular dietary needs of patients with certain physical, physiological, or pathological conditions. These foods may be administered orally or enterally and range from complete defined-formula diets to a single nutrient. Available in liquid or powder form without a prescription, these special foods are, however, used under a doctor's supervision, whether within a hospital or for outpatient care. By contrast, nutrient solutions for parenteral feeding are classified as drugs and are subject to special regulations.

Safety, effectiveness, convenience, and acceptability are the main considerations in using these products. There is a growing interest in providing trained hospital personnel to assess the safety and usefulness of special dietary and medical foods.

ENTERAL AND PARENTERAL FEEDINGS

Although oral ingestion and digestion still constitute the best way to assure the proper nutrient intake of a patient, a number of clinical conditions make the normal route of nourishment unsatisfactory or inadvisable. The two basic artificial methods of feeding a hospitalized patient are enteral and parenteral nutrition.

Enteral feedings are administered directly to the gastrointestinal tract; **parenteral feedings** enter the body by injection directly into blood veins. Enteral feeding may combine oral feeding of regular foods or nutritional supplements with tube feeding with nutritional supplements.

Parenteral feeding may include standard intravenous (IV) therapy and partial or total parenteral nutrition.

Enteral Feedings

In circumstances where oral feeding is difficult, enteral feeding is indicated. Examples include such conditions as head and neck tumors, intestinal diseases, and severe burns. Under these circumstances, feedings may be administered by tube(s) through the nose and throat (nasogastric or nasopharyngeal route); through an artificial opening in the stomach (gastrostomy); or an artificial opening in the upper bowel (jejunostomy).

TABLE 14-13. Foods Permitted and Prohibited in a Soft Diet

Food Types	Foods Permitted	Foods Prohibited
Milk	All milk and milk products without added ingredients; condensed and evaporated milk, chocolate milk and drink; cocoa and hot chocolate; yogurt and whey	Any milk product with prohibited ingredients
Cheese	Cottage cheese, cream cheese, mild cheese, and any cheese not prohibited	Any sharp, strongly flavored cheese; any cheese with prohibited ingredients
Eggs	Poached, scrambled, soft- and hard-cooked eggs; salmonella-free egg powder (pasteurized)	Raw or fried eggs
Breads and equivalents	Breads: white, Italian, Vienna, French, re-fined whole wheat, corn bread, spoon bread, French toast, seedless rye; muffins, English muffins, pancakes, rolls, waffles; melba toast, rusk, zwieback; biscuits, graham crackers, saltines, and other crackers not made with whole grains	Breads: any variety with seeds or nuts Boston brown, pumpernickel, raisin, cracked wheat, buckwheat; crackers: all made with whole grain; rolls: any made with whole grain, nuts, coconut, raisins; tortillas
Cereals	Cooked and refined dry cereals	Dry, coarse cereals such as shredded wheat, all bran, and whole grain
Flours	All varieties except those prohibited	Any made with whole grain wheat or bran
Beverages	All types	None
Meat, fish, poultry	Meats: beef, liver, pork (lean and fresh), lamb, veal; poultry: turkey, chicken, duck, Cornish game hens, chicken livers; fish: all types of fresh varieties, canned tuna and salmon*	Fried, cured, and highly seasoned products such as chitterlings, corned beef, cured and/or smoked products, most processed sausages, and cold cuts; meats with a lot of fat; geese and game birds; most shellfish; canned fish such as anchovies, herring, sardines, and any strongly flavored seafoods
Legumes, nuts	Fine, creamy, smooth peanut butter	Most legumes, nuts, and seeds
Fruits	Raw: avocado, banana; canned or cooked: apples, apricots, cherries, pea-ches, pears, plums, sections of oranges, grapefruits, mandarin oranges without membranes, stewed fruits (except raisins), fruit cocktail, seedless grapes; all juices and nectars	All raw fruits not specifically permitted; all dried fruits; fruits with seeds and skins
Vegetables	All juices; canned or cooked: asparagus, beets, carrots, celery, eggplant, green or wax beans, chopped kale, mushrooms, peas, spinach, squash, shredded lettuce, chopped parsley, green peas, pumpkin; tomato: stewed, pureed, juice, paste	All those not specifically permitted

TABLE 14-13. (continued)

Food Types	Foods Permitted	Foods Prohibited
Fats	Butter, margarine, cream (or substitute), oil, vegetable shortening, mayonnaise, French dressing, crisp bacon, plain gravies, sour cream	Other forms of fats and oils, salad dressings, highly seasoned gravy
Soups	Any made from permitted ingredients: bouillon (powder or cubes), consommé, cream soups; strained soups: gumbos, chowders, bisques	Soups made from prohibited ingredients; split pea and bean soups; highly seasoned soups such as onion
Potatoes	White potatoes: scalloped, boiled, baked, mashed, creamed, au gratin; sweet potatoes: mashed	White potatoes fried, caked, browned, and in salad; yams
Rice and equivalents	Rice (white or brown), macaroni, spaghetti, noodles, Yorkshire pudding	Wild rice, bulgur, fritters, bread stuffing, barley
Sweets	Sugar: granulated, brown, maple, confectioner's; candy: hard, jelly beans, mints, marshmallows, butterscotch, candy corn, chocolate, caramels, fondant, plain fudge, gumdrops; syrups: maple, sorghum, corn; jelly, marmalade, preserves, jams; honey, molasses, apple butter; marshmallow and chocolate sauces	All candies containing nuts, coconut, and prohibited fruits
Desserts	Cake, cookies, custard, pudding, gelatin, ice cream, cobblers, ice milk, sherbet, water ice, cream pie with graham cracker crust; all plain or flavored without large pieces of fruits	Any products containing nuts, coconut, or prohibited fruits
Miscellaneous	Sauces: cream, white, brown, cheese, tomato; vinegar, soy sauce, catsup; all finely ground or chopped spices and herbs served in amounts tolerated by the patient	Spices and sauces that the patient is unable to tolerate, such as red pepper, garlic, curry, mustard; pickles; olives; popcorn, potato chips; Tabasco and Worcestershire sauces

*Cooked tender—may be broiled, baked, creamed, stewed, or roasted.

Although either fluid or semifluid tube feedings may be hospital prepared or commercially purchased, commercial ones are preferred because they reduce the risk of contamination. Considered reasonably nutritious if not completely adequate, tube feedings usually provide about 1 kcal/mL, although the concentration may be adjusted to between 0.5 and 1.5 kcal/mL.

Hospital-prepared tube feedings are normally of two types: *standard* and *standard blenderized*. A sample recipe of a standard hospital-

TABLE 14-14. Sample Meal Plan for a Soft Diet

Breakfast	Lunch	Dinner
Fruit or juice, ½ c	Soup, ½ c	Soup, ½ c
Cereal, ½ c	Meat, poultry, or fish,	Meat, poultry, or fish,
Egg, 1	2–3 oz	2–3 oz
Bacon, 2 strips	Rice or equivalent, ½ c	Potato, ½ c
Toast, 1 sl	Vegetable or salad,	Vegetable or salad,
Butter or margarine, 1 t	½ c	½ c
Jam, preserves, or jelly	Bread or toast, 1 sl	Bread, 1 sl
Milk, 1 c	Butter or margarine, 1 t	Butter or margarine, 1 t
Hot beverage	Dessert	Dessert
Cream	Hot beverage	Milk, 1 c
Sugar	Sugar	Hot beverage
Salt, pepper	Cream	Cream
	Salt, pepper	Sugar
		Salt, pepper

TABLE 14-15. Sample Menu for a Soft Diet

Breakfast	Lunch	Dinner
Orange juice, ½ c	Chowder, strained,	Soup, creamed, ½ c
Farina, ½ c	½ c	Beef, stew meat,
Egg, soft-boiled, 1	Cod, broiled, 2–3 oz	tender, 3–4 oz
Bacon, crisp, 2 strips	White rice, ½ c	Potato, baked, me-
Toast, 1 sl	Toast, 1 sl	dium, 1
Butter or margarine, 1 t	Butter or margarine, 1 t	Asparagus, canned,
Jam, 1–3 t	Pudding, plain, ½ c	½ c
Milk, 1 c	Coffee or tea, 1–2 c	Toast, 1 sl
Coffee or tea, 1–2 c	Sugar, 1–3 t	Butter or margarine, 1 t
Sugar, 1–3 t	Cream, 1 T	Gelatin, flavored, ½ c
Cream, 1 T	Salt, pepper	Coffee or tea, 1–2 c
Salt, pepper		Cream, 1 T
		Sugar, 1–3 t
		Salt, pepper

prepared tube feeding is shown in Table 14-16. The basic ingredients used are milk products. Table 14-17 provides an example of a standard hospital-prepared, blenderized tube feeding. The basic ingredients are regular nutrient-dense foods that have a fluid, semifluid, or very soft texture, such as items used in infant feeding. A standard blenderized tube feeding is usually better tolerated than a standard (commercial) tube-feeding formula. The blenderized feeding uses ingredient ratios that are similar to those of a regular diet.

TABLE 14-16. Standard Hospital Tube Feeding

Ingredient	Measure	Weight (g)	Kcal	Protein (g)	Fat (g)	Carbo-hydrate (g)	Iron (mg)	Vitamin C (mg)
Milk, whole	2 c	488	318	17	17	24	0.2	4.0
Milk, instant, nonfat, dry	1 c	70	250	24	0	35	0.4	5.0
Corn syrup	4¾ T	97.4	280	0	0	71	1.3	0
Egg, powdered, pasteurized*	4 T	30	163	13	12	1	2.3	0
Salt	1 t	5.5	—	—	—	—	—	—
Vitamin preparation	5 mL	—	—	—	—	—	—	—
Total	—	—	1,011	54	29	131	4.2	9.0

Note: Nutrient compositions are adapted from USDA Home and Garden Bulletin No. 72.

Enough water is added to the total ingredients to make 1,000 mL of solution.

*To avoid salmonella contamination, do not use fresh raw eggs. One egg is equivalent to 15 g of powdered eggs.

TABLE 14-17. Standard Blenderized Tube Feeding

Ingredient	Measure	Weight (g)	Kcal	Protein (g)	Fat (g)	Carbo-hydrate (g)	Iron (mg)	Vitamin C (mg)
Milk, evaporated	1½ c	428	517	26.4	29.8	36.6	0.4	4.5
Farina, cooked, enriched	1 c	245	108	3.2	0.2	21.3	12.3	0
Egg, powdered, pasteurized*	6 T	45	243	18.5	18.0	1.5	3.3	0
Liver, pureed	1 jar	100	94	14.0	3.1	2.4	6.8	27.4
Orange juice, fresh	½ c	123	49	0.7	0.2	11.0	0.2	64.0
Carrots, cooked	½ c	77	22	0.6	0.2	4.8	0.5	1.5
Total	—	—	1,033	63.4	51.5	77.6	23.5	97.4

Note: Nutrient compositions are adapted from USDA Home and Garden Bulletin No. 72.

Enough water is added to the total ingredients to make 1,000 mL of solution.

*To avoid salmonella contamination, do not use fresh raw eggs. One egg is equivalent to 15 g of powdered eggs. Cooked egg custard, salmonella-free frozen eggs, or egg yolks processed for infant feeding may also be used.

Although there should be a reasonable content of carbohydrate, fat, and protein, 40 to 50 g of high-quality protein (such as milk casein) per 1,000 mL of formula is acceptable. From 40 to 60 g of fat per 1,000 mL should provide adequate linoleic acid and arachidonic acid. About 90 to 110 g of carbohydrate should be in each 1,000 mL.

Some commercial feedings are inadequate in vitamin C, folic acid, and iron. Supplements may either be added to the feedings or given to the patient separately.

TABLE 14-18. Tube-Feeding Regimen for Programming Patient Tolerance

Progressive Concentration (kcal/mL)	Progressive Feeding Rate (mL/h)*
¼–½	35–50
½–¾	50–75
¾–1	75–100
1	100–130¹
1–1½	

*The period of feeding at each rate varies from a few hours to a few days.
¹ Maximum rate.

Administration: Precautions and Problems

Table 14-18 lists the progressive concentrations and delivery rates for tube feedings. An initial feeding of 150 to 200 mL in 4 to 8 hours is usually tolerated, but every patient must be monitored and evaluated. Once the patient has adapted to the formula and concentration, the feeding may be kept continuous under sanitary supervision.

The physician's prescription for tube feeding should specify: (1) the type of feeding, (2) nutrient modifications, and (3) volume and number of feedings per 24 hours. In addition, whether feedings are to be intermittent or continuous should be stipulated.

The major precautions and problems in the use of tube feedings include: (1) maintaining a record, (2) avoiding contamination, (3) controlling **osmolarity** (concentration), (4) being alert to patient maladjustment, (5) being aware of treatments for diarrhea, and (6) considerations for long-term feeding.

Commercial Nutritional Formulas

Commercial liquid nutritional formulas can be used for both oral and tube feedings. Such preparations are suitable for clinical conditions described earlier and others such as kidney malfunctions and premature birth.

One group of nutritional supplements provides protein and sometimes calories as the major nutrients. Examples include (manufacturers in parenthesis): EMF (Control Drugs), DP High P.E.R. Protein (General Mills), Gevral (Lederle), and Casec (Mead Johnson). A second group of nutritional supplements provides carbohydrate and calories as the major nutrients. Some common brands include: CAL powder (General

Mills), Hycal (Beecham), Controlyte (Doyle), Citrotein (Doyle), Lytren (Mead Johnson), Polycose (Ross), and Sumacal (Hospital Dietetic Products). A third group provides fat and calories as major nutrients; e.g., Lipomul-Oral (Upjohn) and MCT Oil (Mead Johnson). MCT or medium-chained-triglyceride are especially suitable for malabsorption and maldigestion since they are easier to digest and absorb.

A fourth group of nutritional supplements is prescribed for patients with special clinical conditions such as renal failure, carbohydrate intolerance, and phenylketonuria, and to patients requiring sodium-regulated intakes.

A fifth group of commercial formulas is considered nutritionally complete. Examples include Compleat B (Doyle), C.I.B. (Carnation), Sustacal (Mead Johnson), and others.

Commercial formulas have both advantages and drawbacks. Some of the advantages are: (1) reduction of stomach acidity, (2) potency of nutrient content, (3) acceleration of wound healing, (4) reduction of the release of enzymes from the pancreas, (5) facilitation of digestion and absorption, (6) maintenance of low residue in the large intestine as well as a decrease in colon bacteria.

These formulas are easy to order, prescribe, and prepare. They may be frozen on a stick, or used to make ice cream, snow cones, sauces, and puddings. They can also be added to beverages and pastry mixes. Another benefit is that they can be served day or night, either at mealtime or as snacks.

The drawbacks of these formulas are: (1) nutritional composition is fixed, (2) calories are adequate only in large volume, and (3) thorough knowledge of available products is needed to select the appropriate one.

In the last few years most hospitals have used commercial nutritional formulas. However, hospital-prepared oral- or tube-feedings are still preferred by some professionals.

Parenteral Feedings

In some cases, a patient needs to be nourished directly through the bloodstream, bypassing the gastrointestinal system. The nutritional adequacy of parenteral feeding varies from the very temporary standard intravenous (IV) therapy to total parenteral nutrition, which can be nutritionally complete.

Standard IV Therapy

A supportive system of fluids and electrolytes is used in standard intravenous therapy—usually sodium (saline), ammonium chloride, and dex-

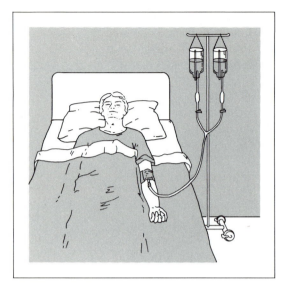

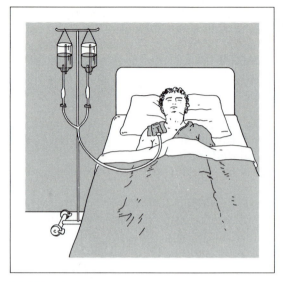

FIGURE 14-2. Conventional intravenous feeding via peripheral veins.

FIGURE 14-3. Total parenteral feeding as administered in a hospital.

trose (5% to 20%) solutions. Used for emergency situations such as the period following difficult childbirth or surgery, this method provides a *minimal* amount of nutrients. The patient is kept on this treatment only for 1 to 2 days to avoid semistarvation. Figure 14-2 illustrates conventional intravenous feeding via peripheral veins.

Total Parenteral Nutrition

Total parenteral nutrition (TPN) provides an adequate amount of calories, protein, fat, carbohydrate, vitamins, and minerals. These nutrients must be administered via a central venous access into an area with rapid blood flow, such as the subclavian vein. At present, TPN is used under various clinical conditions such as kidney failure and cancer.

The use of TPN is increasing because of its many advantages. First, body organs are directly provided with concentrated calories, amino acids, essential fatty acids, vitamins, and minerals, which are completely used without waste. Second, the gastrointestinal tract is permitted to rest and the body has a chance to replenish itself. Third, speedy repair of organs and tissues occurs because of the direct availability of nutrients. TPN can lead to weight gain, a positive nitrogen balance, wound healing, and synthesis of hormones and enzymes—in short, it can hasten recovery.

Other details about TPN may be obtained from the references for this chapter. Figure 14-3 illustrates TPN feeding in a hospital.

STUDY QUESTIONS

1. Discuss the two basic relationships between nutrition and disease.
2. What are the roles of the doctor, the dietitian, and the nurse in the dietary management of a patient?
3. Discuss at least five types of information about a particular patient that are important in individualizing his or her dietary care.
4. Give at least twelve causes of eating problems in hospitalized patients.
5. Around what core does hospital diet planning revolve? Give three examples of slight modifications of this basic diet.
6. What is the traditional four-stage progression from most to least easily tolerated foods? What other stages may now be added or substituted? What approach do some hospitals take instead of routine progressive feeding?
7. When is a clear-liquid diet advised? What essential nutrients does it adequately supply?
8. How does a full-liquid diet differ nutritionally from a clear-liquid diet? How adequate is a modified full-liquid diet? What is it?
9. Describe the consistency of a pureed diet, a mechanical soft diet, and a soft diet. For whom might each be prescribed?
10. Define enteral and parenteral feedings.
11. Discuss the nutritional adequacy of tube feedings in general. What supplements may be necessary?
12. Give some examples of commercial nutritional formulas.

REFERENCES

American Dietetic Association. 1981. *Handbook of clinical dietetics.* New Haven, Conn.: Yale University Press.

American Hospital Association. 1976. *Recording nutritional information in medical records.* Chicago, Ill.

Arbogast, K. K. 1980. *Exchange lists and diet patterns.* New York: Van Nostrand Reinhold.

Aronson, V., and Fitzgerald, B. D. 1980. *Guidebook for nutrition counselors.* North Quincy, Mass.: Christopher Publishing House.

Blackburn, G. L., and Thornton, P. A. 1979. Nutritional assessment of the hospitalized patient. *Med. Clin.* NA 63:1103, 1979.

Ducanis, A. J., and Golin, A. K. 1979. *The interdisciplinary health care team: a handbook.* Rockville, Md.: Aspen Systems Corp.

Grant, J. P. 1980. *Handbook of total parenteral nutrition.* Philadelphia: Saunders.

Hui, Y. H. 1983. *Human nutrition and diet therapy.* Monterey, Calif.: Wadsworth Health Sciences.

Narrow, B. W. 1979. *Patient teaching in nursing practice: a patient and family-centered approach.* New York: Wiley.

Schneider, H., et al., eds. 1984. *Nutritional support in medical practice.* New York: Harper & Row.

15 DIET AND DIABETES MELLITUS

The disease known as **diabetes mellitus,** characterized by body wasting and the excretion of large amounts of glucose-containing urine, was recorded as early as 1552 B.C. During the last two centuries much progress toward understanding the disease has been made. Basic to that understanding is the knowledge that malfunctioning cells in the pancreas are responsible for diabetes. For more than 50 years, chemical insulin has been extracted from animals and used in the treatment of diabetic patients. Insulin can now be synthesized in the laboratory using genetic engineering, but this type of insulin is not yet in general use.

Diet as a part of the management of a diabetic patient has been recognized for a relatively short time. However, its importance cannot be overemphasized. More breakthroughs in treating this disease are expected in the near future.

Simply described, diabetes mellitus is a disease caused by a partially malfunctioning pancreas that provides little or no usable insulin to promote the entry of blood sugar (glucose) into tissues for metabolism. As a result, sugar levels in the urine and blood are higher than normal. (It should be noted that in certain types of diabetes, the patient's pancreas does secrete insulin.)

INCIDENCE AND CAUSES

It is estimated that in the United States alone there are between 4 and 8 million people with diabetes, and the incidence is on the rise. One reason for this increase may be a steady rise in the number of overweight individuals. Although the relationship is not yet understood, the link between obesity and certain types of diabetes has been observed.

Progress in medicine also has increased the incidence of diabetes in the sense that it allows young diabetic patients to live long enough to marry and have children. Since the children of diabetics are at high risk of having the disease, an increasing number of diabetic children are born. At the opposite end of the scale, an increase in the average life span has resulted in a greater number of people over the age of 60, when the more common type of diabetes is most likely to occur.

Diabetes is one of the major contributing causes of death in the United States. Both kidney failure and coronary heart disease are more prevalent among diabetic patients. Among those factors leading to a malfunctioning pancreas, thus possibly to diabetes are: (1) heredity, (2) obesity, (3) sensitivity to insulin, (4) damage to the pancreas.

DIAGNOSIS OF DIABETES

Certain diagnostic tools may be used to determine the presence of diabetes, including studying known clinical symptoms, analyzing blood glucose levels, and urine testing.

Clinical Symptoms

Excessive thirst (polydipsia) and excessive urination (polyuria) may be among the first signs of diabetes. Bedwetting, weight loss, and an increase in appetite are common among children. Patients in whom the disease begins in adulthood are obese. Symptoms also may include loose teeth, sleepiness, and loss of strength. An untreated diabetic or one who fails to comply with medical regimens may become comatose after drinking alcoholic beverages.

Some diabetic patients may experience blurred vision, cataracts, and skin infections. Heart and kidney problems are frequent complications, and impairment of the nervous system (diabetic neuropathy) such as loss of body sensations and reflexes, is not uncommon. In extreme cases, blindness, coma, and even death may occur.

Blood Glucose Level

Increased blood glucose levels (hyperglycemia) can be detected by means of a glucose tolerance test (GTT). By measuring the rate at which glucose disappears from the blood, the GTT can ascertain how much insulin is available in a given patient. Four hypothetical glucose tolerance curves are shown in Figure 15-1.

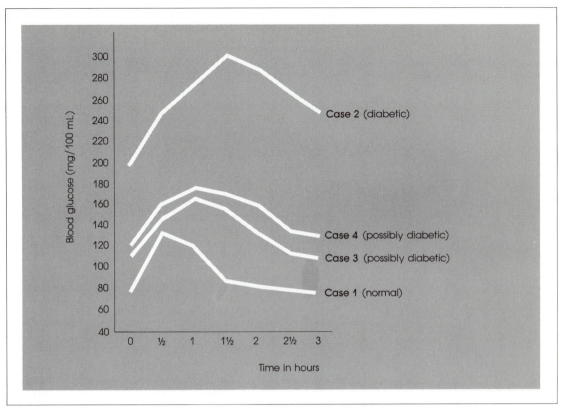

FIGURE 15-1. Four hypothetical glucose tolerance curves.

Urine Testing

An increased glucose level in the urine of a diabetic patient is one indication of diabetes and may be determined by urine tests. The presence of **ketone bodies** in the urine (ketonuria) also may be a sign of the disease.

TREATMENT

The proper classification of a diabetic patient is important in devising appropriate treatment. Diabetes may be categorized into two common types: insulin dependent and insulin independent. Both types are characterized by an abnormal glucose tolerance curve, a high blood glucose level during fasting, and other clinical symptoms. The many differences between these two types are outlined in Table 15-1. A recent new classification of diabetes will not be presented here.

TABLE 15-1. Comparison of Insulin-Dependent and Insulin-Independent Diabetes Mellitus

Criterion	Diabetes Type	
	Insulin dependent	Insulin independent
Age of onset	Under 14, not common among preschoolers; some patients over 40	Over 40, especially over 50; occasionally in children and adolescents
Percent of diabetic population	10% (5% children)	85% to 95%
Onset	Usually sudden with accompanying weight loss	Usually gradual; not diagnosed for years after onset
Disease severity	Usually very severe, especially in adults	Mild to severe
Body weight at time of diagnosis	Usually lean, especially in adults	80% of patients obese
Hyperglycemia severity	Usually severe	Mild to moderate
Serum lipid profile	Usually abnormal	Usually abnormal
Insulin		
Pancreas secretion	Minimal to lacking; an occasional release of insulin	Adequate to insufficient; complete failure not common
Use in therapy	Yes	No, though long-term patients may depend on insulin
Diet therapy required	Yes	Yes
Oral hypoglycemic agents	Less common	More common
Clinical course	Unstable; high and low blood glucose, with symptoms	Usually stable except in severe cases
Proneness to ketoacidosis	Yes, from childhood to adults. More severe in adults.	No, except under unusual stress
Mortality from diabetic ketoacidosis and coma	Possible without medical attention	Not likely
Nutritional needs	Unknown and changing, especially for children	Constant and can be calculated

TABLE 15-1. (continued)

| Criterion | Diabetes Type | |
	Insulin dependent	Insulin independent
Physical activity	Difficult to control	Easy to plan
Role of emotional variations	Great; may influence course of disease	Less; minimal effect on course of disease
Response to infections	More likely; acidosis exhibited quickly with little warning	Acidosis less likely and more predictable
Vascular degeneration	Related to duration of disease	Common
Prognosis	Poor	Good if well controlled

TABLE 15-2. Time Action Characteristics of Commercial Insulin Preparations

Type of Insulin	Example	Onset (h)	Peak of Action (h)	Duration of Action (h)
Short acting	Regular (neutral)	½	1–3	5–10
	Semilente	1	3–5	10–15
Intermediate acting	NPH	2	7–13	24–28
	Lente	2	7–13	24–28
	Globin	2	5–7	18–24
Long acting	Ultralente	6	17–30	≥35
	Protamine zinc	6	15–20	≥35

Insulin Therapy

Insulin-dependent diabetics must continually use insulin. Insulin treatment also is considered mandatory for diabetic patients of all types who experience clinical stresses such as surgery, infection, severe illness, or kidney disease. For these patients, "externally" supplied insulin will help glucose entry into cells for metabolism.

Unfortunately, insulin cannot be taken orally. Although it is administered by subcutaneous injection, insulin may be given by intravenous injection for a more rapid effect. Table 15-2 summarizes the approximate duration of action for most commercial insulin preparations. The patient injects insulin shortly before a meal is to be consumed, when blood glucose levels will be raised by the ingestion of food. Short-acting (regular) insulin may be injected before each meal; longer-acting types may be given once daily. Sometimes a combination may be used.

Oral Hypoglycemic Agents

Oral hypoglycemic agents also can lower blood glucose levels. These substances have limitations, however, and are effective only temporarily in some patients. Questions about the safety of these agents have removed all but one type—the sulfonylureas—from the prescription counter. Although sulfonylureas rarely produce side effects, they may lead to heart disease when used for a prolonged period.

MEDICAL MANAGEMENT OF DIABETES

The most important factor in treating a diabetic patient is to establish goals and priorities according to the needs of the individual. Stabilizing the condition of the patient is an initial goal. For example, blood glucose levels should be normalized and tolerance to glucose restored. Sensitivity to insulin also should be brought under control. Body weight should be stabilized and clinical complications caused by diabetes treated.

Diet, insulin, and oral hypoglycemic agents all play important roles in managing a diabetic patient. As already indicated, the extent to which these tools are used or are effective vary from patient to patient. A carefully planned diet that is faithfully adhered to allows most diabetic patients to control their condition without resorting to insulin or oral drugs. Insulin use depends on blood glucose stability.

Before oral hypoglycemic agents are prescribed, the patient's insulin secretion status and glucose tolerance should be determined. Potential side effects also should be considered.

The health history of a patient is essential in establishing a good management program. Information included should be: general eating habits, employment details, family history, physical activities and living conditions, health problems, and body weight history. Also see Chapter 14.

Dietary Care

Diet therapy for the diabetic patient is very important. The factors to be considered include:

- **Caloric intake.** The total number of calories must be regulated according to the activity level of the patient to achieve and maintain ideal body weight.

- **Essential nutrients.** The appropriate balance and quantity of nutrients for optimal body functions should be provided for all types of diabetic patients.
- **Blood and urine glucose.** Food should be supplied at a rate consistent with the availability of insulin to maintain proper glucose levels.
- **Complications.** Every effort should be made to control the complications of diabetes or clinical symptoms of other conditions.

Table 15-3 describes the overall dietary care for the two major types of diabetes. A rigid diet need not be followed if patients are cooperative and willing to make adjustments for exercise, illness, work schedules, and eating out.

Caloric Need

The method of determining caloric need developed by the American Diabetes Association (ADA) is widely used and accepted. It assumes that an adult's basal caloric need is 10 kcal/lb of ideal body weight, so that the basal caloric need for a man weighing 154 lb (70 kg) is $154 \times 10 = 1,540$ kcal and that for a woman weighing 128 lb (58.1 kg) is $128 \times 10 = 1,280$ kcal. After the basal caloric need is determined, the amount of energy used in physical activity must be calculated (see Table 15-4).

For a child the caloric need is determined by either the latest RDAs or the age rule. According to the age rule, 1,000 kcal/day should be allowed for a 1-year-old, with an additional 100 kcal for each year over 1 up to adolescence. Pregnant diabetics and nursing mothers require an additional 300 or 500 kcal/day, respectively.

Carbohydrate, Protein, and Fat

The overall distribution of carbohydrate, protein, and fat in a diabetic diet is fairly similar to that of the general American public (see Table 15-5). Such a diet allows a diabetic patient to eat more or less what everyone else does.

About 40 to 50 percent of the total calories consumed by Americans come from *carbohydrates*. Diabetic patients are fed a similar quantity, depending on their blood and urine glucose levels and the ability of the pancreas to secrete insulin. The actual amount of carbohydrate consumed is usually between 100 and 300 g. Less than 100 g will produce starvation ketosis, while an amount over 300 g will overtax the pancreas.

Although insulin-dependent diabetics experience greater restrictions than insulin-independent patients, most diabetics are allowed some control over their total intake of simple sugars. About 10 to 15 percent of the carbohydrate calories should be simple sugars, with the rest from

TABLE 15-3. Nutritional and Dietary Care of the Two Major Types of Diabetic Patients

| | Diabetes Type | |
| | Insulin dependent (lean) | Insulin independent (obese) |
Criterion		
Overall diet prescription		
Regulation	Yes	Yes
Predictability	Yes	Not so important
Rigidity	No	No
Total caloric intake	Adjusted to maintenance and activity; constant and consistent from day to day	Must be reduced; variable to achieve ideal weight
Daily intake of relative amounts of carbohydrate, protein, and fat	Constant and consistent from day to day	Usually not important
Four to six daily feedings	Highly recommended	Recommended if patient can adhere to limited caloric intake, otherwise not recommended
Coordination of meal and insulin injection times	Highly recommended	Not applicable
Dietary compensation for regular and unscheduled exercises	Very important	Not important
Dietary compensation for occasions of low blood glucose	Must eat food	Usually no measures needed
Nutritional compensation for sickness	Frequent parenteral feedings of dextrose to abort ketosis	Usually no measures needed since ketosis is unlikely

complex sources. Individual needs and tastes can be met by adjusting daily planning menus.

Protein contributes from 12 to 25 percent of a diabetic patient's total daily calories. The average amount of protein recommended is 80 to 100 g per day, although patients usually eat more. Protein intake should not drop below 60 to 70 g per day.

The suggested *fat* intake for diabetics is 30 percent of total calories,

TABLE 15-4. American Diabetes Association Method to Calculate Daily Caloric Need

Physical Activity	Total Calories Needed
Sedentary	Basal calories + (desirable body weight × 3)
Moderate	Basal calories + (desirable body weight × 5)
Strenuous	Basal calories + (desirable body weight × 10)

TABLE 15-5. Contents of a Regular Diet and Diabetic Diets for Adults and Children

Diet	Daily Permitted Caloric Intake (%)				
	Carbohydrate		Fat[‡]	Protein	Alcohol
	Complex[*]	Simple[†]			
Regular	20–40	25–35	35–45	10–20	0–15
Diabetic					
Adult	30–45	5–15	20–35	12–25	0–5
Children	30–40	5–15	35–40	18–23	0

Note: Ranges of values serve as a guide. Each practitioner's prescription varies.

[*] Includes starch and fibers.

[†] For nondiabetic diets, includes monosaccharides and disaccharides from all sources. For diabetic diets, includes monosaccharides and disaccharides from natural sources such as fruits, fruit juices, and milk.

[‡] A regular diet contains a ratio of saturated to unsaturated fats of about 2–3:1; a diabetic diet, 1:1–3.

with one third of them consumed as saturated and two thirds as unsaturated fats. Saturated fats and cholesterol may lead to atherosclerosis and related complications.

Approximate amounts of carbohydrate, protein, and fat must be determined for the individual by the physician. The American Diabetes Association uses a method involving percentage estimates. Of the total daily calories needed, about 20 percent will be contributed by protein,

TABLE 15-6. Outline of the 1976 American Diabetes Association Exchange Lists

Food Exchange List	Food Group	Contribution per Exchange of Food Group			
		kcal	Protein (g)	Carbohydrate (g)	Fat (g)
1	Milk	80	8	12	Trace
2	Vegetables	25	2	5	0
3	Fruits	40	0	10	0
4	Bread	70	2	15	0
5	Meat				
	Lean	55	7	0	3.0
	Medium	80	7	0	5.5
	Fat	100	7	0	8.0
6	Fat	45	0	0	5.0

50 percent by carbohydrate, and 30 percent by fat. In calculating the respective weights needed for the three nutrients, the following equivalents are used: 1 g protein = 4 kcal; 1 g fat = 9 kcal; 1 g carbohydrate = 4 kcal. An example of the calculations for a daily intake of 1,800 kcal is:

Protein: 20% total calories = 360 kcal/[4 kcal/g] = 90 g

Carbohydrate: 50% total calories = 900 kcal/[4 kcal/g] = 225 g

Fat: 30% total calories = 540 kcal/[9 kcal/g] = 60 g

Using the Food Exchange Lists

Many food selection methods are available, based on the daily number of calories needed by the patient and the relative amounts of carbohydrate, protein, and fat permitted. One system used extensively in the United States is the Food Exchange List system developed specifically for diabetic patients.

There are six exchange lists, each containing one group or category of food. Within each list are possible exchanges among the listed foods, and each exchange contributes similar amounts of calories, carbohydrate, fat, and protein. Table 15-6 summarizes the nutrient contributions of the items in each of the six exchange lists. The different types of foods contained within each list are described in Table 15-7. The actual exchange lists appear in Tables 15-8 to 15-15.

The exchange lists in Tables 15-6 to 15-15 are based on material in the *Exchange Lists for Meal Planning* prepared by Committees of the

TABLE 15-7. Types of Food Included in the Exchange Lists

Food Exchange List	Food Group	Food Types
1	Milk	Nonfat fortified milk and products; low-fat fortified milk and products; whole milk and products*
2	Vegetables	Various raw and cooked vegetables excluding starchy vegetables
3	Fruits	Various fresh, dried, canned, frozen, and cooked fruits†
4	Bread	Bread, cereal, starchy vegetables
5	Meat	Red meat, poultry, fowl, seafood, meat alternates
6	Fats	Butter, margarine, dressings, nuts, others

*Used with adjustments.
†All processed products are unsweetened.

TABLE 15-8. List 1: Milk Exchanges (Includes Nonfat, Low-fat, and Whole Milk)

Nonfat fortified milk	
Skim or nonfat milk	1 cup
Powdered (nonfat dry, before adding liquid)	⅓ cup
Canned, evaporated skim milk	½ cup
Buttermilk made from skim milk	1 cup
Yogurt made from skim milk (plain, unflavored)	1 cup
Low-fat fortified milk	
1% fat fortified milk (omit ½ fat exchange)	1 cup
2% fat fortified milk (omit 1 fat exchange)	1 cup
Yogurt made from 2% fortified milk (plain, unflavored) (omit 1 fat exchange)	1 cup
Whole milk (omit 2 fat exchanges)	
Whole milk	1 cup
Canned, evaporated skim milk	½ cup
Buttermilk made from skim milk	1 cup
Yogurt made from whole milk (plain, unflavored)	1 cup

Note: One exchange of milk contains 12 g of carbohydrate, 8 g of protein, a trace of fat, and 80 kilocalories. This list shows the kinds and amounts of milk or milk products to use for one milk exchange. Those which appear in **bold type** are **non-fat**. Low-fat and whole milk contain saturated fat.

American Diabetes Association, Inc. and The American Dietetic Association in cooperation with the National Institute of Arthritis, Metabolism and Digestive Diseases and the National Heart and Lung Institute, National Institutes of Health, Public Health Service, U.S. Department of Health, Education and Welfare.

Using the exchange system is not a simple task. To help you use the exchange system, step-by-step instructions for determining a patient's daily food needs from the Food Exchange Lists follow:

Step 1 determines the caloric need of the patient and the apportionment of calories contributed by protein, carbohydrate, and fat. We demonstrate an example for a patient requiring 1,800 kcal daily. For Step 1 (see calculations above):

TABLE 15-9. List 2: Vegetable Exchanges

Asparagus	Greens:
Bean sprouts	Mustard
Beets	Spinach
Broccoli	Turnip
Brussels sprouts	Mushrooms
Cabbage	Okra
Carrots	Onions
Cauliflower	Rhubarb
Celery	Rutabaga
Eggplant	Sauerkraut
Green pepper	String beans, green or yellow
Greens:	Summer squash
Beet green	Tomatoes
Chard	Tomato juice
Collard	Turnips
Dandelion	Vegetable juice cocktail
Kale	Zucchini

The following raw vegetables may be used as desired:

Chicory	Lettuce
Chinese cabbage	Parsley
Endive	Radishes
Escarole	Watercress

Starchy vegetables are found in the Bread Exchange List.

Note: One exchange of vegetables contains about 5 g of carbohydrate, 2 g of protein, and 25 kilocalories. This list shows the kinds of vegetables to use for one vegetable exchange. One exchange is ½ cup.

Protein	90 g
Carbohydrate	225 g
Fat	60 g

Step 2 determines the number of exchanges of nonfat milk, vegetables, and fruit needed by the patient. This determination varies with the physician and the patient, but for our hypothetical patient we shall use the figures of 2, 2, and 5—that is, 2 exchanges (servings) of nonfat milk, 2 of vegetables, and 5 of fruit. If mono- or disaccharides must be limited, fruits may have to be restricted. Serving sizes should be consistent. Yellow and dark green vegetables should be included every day as well as a good source of vitamin C. Table 15-16 shows the protein, carbo-

TABLE 15-10. List 3: Fruit Exchanges

Apple	1 small	Mango	½ small
Apple juice	⅓ cup	Melon	
Applesauce (unsweetened)	½ cup	Cantaloupe	¼ small
Apricots, fresh	2 medium	Honeydew	⅛ medium
Apricots, dried	4 halves	Watermelon	1 cup
Banana	½ small	Nectarine	1 small
Berries		Orange	1 small
Blackberries	½ cup	Orange juice	½ cup
Blueberries	½ cup	Papaya	¾ cup
Raspberries	½ cup	Peach	1 medium
Strawberries	¾ cup	Pear	1 small
Cherries	10 large	Persimmon, native	1 medium
Cider	⅓ cup	Pineapple	½ cup
Dates	2	Pineapple juice	⅓ cup
Figs, fresh	1	Plums	2 medium
Figs, dried	1	Prunes	2 medium
Grapefruit	½	Prune juice	¼ cup
Grapefruit juice	½ cup	Raisins	2 T
Grapes	12	Tangerine	1 medium
Grape juice	¼ cup		

Cranberries may be used as desired if no sugar is added.

Note: One exchange of fruit contains 10 g of carbohydrate and 40 kilocalories. This list shows the kinds and amounts of fruits to use for one fruit exchange.

hydrate, and fat distributions of nonfat milk, vegetables, and fruits to our hypothetical patient.

Step 3 determines the grams of carbohydrate contributed by the nonfat milk, vegetable, and fruit exchanges. In our example the total is 84 g, as shown in Table 15-16.

Step 4 determines the number of bread exchanges permitted the patient. If the patient is allowed 225 g of carbohydrate (Step 1), and 84 g have already been assigned (Step 3), then 141 g (225 g − 84 g = 141 g) are left to be assigned. Since meat and fat contain little carbohydrate, these 141 g can be allocated to bread. If 1 exchange of bread contains 15 g of carbohydrate (Table 15-6), the number of exchanges of bread permitted the patient is 141 ÷ 15 = 9⅖, rounded off to 9. The nutrient contribution of 9 exchanges of bread is shown in Table 15-17.

Step 5 determines the grams of protein contributed by the nonfat milk, vegetable, fruit, and bread exchanges. The amount of protein is 38 g as shown in Table 15-17.

Step 6 determines the number of meat exchanges permitted the patient. The patient is allowed 90 g of protein (Step 1), and 38 g have al-

TABLE 15-11. List 4: Bread Exchanges (Includes Bread, Cereal, and Starchy Vegetables)

Bread		**Dried beans, peas, and lentils**	
White (including French and Italian)	1 sl	**Beans, peas, lentils (dried and cooked)**	½ cup
Whole wheat	1 sl	**Baked beans, no pork (canned)**	¼ cup
Rye or pumpernickel	1 sl	**Starchy vegetables**	
Raisin	1 sl	**Corn**	⅓ cup
Bagel, small	½	**Corn on cob**	1 small
English muffin, small	½	**Lima beans**	½ cup
Plain roll, bread	1	**Parsnips**	⅔ cup
Frankfurter roll	½	**Peas, green (canned or frozen)**	½ cup
Hamburger bun	½	**Potato, white**	1 small
Dried bread crumbs	3 T	**Potato (mashed)**	½ cup
Tortilla, 6″	1	**Pumpkin**	¾ cup
Cereal		**Winter squash, acorn, or butternut**	½ cup
Bran flakes	½	**Yam or sweet potato**	¼ cup
Other read-to-eat unsweetened cereal	¾ cup	Prepared foods	
Puffed cereal (unfrosted)	1 cup	Biscuit 2″ dia.	
Cereal (cooked)	½ cup	(omit 1 fat exchange)	1
Grits (cooked)	½ cup	Cornbread, 2″ x 2″ x 1″	
Rice or barley (cooked)	½ cup	(omit 1 fat exchange)	1
Pasta (cooked),	½ cup	Corn muffin, 2″ dia.	
Spaghetti, noodles, macaroni		(omit 1 fat exchange)	1
Popcorn (popped, no fat added)	3 cups	Crackers, round butter type	
Cornmeal (dry)	2 T	(omit 1 fat exchange)	5
Flour	2½ T	Muffin, plain small	
Wheat germ	¼ cup	(omit 1 fat exchange)	1
Crackers		Potatoes, french fried, length 2″ to 3½″	
Arrowroot	3	(omit 1 fat exchange)	8
Graham, 2½″ sq.	2	Potato or corn chips	
Matzoh, 4″ × 6″	½	(omit 2 fat exchanges)	15
Oyster	20	Pancake, 5″ × ½″	
Pretzels, 3⅛″ long × ⅛″ dia.	25	(omit 1 fat exchange)	1
Rye wafers, 2″ × 3½″	3	Waffle, 5″ × ½″	
Saltines	6	(omit 1 fat exchange)	1
Soda, 2½″ sq.	4		

Note: One exchange of bread contains 15 g of carbohydrate, 2 g of protein, and 70 kilocalories. This list shows the kinds and amounts of **breads**, **cereals**, **starchy vegetables**, and prepared foods to use for one bread exchange. Those which appear in **bold type** are **low-fat**.

ready been assigned (Step 5). This patient is left with 90 − 38, or 52 g of protein to be obtained from other foods. Since fat contains no protein, we can assign all 52 g to meat. Since 1 exchange of meat contains 7 g of protein, the number of exchanges of meat permitted the patient is 52 ÷ 7 = 7²⁄₇, rounded up to 8. The nutrient contribution of 8 exchanges of meat is shown in Table 15-18.

Step 7 determines the grams of fat contributed by the nonfat milk,

TABLE 15-12. List 5: Meat Exchanges (Lean Meat)

Beef:	**Baby beef (very lean), chipped beef, chuck, flank steak, tenderloin, plate ribs, plate skirt steak, round (bottom, top), all cuts rump, sirloin, tripe**	1 oz
Lamb:	**Leg, rib, sirloin, loin (roast and chops), shank, shoulder**	1 oz
Pork:	**Leg (whole rump, center shank), ham, smoked (center slices)**	1 oz
Veal:	**Leg, loin, rib, shank, shoulder, cutlets**	1 oz
Poultry:	**Meat (without skin) of chicken, turkey, Cornish hen, guinea hen, pheasant**	1 oz
Fish:	**Any fresh or frozen**	1 oz
	Canned salmon, tuna, mackerel, crab, and lobster	¼ cup
	Clams, oysters, scallops, shrimp	5 or 1 oz
	Sardines, drained	3
Cheeses containing less than 5% butterfat		1 oz
Cottage cheese, dry and 2% butterfat		¼ cup
Dried beans and peas (omit 1 bread exchange)		½ cup

Note: One exchange of lean meat (1 oz) contains 7 g of protein, 3 g of fat, and 55 kilocalories. This list shows the kinds and amounts of **lean meat** and other protein-rich foods to use for one low-fat meat exchange. To plan a diet low in saturated fat, select only those exchanges that appear in **bold type**.

TABLE 15-13. List 5: Meat Exchanges (Medium-fat Meat)

Beef:	Ground (15% fat), corned beef (canned), rib eye, round (ground commercial)	1 oz
Pork:	Loin (all cuts tenderloin), shoulder arm (picnic), shoulder blade, Boston butt, Canadian bacon, boiled ham	1 oz
Liver, heart, kidney, and sweetbreads (these are high in cholesterol)		1 oz
Cottage cheese, creamed		¼ cup
Cheese:	Mozzarella, Ricotta, farmer's cheese, Neufchatel,	1 oz
	Parmesan	3 T
Egg (high in cholesterol)		1
Peanut butter (omit 2 additional fat exchanges)		2 T

Note: For each exchange of medium-fat meat omit ½ fat exchange. This list shows the kinds and amounts of medium-fat meat and other protein-rich foods to use for one medium-fat meat exchange. To plan a diet low in saturated fat, select only those exchanges that appear in **bold type**.

TABLE 15-14. List 5: Meat Exchanges (High-fat Meat)

Beef:	Brisket, corned beef (brisket), ground beef (more than 20% fat), hamburger (commercial), chuck (ground commercial), roasts (rib), steaks (club and rib)	1 oz
Lamb:	Breast	1 oz
Pork:	Spare ribs, loin (back ribs), pork (ground), country style ham, deviled ham	1 oz
Veal:	Breast	1 oz
Poultry:	Capon, duck (domestic), goose	1 oz
Cheese:	Cheddar types	1 oz
Cold cuts		4½″ × ⅛″ slice
Frankfurter		1 small

Note: For each exchange of high-fat meat omit 1 fat exchange. This list shows the kinds and amounts of high-fat meat and other protein-rich foods to use for one high-fat meat exchange.

vegetable, fruit, bread, and meat exchanges. This amount is 24 g, as shown in Table 15-18.

Step 8 determines the number of fat exchanges permitted the patient. The patient is permitted 60 g of fat (Step 1), and 24 g have already been assigned (Step 7), leaving 36 g of fat (60 − 24 g) to consume. Since 1 exchange of fat contains 5 g of fat, the number of fat exchanges permitted the patient is 36 ÷ 5 = 7⅕, rounded off to 7. The nutrient contribution of 7 exchanges of fat is shown in Table 15-19, which summarizes the total food exchanges in a 1,800-kcal diet for our hypothetical diabetic patient. The number of exchanges obtained are used to apportion the foods into breakfast, lunch, dinner, and a snack meal, as shown in Table 15-20. Two sample menus for these meal plans are shown in Table 15-21.

Although the Food Exchange Lists developed by the American Diabetes Association are widely used, some physicians feel that this method is too complicated and limited. Several other methods are discussed in the references for this chapter.

Meal Planning

The patient's need for insulin determines the type and amount of food served at each meal. While the distribution of nutrients may be accomplished in a number of ways, for convenience the following discussion assumes that if each nutrient (protein, carbohydrate, and fat) is assigned a specific number of calories, then the nutrients will be distributed proportionately among each meal (breakfast, lunch, dinner,

TABLE 15-15. List 6: Fat Exchanges

Margarine, soft, tub, or stick*	1 t
Avocado (4" in diameter)†	⅛
Oil, corn, cottonseed, safflower, soy, sunflower	1 t
Oil, olive†	1 t
Oil, peanut†	1 t
Olives†	5 small
Almonds†	10 whole
Pecans†	2 large whole
Peanuts†	
Spanish	20 whole
Virginia	10 whole
Walnuts	6 small
Nuts, other†	6 small
Margarine, regular stick	1 t
Butter	1 t
Bacon fat	1 t
Bacon, crisp	1 strip
Cream, light	2 T
Cream, sour	2 T
Cream, heavy	1 T
Cream cheese	1 T
French dressing‡	1 T
Italian dressing‡	1 T
Lard	1 t
Mayonnaise‡	1 t
Salad dressing, mayonnaise type‡	2 t
Salt pork	¾-inch cube

Note: One exchange of fat contains 5 g of fat and 45 kilocalories. This list shows the kinds and amounts of fat-containing foods to use for one fat exchange. To plan a diet low in saturated fat, select only those exchanges that appear in **bold type**. They are **polyunsaturated**.

*Made with corn, cottonseed, safflower, soy, or sunflower oil only.

†Fat content is primarily monounsaturated.

‡If made with corn, cottonseed, safflower, soy, or sunflower oil, can be used on fat modified diet.

and snacks). Table 15-22 shows different ways of dividing the daily calories according to patient status.

Insulin-independent patients usually have stable blood glucose levels and do not require oral hypoglycemic agents. These patients are permitted liberal meal planning. Meal planning for insulin-dependent patients need not be too restrictive. Both the type of insulin used and the intervals at which it is administered can enhance flexibility. For example, if the patient wants an afternoon snack, intermediate-acting insulin can be used so that its action time coincides with the snack time.

TABLE 15-16. Amount of Carbohydrate Calculated from Milk, Vegetable, and Fruit Exchanges

Food List	No. of Exchanges	Protein (g)	Carbohydrate (g)	Fat (g)
Nonfat milk*	2	16	24	0
Vegetables†	2	4	10	0
Fruits‡	5	0	50	0
Total	—		84	—

*From Table 15-6, we see that 2 exchanges of nonfat milk provide 2 × 8 = 16 g of protein, 2 × 12 = 24 g of carbohydrate, and 2 × trace = 0 g of fat.

†From Table 15-6, we see that 2 exchanges of vegetables provide 2 × 2 = 4 g of protein, 2 × 5 = 10 g of carbohydrate, and 2 × 0 = 0 g of fat.

‡From Table 15-6, we see that 5 exchanges of fruits provide 5 × 0 = 0 g of protein, 5 × 10 = 50 g of carbohydrate, and 5 × 0 = 0 g of fat.

TABLE 15-17. Amount of Protein Calculated from Milk, Vegetable, Fruit, and Bread Exchanges

Food List	No. of Exchanges	Protein (g)	Carbohydrate (g)	Fat (g)
Nonfat milk	2	16	24	0
Vegetables	2	4	10	0
Fruits	5	0	50	0
Bread*	9	18	135	0
Total		38	—	—

*From Table 15-6, we see that 9 exchanges of bread provide 9 × 2 = 18 g of protein, 9 × 15 = 135 g of carbohydrate, and 9 × 0 = 0 g of fat.

TABLE 15-18. Amount of Fat Calculated from Milk, Vegetable, Fruit, Bread, and Meat Exchanges

Food List	No. of Exchanges	Protein (g)	Carbohydrate (g)	Fat (g)
Nonfat milk	2	16	24	0
Vegetables	2	4	10	0
Fruits	5	0	50	0
Bread	9	18	135	0
Meat, lean*	8	56	0	24
Total		—	—	24

*From Table 15-6, we see that 8 exchanges of lean meat provide 8 × 7 = 56 g of protein, 8 × 0 = 0 g of carbohydrate, and 8 × 3 = 24 g of fat.

TABLE 15-19. Total Food Exchanges in an 1,800-kcal Diet for a Diabetic Patient

Food List	No. of Exchanges	Protein (g)	Carbohydrate (g)	Fat (g)	kcal*
Nonfat milk	2	16	24	0	160
Vegetables	2	4	10	0	50
Fruits	5	0	50	0	200
Bread	9	18	135	0	630
Meat, lean	8	56	0	24	440
Fat†	7	0	0	35	315
Total		94	219	59	1,795

*Calories are obtained by using the following equivalencies: 1 g protein = 4 kcal; 1 g of carbohydrate = 4 kcal; 1 g fat = 9 kcal.

† From Table 15-6, we see that 7 exchanges of fat provide 7 x 0 = 0 g of protein, 7 x 0 = 0 g of carbohydrate, and 7 x 5 = 35 g of fat.

Variations in Routine

Diabetics, especially those using insulin, must guard against variations in routine that could cause large swings in blood glucose levels. Three common situations that might arise are changes in physical activity, eating out, and meal delays.

Exercise

Any form of exercise, whether mild or strenuous, can lower blood glucose and cause hypoglycemia. The diabetic must have access to a readily available form of carbohydrate to compensate for the extra blood glucose used during exercise. Mild exercise requires 5 to 10 extra grams of glucose, moderate exercise 10 to 25, and intense exercise 25 to 50. Carefully planning patient diets in regard to insulin usage and regular exercise is important. For example, if a diabetic patient uses insulin and intends to exercise strenuously for an hour, he or she should eat some form of carbohydrate either before or during the exercise. However, the amount of carbohydrate consumed must be considered as part of the patient's diet. This is especially important if the patient's physical exertions are unplanned. Unintentional overconsumption of carbohydrate may eventually cause fluctuation in the blood sugar level and lead to patient discomfort.

Eating Out and Meal Delays

Eating in a restaurant, at a picnic, or at a friend's house poses problems for diabetic patients because the ingredients and quantities of the food consumed are unknown. The most fortunate patients are thin diabetics

TABLE 15-20. Distribution of Food Exchanges over Meals Using the Number of Exchanges Given in Table 15-19

Exchange List	No. of Exchanges
Breakfast	
Nonfat milk	½
Vegetable	0
Fruit	1
Bread	2
Meat, lean	1
Fat	3
Lunch	
Nonfat milk	½
Vegetable	1
Fruit	1
Bread	2
Meat, lean	2
Fat	2
Dinner	
Nonfat milk	0
Vegetable	1
Fruit	1
Bread	3
Meat, lean	3
Fat	2
Bedtime Snack	
Nonfat milk	1
Vegetable	0
Fruit	2
Bread	2
Meat, lean	1
Fat	2

TABLE 15-21. Sample Menus for Exchange Distribution of Table 15-20

Breakfast
Oatmeal, ½ c
Light cream, 4 T
Toast, whole wheat, 1 sl
Margarine, 1 t
Cantaloupe, small, ¼
Cottage cheese, ¼ c
Milk, skim, ½ c
Coffee or tea

Lunch
Turkey sandwich:
    Bread, whole wheat,
      2 sl
    Margarine, 1 t
    Turkey, 2 oz
String beans, ½ c
Margarine, 1 t
Yogurt, skim milk, ½ c
Grapefruit juice, ½ c
Salt, pepper
Coffee or tea

Dinner
Tomato juice, ½ c
Green salad
    Lettuce
    Radish
    Italian dressing, 1 T
Salmon, broiled, 3 oz
Bagel, small, 1
Cream cheese, 1 t
Green peas, ½ c
Apple, small, 1
Salt, pepper, lemon
Coffee or tea

Snack
Apple juice, ⅓ c
Bran flakes, ½ c
Raisins, 2 T
Milk, skim, ½ c
Biscuit, plain, small, 1
Margarine, 1 t
Chicken, 1 oz
Milk, skim, ½ c

Breakfast
Yogurt, skim milk, ½ c
Pineapple, chunks, ½ c
Ham, 1 oz
Biscuits, 2
Butter, ½ t
Coffee or tea

Lunch
Salad:
    Lettuce wedge, 1
    Radish, sliced, 1
    Tomato, sliced, ½ c
    Crab, canned, ¼ c
    Shrimp, 1 oz
    French dressing, 1 T
Matzo, 4" × 6", 1
Butter, 1 t
Peach, 1
Buttermilk, skim, ½ c
Salt, pepper
Coffee or tea

Dinner
Beef, tenderloin, 3 oz
French fries, 8
Vegetable medley:
    Zucchini, cooked, ½ c
    Corn, cooked, ⅓ c
Bread, rye, 1 sl
Margarine, 1 t
Honeydew, ⅛
Salt, pepper
Coffee or tea

Snack
Banana, 1
Graham crackers, 2½ in.
    square, 4
Cream cheese, 2 T
Chicken, leg, cold, 1 oz
Milk, skim, 1 c

TABLE 15-22. Distributions of Calories over Meals

Patient Status	Daily Caloric Distribution in Proportion					
	Breakfast	Midmorning snack	Lunch	Midafternoon snack	Dinner	Bedtime snack
No insulin needed; blood glucose level stable; usually no oral hypoglycemic agents needed	3/10 1/3	— —	3/10 1/3	— —	4/10 1/3	— —
Insulin needed; blood glucose level stable; usually no oral hypoglycemic agents needed	3/10 2/7 1/6 2/7	— — — —	3/10 2/7 2/6 2/7	— 1/7 1/6 —	3/10 2/7 2/6 2/7	1/10 — — 1/7
Insulin needed; variable blood glucose level throughout the day	2/10 1.6/10	1/10 1.6/10	2/10 1.6/10	1/10 1.6/10	3/10 2/10	1/10 1.6/10

who require no insulin—they need only be aware of the amount of food eaten and whether it contains carbohydrate, protein, or fat. Eating on special occasions poses few problems for them. It is advisable for overweight diabetics requiring no insulin to lose weight before eating out of the home; eating out too frequently can interfere with weight loss. Patients who depend on insulin and are not obese should plan ahead for each occasion. For example, they should incorporate foods served at a picnic into their diet prescription. Risks posed by eating out can also be reduced by learning to estimate the quantity and nutrient content of foods served and increasing the frequency of urine testing.

Meal delays or a simple lack of food can create problems for diabetic patients. They should know what to do if no food is available for a certain period of time. One quick remedy is to carry some form of simple carbohydrate. For example, hard candies will provide small amounts of sucrose and prevent hypoglycemia for ½ to 2½ hours. Nondiet soft drinks can also be used. The amount of simple sugars consumed in these instances should be 10 to 35 g.

PATIENT EDUCATION

The success of the diet and of the treatment with insulin and oral drugs largely depends on the cooperation of the diabetic patient. A comprehensive and successful diabetic management program, therefore, must always include patient education. When teaching a patient, some special points should be kept in mind.

1. Teaching an individual patient instead of a group is more effective.
2. If group education is used, patients should be sorted by the type of diabetes—for example, young diabetics, insulin-independent diabetics, and obese patients using insulin.
3. The patient's history should be studied to ensure that the patient does not receive contradictory information.
4. A close friend or relative should be familiar with the information provided the patient.

The characteristics of the disease should be explained as well as the role of insulin, diet, drugs, and exercise. Diet instructions, including specific diet prescriptions and ways of making them work, should be written down. Patients should be taught what foods are permitted and forbidden, recommended serving sizes, feeding schedules, flexibility of meal planning, advisability of drinking alcohol, and any other information that will encourage them to cooperate in controlling their condition.

Some clinics teach certain patients to test their own urine regularly to monitor their clinical status. Some patients are now being taught to determine their blood glucose level. For further information, check the references at the end of this chapter.

Some teaching aids and counseling services for diabetes include: local, city, and county diabetic programs; private and public diabetic clinics; professional sources of materials, such as drug companies; recipes and cookbooks; and food models, films, and slides.

STUDY QUESTIONS

1. What is diabetes mellitus? Why is the incidence of this disease on the rise? What complications are often associated with it?
2. What are the clinical symptoms of diabetes mellitus? Briefly describe the laboratory tests used to confirm diabetes in a patient?
3. What are the different types of insulin preparations currently available in the United States for diabetic patients?
4. Explain briefly how a Food Exchange List works. Use specific examples from the tables in the text to illustrate your explanation. Calculate the daily exchange requirements of one of your diabetic patients. Follow the calculations in this chapter.
5. What two factors must be taken into account in meal planning for insulin-dependent diabetics? Briefly describe variations in routine

that must be considered in dietary planning for diabetics. How does each of these factors alter caloric and/or nutrient intake?
6. When educating a diabetic patient, what points should be especially emphasized? How can a positive attitude be encouraged?

REFERENCES

Arky, R. A. 1984. Prevention and therapy of diabetes mellitus. In *Present knowledge of nutrition,* 5th ed. Washington, D. C.: The Nutrition Foundation.

Brownlee, M., ed. 1981. *Handbook of diabetes mellitus.* Vol. 1. Etiology/hormone physiology. Vol. 2. Islet cell function/insulin action. Vol. 3. Intermediary metabolism and its regulation. Vol. 4. Biochemical pathology. New York: Garland STPM Press.

Cohen, S. 1980. Programmed instruction: controlling diabetes mellitus. *Am. J. Nurs.* 80:1827.

Craig, O. 1981. *Childhood diabetes and its management.* 2nd ed. Boston: Butterworths.

Crofford, O. 1975. *Report of the national commission on diabetes to the Congress of the United States.* USDHEW pub. no. (NIH) 76-1018. Washington, D. C.: Government Printing Office.

Drug Therapy. 1981. On the present status of the treatment of diabetes. 11:41.

Rifkin, H., et al., eds. 1981. *Diabetes mellitus,* vol. V. Bowie, Md.: R. J. Brady.

Schulman, P. K. 1980. Diabetes in pregnancy: nutritional aspect of care. *J. Amer. Dietet. Assoc.* 76:585.

Sims, D. F., ed. 1980. *Diabetes: reach for health and freedom.* St. Louis, C. V. Mosby.

Traisman, H. S. 1980. *Management of juvenile diabetes mellitus.* 3rd ed. St. Louis: C. V. Mosby.

16 OBESITY

People of both sexes and of all ages, from infancy to old age, can be affected by the accumulation of excess body weight. The human body contains fat, water, muscle mass, and cell solids. Changes in body weight reflect an increase or decrease in quantity of any of these compounds. For example, an accumulation of fat may result in obesity. Although obesity cannot be "cured," it can be controlled.

Beginning with some basic definitions, this chapter examines the disadvantages of being obese and current theories on the causes of obesity. The rest of the chapter deals with ways of losing weight and the obstacles and hazards in doing so. Information about methods of determining desirable body weight and individual energy needs is presented in Chapter 4.

FACTS ABOUT OBESITY

Although the term "overweight" simply means the condition of weighing more than the ideal or desirable body weight, in this chapter it is used interchangeably with "obesity." **Obesity** is also an overweight condition, but one that results from an accumulation of fat rather than large bone structure or excess muscle or water. A person who weighs more than his ideal weight by 15 to 25 percent owing to excess fat is said to be obese.

A constant small accumulation of calories from overeating over a long period causes obesity. There is no cure; however, knowing the relationship between caloric intake and energy expenditure facilitates the process of weight control.

Body fat includes some water and nonfat cell components, as follows:

$$1 \text{ lb pure fat} = 454 \times 9 \text{ kcal/g} = 4{,}086 \text{ kcal}$$
$$1 \text{ lb body fat} = 85\% \text{ fat} + 15\% \text{ water and cell components}$$
$$= 85/100 \times 4{,}086 \text{ kcal}$$
$$= 3{,}473 \text{ kcal (or approximately 3,500 kcal)}$$

To simplify this formula, we can say that there are 7.7 kcal (that is, $3{,}500 \div 454$) per gram of body fat.

For each 3,500 kcal we eat above what we expend as energy, we gain approximately 1 lb of weight. Chapter 4 contains more detailed information about the relationship between body weight and energy expenditure. As an example of how easy it is to gain weight, suppose that a woman begins to consume an extra ¾ cup of celery soup and one slice of toast as an afternoon snack, and that she does this three times a week. If her other meals and activities remain unchanged, this woman will gain 8 to 9 lb of body fat within 1 year.

Most women begin to gain weight after age 20, with further gains occurring during pregnancy and after menopause. Men usually gain weight between the ages of 25 and 40. Adult males can lose weight slightly more easily than females. From 20 to 25 percent of Americans over 30 years old are 10 to 25 percent above their desirable body weights.

CONSEQUENCES AND CAUSES OF OBESITY

An obese person has more problems, health-related and otherwise, than a person with normal weight. Medical complications that may affect people more than 15 percent overweight include: (1) higher morbidity and mortality, (2) respiratory difficulties, (3) cardiovascular diseases, (4) kidney diseases, (5) diabetes mellitus, (6) increased risks during surgery, (7) alimentary tract disorders, (8) increased risk of toxemia and prolonged labor and delivery during pregnancy, (9) arthritis in the joints, and (10) chronic illnesses.

Certain nonmedical complications also may result from overweight. One of these is the psychological maladjustment of feeling different or viewing oneself as inferior to others because of rejection, discrimination, and frustration. Minor aches and pains from carrying too much weight add to these problems. Even the cost of living is higher, since the cost of clothes, food, and travel is affected by one's size.

No satisfactory answers have emerged to explain why some people overeat to the point of obesity, despite the many disadvantages of carrying excess body fat. Table 16-1 summarizes some current thoughts on the possible causes of obesity.

TABLE 16-1. Some Proposed Causes of Obesity

Factor	Analysis
Genetics	
Body build by birth	All types: round, plump, thin, fragile, heavily muscular. For example, a person born thin, fragile, and linear may grow up to be a small person and underweight.
Familial traits	If parents are obese, their children have a higher chance of being obese.
Defective hunger and satiety center	Hypothalamus does not respond normally. Usually, it responds to hunger and informs the person to stop eating when full. Its failure to do so results in obesity.
Defective body metabolism	Defects in an obese person: inability to release energy efficiently (from ATP, for example), reduced lipase (enzyme) activity to mobilize fat, and overactive fat storage enzyme system.
Body fat cell type	An obese person may be born with a large number of fat cells or a special type of fat cell that can hypertrophy easily.
Anthropological factors	
Cultural acceptance	Obesity is considered good fortune or a beautiful attribute in many countries.
Food and hospitality	The expression of hospitality through food and drink makes food more available. In an affluent society like the United States, this increases food consumption.
Eating habits	
Overeating	Obese people like to eat. They eat more calories than they expend.
Meal pattern	Eating three meals a day may predispose some individuals to deposit more fat. Nibbling the same quantity of food throughout the day may enable the body enzyme system to use the calories more efficiently, and less fat is deposited.
Childhood conditioning	
Infancy eating maladjustment	Solid foods given too early, excess high-caloric density milk, and excess food consumption all may result in large weight gain. A big baby (from too much fat) is not necessarily a healthy baby.
Overeating	A fat child can grow into an obese adult.
Psychological factors	
Eating as an emotional outlet	If the person wants to stay away from food, he or she must be convinced to use another means of emotional support.
Eating to allay anxiety, tension, frustration, and insecurity	The greater the level of anxiety, tension, frustration, or insecurity, the more food a person eats and the more likely he or she is to gain weight.
Eating as a substitute or demonstration of love and affection	The relationship between family members is expressed with food. To show love and affection, one person serves more food to another. Or to replace loss of love and affection, a person eats more or is served more food.
Eating as a substitute for whatever is missing (e.g., no job)	In this context, eating is similar to excess alcohol drinking and heavy smoking.
Physiological factors	
Hormones	Hypothyroidism or decreased metabolism may result in weight gain and therefore obesity.
Basal metabolic rate	BMR decreases with age, while the caloric consumption is undiminished and there is a decrease (or no increase) in daily activity.
No exercise or activity	Eating a lot of foods without a good exercise program results in obesity.
Environmental factors	
Trauma and emotion	Certain individuals are susceptible to traumatic and emotional experiences and will eat more food.

TABLE 16-1. (continued)

Factor	Analysis
Family eating habits	One develops an overeating habit if parents and other members in the family eat too much.
Sedentary job	Some jobs require constant sitting, with minimal movement.
Abundance of foods	Obesity is more common in affluent societies.
Advertisements	A person is conditioned to the type of foods advertised on television and in magazines, most of which are high in calories.
Living comfort	Comfortable ambient temperature, light clothing, minimal shivering, and lack of heavy work all contribute to reduced expenditure of calories.
Convenience of food preparation	Minimal preparation time and labor. Less activity, more food consumed.
Smoking or alcohol	When a person tries to stop smoking or drinking, he or she may eat more and gain weight.

LOSING WEIGHT

In 1958, Dr. A. J. Stunkard of Stanford University stated: "Most obese persons will not stay in treatment for obesity. Of those who stay in treatment, most will not lose weight and of those who do lose weight, most will regain it." Although this statement is still true, the number of obese individuals who manage to lose and maintain the ideal body weight is increasing.

Obstacles to Weight Loss

Losing weight is difficult both because we like to eat and because common problems are always present as stumbling blocks. One of these is our lifelong eating habits, which are difficult to change. A second problem is the discouragingly slow results of attempting to lose weight. For example, if a person who is 50 to 100 pounds overweight loses 1 or 2 pounds a week, it may take 1 to 2 years to reach the desired goal. Still another deterrent to successful dieting may be the relationship between the physician and the patient, usually because of unrealistic expectations on one or both sides.

Studies show that overweight individuals who are charged a fee for medical advice and a low-caloric diet are more likely to regard them seriously. Free advice about how to lose weight often goes unheeded. Also, the earlier an obese person seeks medical advice, the easier it is to lose weight.

Once the excess weight has been lost, the other half of the battle begins: maintaining that ideal weight. The best way to keep body weight within normal range is to eat a proper diet, exercise regularly, and develop good eating habits—in short, to strike a balance between caloric intake and expenditure.

General Considerations

A sensible approach to weight loss should include the following considerations: (1) a goal of slow and steady decrease in weight of 1 to 2 pounds a week, (2) regular daily exercise, (3) anticipation of "plateaus" when weight loss temporarily stops, (4) following weight loss with a weight maintenance program, and (5) developing a positive attitude toward oneself.

Advice and treatment of the obese patient should be sensitive and supportive. Embarrassing and discouraging attitudes must be avoided. The increase in certain health risks posed by obesity should not be used to frighten patients.

In addition to benefiting from a positive approach to weight loss, the patient is more likely to succeed if the details of the treatment are carefully explained. Anticipated obstacles as well as projected goals should be clearly defined.

SCIENTIFIC METHODS OF WEIGHT REDUCTION

There are various treatment methods aimed at reducing body weight. Table 16-2 summarizes these methods and analyzes each briefly. Each method also is discussed below.

Reduced Caloric Intake

The most obvious way to lose weight is to eat less. The sections that follow give the general characteristics of a successful weight-loss diet and four methods of planning a reduced-calorie eating regimen.

Characteristics of a successful diet

A successful weight reduction diet should be:

1. *Nutritionally adequate but low in calories.* The individual's RDAs serve as a guideline to plan an appropriate diet. Three or four meals daily are recommended, each providing 250 to 350 kcal and some carbohydrate, protein, and fat. Total consumption of fat and carbohydrate should be small to moderate, with a liberal protein distribution.
2. *Appetizing and simple to prepare.* A diet that can be integrated into

TABLE 16-2. Some Scientific Methods of Reducing Weight

Treatment Method	Analysis
Reduced caloric intake	If done without medical supervision, caloric intake should not be less than 1,200 kcal per day. May be accomplished with the help of a doctor, nurse, dietitian, nutritionist, or other allied health personnel.
Increased exercise	May be accomplished by oneself or with the supervision of a doctor, exercise physiologist, or other similarly trained personnel.
Behavioral modification	May be accomplished by oneself or with one-to-one or group counseling with a trained therapist, clinical psychologist, or psychiatrist.
Group program	May be accomplished by organizing one's own group weight reduction program, joining national groups, and participating in commercially supervised (nonclinical) weight reduction enterprises.
Hypnosis	May be achieved under the care of a clinical hypnotist or by learning self-hypnosis.
Jaw wiring or lock-jaw	Some success when conducted by experienced medical personnel.
Forced exercise	Some success when performed under the direct supervision of a physician.
Drug therapy	Overall effectiveness is not sure. Physician's prescription required.
Surgery	Some success, although some techniques are accompanied by severe side effects: high morbidity and mortality.
Starvation or fasting	1. Semistarvation. Reduction of dietary intake to 500–1,200 kcal per day requires the direct supervision of a physician. 2. Protein-sparing modified fast. Requires the direct supervision of a physician. 3. Total starvation. Requires the direct supervision of a physician.
Comprehensive medical weight reduction program	Some success. Must be conducted under direct medical supervision.

the entire family's eating routine and will not soon become boring is most likely to be followed.

3. *Carefully planned.* Successful dieting requires organization and planning; attention to detail can increase and/or enhance weight loss. For example, cooking stews, soups, and casseroles in advance allows them to be refrigerated and the solid fat skimmed off. Keeping celery and carrot sticks handy lessens the temptation to reach for more calorie-costly snacks. Fresh fruit or fruit canned in its own juice makes a delicious and satisfying dessert.

People attempting to lose weight should learn about basic nutrition and new eating habits. Dieters should begin to recognize those circumstances under which they are most likely to overeat. Meals eaten away from home, for example, may require special planning.

TABLE 16-3. A Core Eating Plan Providing 1,000 to 1,500 kcal Per Day

Food type	Serving	Approximate Caloric Contribution	Remarks
Milk	2–2½ c	Skim milk: 170–255 kcal Whole milk: 330–495 kcal	If interested in cheeses, ice cream, cream, and other dairy products, make calculations and replace.
Meat	4–6 oz	200–500 kcal for fish, poultry, meat (baked, boiled, roasted, broiled), all visible fat trimmed	If interested in eggs and shellfish, make calculations and replace.
Fruits	2–5	80–250 kcal, fruits or fruit juices, unsweetened	Make sure to include citrus fruits or a source of vitamin C.
Vegetables	2–5	20–250 kcal, with at least 1 serving of a dark green leafy vegetable	Many varieties have virtually zero calories. Exclude peas, corns, beans, and potatoes.
Grain	2–4	50–350 kcal	Include potatoes, peas, beans, and corn.
Fats	1–3	100–300 kcal	
Free foods	No limit	Coffee, tea, lemon juice, celery, spices, condiments, consommé, bouillon and others. Very little calorie contribution.	

Many sources of help are available to the dieter. Free classes are often presented by adult schools, colleges, and churches. Books and publications on food preparation, dieting, menus, calories, and nutrition may be obtained in most public libraries. Also, new friends and activities can limit one's dependency on food.

Calorie Counting

Consult Chapter 4 for methods of determining ideal body weight and daily caloric need according to activity level. Those figures provide guidelines for establishing a safe starter diet. Eating less than 1,000 to 1,200 kcal per day should be under medical supervision.

Once the number of calories has been determined, the next step is to plan a diet that is both successful and convenient. There are four main ways: following a core eating plan, compiling a long list of menu plans, using an accepted commercial weight reduction plan, and using the food exchange system developed by the American Diabetes and Dietetic Associations. These methods are described below.

Core eating plan. A core eating plan tells the dieter the approximate number of servings of each category of food he or she can eat daily. Table 16-3 provides a core eating plan of 1,000 to 1,500 kcal per day, depend-

TABLE 16-4. Examples of Food Items Included in the Core Eating Plan

Food Type	Servings Providing Equivalent Amount of Calories
Milk	1 c skim milk, ½ c whole milk, ⅔ c cheddar cheese
Meat	1 oz meat, 1 egg, ¼ c salmon, 3 sardines, 5 oysters
Fruits	½ c applesauce, 1 medium nectarine, ⅔ c blueberries, 1 small pear
Vegetables	½ c spinach, 1 medium artichoke, ½ c chard, ½ c cooked cabbage, 1 small cucumber, ½ c cooked mustard greens
Grain	1 sl bread, ½ c cooked cereal, ½ c cooked noodles or rice, 2 graham crackers, ½ c peas, ½ c cooked dried beans, ½ c mashed potato
Fats	½ T butter, margarine, or oil; 1 sl bacon; 1 T French dressing

ing on the number of servings of each food type consumed. Table 16-4 provides a few examples of food servings that give an approximately equivalent amount of calories within the food type. The appendix provides a number of examples of each food type. Table 16-5 uses the information in Tables 16-3 and 16-4 and appendix to develop a daily menu plan of approximately 1,400 kcal.

Preplanned menus. Menus preplanned for a certain calorie level simplify the process of meal planning for the dieter. Such menus are available from a variety of sources, such as nutrition textbooks, or may be developed by the dieter personally. The person follows the meal plans exactly and repeats them weekly. Tables 16-6 and 16-7 provide daily menus for one week at a caloric level of 1,500 kcal. Tables 16-8 and 16-9 provide daily menus for one week at a caloric level of 1,200 kcal.

Commercial diet reduction regimens. Several diet plans have been successful in helping obese people lose weight. Two of the most popular are the *Wise Woman's Diet* (by *Redbook* magazine) and *Weight Watchers Menu Plans* (by Weight Watchers International). High cost and time-consuming preparation are two notable drawbacks, however.

TABLE 16-5. A 1,400-kcal Menu Plan

Breakfast	Lunch	Dinner
½ pink grapefruit	½ c cottage cheese on lettuce	3 oz breaded, baked haddock
½ c oatmeal	and carrot sticks	½ c asparagus spears
1 poached egg	1 c vegetable beef soup	1 baked potato
1 sl whole wheat toast	4 saltine crackers	1 sl French bread
1 t margarine	1 c sliced strawberries	1 t margarine
1 c skim milk	1 c skim milk	1 plum
Salt, pepper	Salt, pepper	10 grapes
Coffee or tea	Coffee or tea	1 c skim milk
		Salt, pepper
		Lemon
		Coffee or tea

The American Diabetes/Dietetic Food Exchange System. Food products are divided into six lists: (1) milk, (2) vegetables, (3) fruits, (4) bread, (5) meat, and (6) fats. Within each list foods with similar caloric content are grouped together and are interchangeable. These lists are presented in detail in Chapter 15. Table 16-10 presents meal plans using the Food Exchange System for 12 different caloric levels. Table 16-11 translates the exchanges into a simple menu for 1,200 kcal.

Increased Exercise

The more we exercise, the better the chance of losing weight. Although vigorous exercise may stimulate hunger, running or jogging 1 to 2 miles daily probably will not increase the appetite to the detriment of a diet regimen.

Exercise affects individuals in different ways. Some people tire easily, while others become dizzy because of hypotension. All obese people must be careful to avoid back injuries. Patients with certain clinical conditions, such as hypertension, should not indulge in heavy exercise.

Behavioral Modification

It is important for an obese patient to learn new eating habits. The patient's personal history and his or her eating and activity patterns are used to identify problem areas and set realistic goals for weight loss.

Modifying eating habits involves changing the amount and types of food eaten as well as the frequency of eating. For example, the *amount* of food may be reduced by eating in small bites and counting each mouthful. The *types* of food may be controlled by shopping for groceries on a

TABLE 16-6. Daily 1,500-kcal Menu Plans for Monday to Friday

Monday	Tuesday	Wednesday	Thursday	Friday
Breakfast	**Breakfast**	**Breakfast**	**Breakfast**	**Breakfast**
½ c pineapple juice	½ c grape juice	½ c grapefruit juice	½ c apricot nectar	½ c orange juice
1 hard-cooked egg	½ c Cream of	⅛ honeydew melon	¾ c shredded	½ c cottage cheese
1 toasted bagel	Wheat	1 poached egg	wheat biscuits	2 pear halves,
2 t margarine	Cinnamon	1 sl whole wheat	(spoon size)	canned in water
½ banana	2 T raisins	toast	½ c skim milk	1 sl toasted rye
Salt, pepper	1 sl bacon	1 t margarine	½ sliced banana	bread
Coffee or tea	1 sl whole wheat	2 sl bacon	2 sausage links	1 t margarine
	bread	Salt, pepper	Salt, pepper	2 sl bacon
Lunch	1 t margarine	Coffee or tea	Coffee or tea	Salt, pepper
2 oz chicken	Salt, pepper			Coffee or tea
2 sl whole wheat	Coffee or tea	**Lunch**	**Lunch**	
bread		2 oz turkey	2 oz chicken	**Lunch**
1 t margarine	**Lunch**	½ c asparagus	½ c green beans	2 T peanut butter
1 t mayonnaise	2 oz lean beef	1 t mayonnaise	½ c cooked carrots	2 sl French bread
1 c mixed cooked	½ c cooked	3 sq. in. cornbread	½ c rice	6–8 carrot sticks
carrots, broccoli,	mushrooms	1 t margarine	2 t margarine	½ c cooked kale
cauliflower	½ c Swiss chard	1 c lettuce salad	½ c ice milk	1 pear
1 pear	½ c baked beans	with lemon juice	1 c sliced	1 c skim milk
1 c skim milk	1 sl rye bread	1 orange	strawberries	Salt, pepper
Salt, pepper	1 t margarine	1 c skim milk	1 c skim milk	Coffee or tea
Coffee or tea	1 apple	Salt, pepper	Salt, pepper	
	1 c skim milk	Coffee or tea	Coffee or tea	**Dinner**
Dinner	Salt, pepper			3 oz chicken
3 oz lean beef	Coffee or tea	**Dinner**	**Dinner**	½ c rice
½ c cooked kale		1 c lettuce salad	3 oz roast beef	1 c cooked zucchini
½ c cooked beets	**Dinner**	1 c canned salmon	½ c asparagus	onion
1 sl French bread	3 oz halibut	1 T French dressing	½ c cooked	½ c ice milk
1 t margarine	½ c peas	½ c green beans	summer squash	⅔ c frozen
½ c sliced	2–3 carrot strips	1 sl French bread	1 sl rye bread	blueberries
strawberries	1 hard roll	1 t margarine	1 t margarine	1 c skim milk
1 c skim milk	1 t margarine	1 peach	1 apple	Salt, pepper
Salt, pepper	1 orange	1 c skim milk	1 c skim milk	Coffee or tea
Coffee or tea	1 c skim milk	Salt, pepper	Salt, pepper	
	Salt, pepper	Coffee or tea	Coffee or tea	
	Coffee or tea			

full stomach. The *frequency* of eating may be modified by confining meals to a specific time and place. A special low-calorie diet is not necessarily involved.

Weight reduction by behavioral modification may involve both positive and negative reinforcement. If the patient fails to change undesirable eating habits, for example, he or she may have to pay a "fine" or forfeit. On the other hand, a patient's success may be reinforced by a reward such as a movie or concert. Behavioral modification acknowl-

TABLE 16-7. Daily 1,500-kcal Menu Plans for Saturday and Sunday

Saturday	Sunday
Breakfast	**Brunch**
½ c tomato juice	½ c orange juice
1 muffin	Omelet
1 t margarine	2 eggs
¼ medium cantaloupe	1 oz cheddar cheese
1 scrambled egg	Mushrooms
1 sausage link	Onion
Salt, pepper	1 sl French bread,
Coffee or tea	toasted
	1 t margarine
	½ grapefruit
Lunch	1 sl bacon
2 sl whole wheat bread	1 c skim milk
1 sl tomato	Salt, pepper
2 oz cheddar cheese	Coffee or tea
1 t mayonnaise	
½ c cooked carrots	**Snack**
1 apple	1 pear
1 c skim milk	½ c grapefruit juice
Salt, pepper	
Coffee or tea	
	Dinner
	3 oz roast pork (lean)
Dinner	½ c sauerkraut
3 oz turkey	½ c peas
½ c green beans	1 sl whole wheat bread
1 small baked potato	1 t margarine
1 T sour cream	1 baked banana with
½ c green salad with	cinnamon
lemon juice	1 t margarine
1 orange	1 c skim milk
1 c skim milk	Salt, pepper
Salt, pepper	Coffee or tea
Coffee or tea	

edges each step toward the desired goal. See references for this chapter for more information on methods of losing weight through behavior modification.

Group Programs

Several self-help group programs, such as Weight Watchers and TOPS, are fairly successful in encouraging overweight people to help one another lose weight. These groups have certain things in common, including: (1) regularly scheduled meetings; (2) lectures, presentations,

TABLE 16-8. Daily 1,200-kcal Menu Plans for Monday to Friday

Monday	Tuesday	Wednesday	Thursday	Friday
Breakfast	**Breakfast**	**Breakfast**	**Breakfast**	**Breakfast**
½ c grapefruit juice	1 orange	1 c strawberries	2 canned peach	½ c tomato juice
1 poached egg	½ c oatmeal	4 T milk	halves (water	1 sl whole wheat
1 sl whole wheat	4 T milk	1 sl toast	packed)	toast
toast	1 3″ sausage link	2 T peanut butter	½ c cottage cheese	1 sl American
1 t margarine	Salt, pepper	Coffee or tea	1 muffin	cheese
Salt, pepper	Coffee or tea		1 t margarine	1 scrambled egg
Coffee or tea		**Lunch**	Coffee or tea	Salt, pepper
	Lunch	½ c cooked carrots		Coffee or tea
Lunch	1 c lettuce salad	½ c rice	**Lunch**	
Sandwich	with lemon juice	2 oz broiled chicken	6–8 carrot and	**Lunch**
2 sl whole wheat	½ c beet greens	10 pretzel sticks	celery sticks	½ c cauliflower
bread	1 hot dog	1 sl watermelon	1 c lettuce salad	½ c cabbage
2 oz cheddar	1 bun	1 c skim milk	½ c tuna (water	2 oz lean roast beef
cheese	1 t mayonnaise	Salt, pepper	packed)	2 sl whole wheat
1 sl tomato	½ banana	Coffee or tea	1 T French dressing	bread
⅛ avocado	1 c skim milk		5 saltine crackers	1 t mayonnaise
½ c cooked	Salt, pepper	**Dinner**	3 apricots	1 apple
broccoli	Coffee or tea	½ c turnip greens	½ c ice milk	1 c skim milk
1 apple		½ c summer squash	Salt, pepper	Salt, pepper
1 c skim milk	**Dinner**	3 oz lean beef	Coffee or tea	Coffee or tea
Salt, pepper	½ c cooked carrots	1 sl French bread		
Coffee or tea	½ c cooked	1 t margarine	**Dinner**	**Dinner**
	mushrooms	1 peach	½ c spinach	1 c green salad
Dinner	1 small baked	1 c skim milk	½ c cauliflower	½ c green beans
½ c asparagus	potato	Salt, pepper	½ c noodles	3 oz halibut with
½ c peas	3 oz chicken	Coffee or tea	3 oz turkey	lemon juice
½ c rice	3 apricots		½ c pineapple	1 cornmeal muffin
3 oz baked bluefish	1 c skim milk		chunks	1 orange
with lemon	Salt, pepper		1 c skim milk	1 c skim milk
⅔ c blueberries	Coffee or tea		Salt, pepper	Salt, pepper
1 c skim milk			Coffee or tea	Coffee or tea
Salt, pepper				
Coffee or tea				

or discussions on topics of general interest to overweight individuals; (3) payment of dues; and (4) recognition of a successful weight reduction effort.

Members of these groups are expected to follow a special low-calorie diet and engage in a regular exercise program. Such self-help groups are believed to be more effective in helping people lose weight than most physicians and clinics.

TABLE 16-9. Daily 1,200-kcal Menu Plans for Saturday and Sunday

Saturday	Sunday
Breakfast	**Brunch**
½ c unsweetened applesauce	½ c orange juice
1 oz lean ham	1 sl whole wheat toast
2 2½ in.-square graham crackers	1 t margarine
1 T cream cheese	1 sausage link
Salt, pepper	1 sl quiche
Coffee or tea	¼ cantaloupe
	Salt, pepper
	Coffee or tea
Lunch	**Dinner**
2 oz turkey	½ c winter squash
½ c baked beans	½ c peas and mushrooms
1 c green salad	3 oz lean roast pork
1 T French dressing	1 hard roll
10 cherries	1 t margarine
1 c skim milk	1 baked apple with cinnamon
Salt, pepper	1 c skim milk
Coffee or tea	Salt, pepper
	Coffee or tea
Dinner	
½ c beets	
1 artichoke	
½ c mashed potatoes made with milk only	
3 oz chicken	
1 sl watermelon	
1 c skim milk	
Salt, pepper	
Coffee or tea	

Hypnotism

Claims have been made that hypnotism can help people lose weight. The therapist first establishes a relationship of trust with the patient, develops the patient's confidence in hypnotism, and familiarizes him or her with the procedures. After several sessions, hypnosis is induced; suggestions can be made during the trance stage that may affect the patient's attitude toward food. For example, the patient may be encouraged to chew gum instead of candy or told to transfer overeating activity to some form of exercise.

TABLE 16-10. Using the Food Exchange Lists to Prepare Menu Plans at 12 Different Caloric Levels

Food type	Food Exchange List	Number of Exchanges Assigned to the Daily Permitted Number of Kilocalories											
		600	800	900	1,000	1,100	1,200	1,300	1,400	1,500	1,600	1,700	1,800
Breakfast													
Meat (medium fat)	5	1	1	1	1	1	1	1	1	1	1	1	1
Vegetables	2	0	0	0	0	0	0	0	0	0	0	0	0
Fruits	3	1	1	1	1	1	1	1	1	1	1	1	1
Bread	4	½	1	1	1	1	1	1	1	1	1	1	1
Milk (nonfat)	1	½	½	½	1	1	1	1	1	1	1	1	1
Fats	6	0	0	0	0	0	1	1	1	1	1	1	1
Lunch													
Meat (medium fat)	5	2	2	2	2	2	2	2	2	2	2	2	2
Vegetables*	2	1	1	1	1	1	1	1	1	1	1	1	1
Fruits	3	1	1	1	1	2	2	2	1	2	2	2	1
Bread	4	½	0	1	1	1	2	1	2	2	2	2	2
Milk (nonfat)	1	0	½	½	½	½	½	½	½	½	½	½	½
Fats	6	0	0	0	0	0	0	1	1	1	2	2	2
Dinner													
Meat (medium fat)	5	2	2	2	2	2	2	2	3	3	3	3	3
Vegetables*	2	1	1	1	1	1	1	1	1	1	1	1	1
Fruits	3	1	1	1	1	1	1	1	1	1	1	1	2
Bread	4	0	1	0	0	1	1	2	2	2	2	2	2
Milk (nonfat)	1	0	0	½	½	½	½	½	½	½	½	1	1
Fats	6	0	0	0	0	0	0	1	1	2	2	2	2

*One of the two daily servings of vegetables must be raw and have few calories (see the exchange lists in Chapter 15).
Adapted from A. Dean, Home and Family Series, Extension Bulletin E-782, Cooperative Extension Service, Michigan State University and the Food Exchange Lists of the American Diabetes Association. The exchange lists are based on material in the *Exchange Lists for Meal Planning* prepared by Committees of the American Diabetes Association, Inc., and The American Dietetic Association in cooperation with the National Institute of Arthritis, Metabolism and Digestive Diseases and the National Heart and Lung Institute, National Institutes of Health, Public Health Service, U.S. Department of Health and Human Services.

These and similar suggestions are made repeatedly to reinforce the message that weight loss is desirable. Some patients even learn how to hypnotize themselves.

Forced Exercise

The patient is required to perform a specified amount of exercise under medical supervision. Exercises might include running on a treadmill or riding a stationary bicycle. Not only do some patients lose weight but both muscle tone and respiratory functions are improved.

Certain factors should be considered when implementing forced ex-

TABLE 16-11. Sample Menu for a 1,200-kcal Diet Using the Exchanges in Table 16-10.

Breakfast	Lunch	Dinner
½ c orange juice	2 small boiled frankfurters	2 oz broiled hamburger
1 poached egg	½ c cooked green	½ c cooked summer squash
1 sl toast	beans	Sliced tomato on lettuce
1 t margarine	1 sl whole wheat toast	½ c cooked rice
1 c skim milk	1 medium tangerine	1 small apple
Salt, pepper	1 small banana	12 grapes
Coffee or tea	½ c skim milk	½ c skim milk
	Salt, pepper	Salt, pepper
	Coffee or tea	Coffee or tea

ercises, however. There should be appropriate medical supervision and a slow, gradual implementation of the exercise program. Patients should combine exercise with a diet of 900 to 1,000 kcal per day. Personality changes may occur and should be monitored. Injuries to the back and joints are not uncommon.

Surgery

One popular surgical technique for treating obesity is gastrointestinal bypass. For some patients, this procedure is risky with complications and death.

There are two types of gastrointestinal bypass. One involves closing off part of the stomach by stapling and is reversible. The other removes part of the small intestine and is usually irreversible. In either case, the amount of food digested and absorbed is reduced. Stomach stapling is the less hazardous procedure and is more popular. Figure 16-1 shows a patient before and after intestinal bypass surgery. More information about surgical procedures is available in references for Chapter 20 and this chapter.

Starvation (Fasting)

Partial or complete avoidance of food is one of the oldest methods of losing weight. Reducing caloric intake to less than 1,200 kcal per day requires a doctor's supervision, however. It is especially important to monitor fluid and electrolyte levels, mineral and vitamin balance, and cardiovascular functions. Although fasting has proved successful, sudden death in a small number of patients has been reported.

Recently a program called "modified fasting" was developed by a

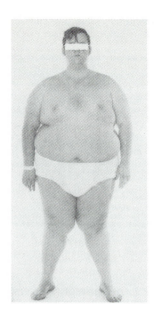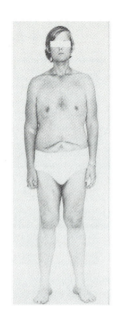

FIGURE 16-1. A 20-year-old patient before (left, at 400 lb) and 2 years after (right, at 210 lb) intestinal bypass. (From H. W. Scott et al., *South Med. J.* 69 [1976]: 789)

group of physicians. In addition to providing a high-quality liquid protein diet, the program includes regular exercise, nutrition education, counseling, and an emphasis on maintenance of weight loss.

Despite the availability of commercial protein preparations, such substances are not recommended for use without medical supervision. More than 20 deaths have resulted from this regimen, though the reasons for death remain unknown.

Weight Reduction Clinics

There are many authentic, reputable, and fairly successful weight reduction clinics. These programs may contain any or all of the following treatment procedures: (1) a comprehensive patient history, (2) an individualized and slowly implemented diet, (3) appropriate drug therapy, (4) a well-designed exercise program, (5) limited fasting, (6) modification of eating habits. Such clinics are under the supervision of medically qualified individuals.

Conscientious patients can lose weight in these programs. However, there are some basic problems. One is high cost. Another is the time required to make the program work. A third consideration is the psychological factors involved, factors that act as barriers to all weight reduction plans—that is, the patience and willpower required to lose weight, unwillingness to change lifelong habits, and the difficulty of maintaining normal weight.

GENERAL ADVICE FOR WEIGHT LOSS

First, when using a diet to lose weight, check its authenticity and accuracy. Consult your physician, public health nutritionist, hospital dietitian, or an academic specializing in the field.

Second, when using any over-the-counter drugs, check their effectiveness and safety. Seek medical supervision if so advised on the label. Consult *Consumer Reports,* your physician, or an academic specialist in pharmacology and related fields. Never take a prescription drug obtained illegally without full awareness of its safety and effectiveness.

Third, do not believe any advertisement promoting a diet, drug, device, regimen, or other procedure that *guarantees* weight loss. At present, there is no known method that can guarantee weight loss with absolute safety.

Fourth, exercise—but take precautions. The exercise program must be appropriate for *you* (age, sex, and medical conditions). Proper professional advice must be sought or a professionally written manual for physical activity must be followed.

Fifth, at present, avoid most mechanical devices for losing weight, which can be harmful. Body trappings, for example, can impair circulation.

Finally, before adopting any diet or weight loss program, be sure that you are in normal health. Many diets, drugs, and exercise programs are all right for normal, healthy people. If at all feasible, inform your physician of what you are doing and ask him or her to help check your progress or check your health before beginning any program. If you are unable to consult your doctor, talk to other health professionals such as nutritionists. If they work in a health clinic, they will provide advice and assistance as a public service and usually do not charge a fee.

The most effective way to lose weight is to combine at least a minimal amount of daily activity, learning the basics of good nutrition, retraining eating habits, and following a sensible and practical low-calorie diet.

STUDY QUESTIONS

1. What is the difference between the terms *overweight* and *obese*?
2. How many excess kilocalories (energy not spent) does it take to gain 1 lb of body fat?
3. Name at least six medical problems for which people more than 15% overweight run a higher–than–normal risk. What are some nonmedical problems associated with obesity?

4. What five considerations are essential to any successful weight loss program?
5. What assumptions underlie the behavioral modification approach to weight loss? Describe some techniques for reducing stimulus control of eating.
6. Is fasting recommended for those who are obese or only slightly overweight? What is a modified fasting program?
7. Compile a list of diet books that were popular during the last 2 years.
8. Compile a list of diet aids that were popular during the last 2 years.

REFERENCES

Better Homes & Gardens. 1980. *Eat and stay slim*. Des Moines, Iowa: Meredith, Consumer Book Division.

Bray, G. A., ed. 1980. *Obesity: comparative methods of weight control*. Westport, Conn.: Technomic Publishing.

Edelstein, B. 1980. *The woman doctor's diet for teen-age girls*. Englewood Cliffs, N. J.: Prentice-Hall.

Kornguth, M. L. 1981. Obesity: nursing management. *Am. J. Nurs.* 81:553.

Langford, R. W. 1981. Teenagers and obesity. *Am. J. Nurs.* 81:556.

Powers, P. S. 1980. *Obesity, the regulation of weight*. Baltimore: Williams & Wilkins.

Stern, J. S., and Denenberg, R. V. 1980. *How to stay slim and healthy on the fast food diet*. Englewood Cliffs, N. J.: Prentice-Hall.

Stunkard, A. J., ed. 1980. *Obesity*. Philadelphia: Saunders.

Thompson, C. I. 1980. *Controls of eating*. Jamaica, N. Y.: Spectrum Publications.

White, J. H., and Schroeder, M. A. 1981. Obesity: nursing assessment. *Am. J. Nurs.* 81:550.

17 DIET AND CARDIOVASCULAR DISEASES

In the highly developed countries of the world, heart disease has reached epidemic proportions. Although in the United States there has been a recent decline in the number of deaths from heart-related illnesses, heart disease is still a major killer.

The heart and circulatory system are associated with a number of clinical problems including atherosclerosis, hypertension, and congestive heart failure. Each of these pathological disorders is discussed below with a special emphasis on diet therapy.

ATHEROSCLEROSIS AND RELATED CONDITIONS

Definitions

The major pathological condition that leads to a diseased heart is *arteriosclerosis*—a term used to describe a thickening of the artery walls. **Atherosclerosis**—a thickening of the artery walls accompanied by the formation of fatty deposits on the innermost layer of the arteries—is the major villain in heart disease.

Under normal conditions, the *lumina,* or passages, of the blood vessels are open and clear, allowing blood to flow easily through them. If the process of atherosclerosis has begun, however, fatty deposits called *plaques* form on artery walls. This plaque formation continues to build, gradually causing blood vessels to narrow and reducing the flow of blood. If the blood flow in a coronary artery stops altogether, heart muscle cells die of *ischemia,* a lack of oxygen.

Clinical Complications

Atherosclerosis is the main cause of heart disease, stroke, gangrene, and aneurysm (a sac formed by partial artery or vein dilatation). Kidney failure and high blood pressure may also result. *Angina pectoris* is a condition in which the patient suffers chest pain caused by inadequate blood supply to the heart muscle. Still another complication is myocardial infarction, in which blockage of the heart's blood supply results in the death of heart muscle cells.

Diet Therapy and the Heart Patient

The dietary care of a heart patient has two phases: acute and rehabilitative. For a patient confined to an intensive care unit (ICU), dietary care is a small part of the medical management. Some important considerations are as follows.

Patients who are fed either a liquid diet or only a small quantity of food over a period of time may, in some cases, actually suffer from malnutrition. Patients who have been overfed, on the other hand, may develop such symptoms as profuse sweating, breathing difficulties, fast heartbeat, palpitation, and arrhythmia.

Because excess fluid may distend the abdomen and exert pressure on the heart, fluid intake is usually limited to less than 2 cups per meal, preferably 1 to 1½ cups. Weak tea and coffee are sometimes permitted, but in general foods and drinks that contain caffeine and other stimulants are excluded.

Foods should be served at room temperature or as specified by the physician. The food should be soft and tender and contain no roughage, stimulants, or irritants. Canned or cooked fruits and vegetables, puddings, gelatin, cooked cereals, plain bread, lean meat, poultry, and fish are usually included in the diet.

The amount of sodium restriction should depend on the clinical condition of the patient. The patient's blood chemistry and urine must be studied carefully before the physician can make a decision. Caution is needed, since low sodium intake may upset a patient's electrolyte balance. Information on how to plan a sodium-restricted diet is presented later in this chapter.

During the rehabilitative phase, most physicians advocate a prudent diet (low fat) which is discussed below.

Causes

It has already been established that plaque formation leads to coronary heart disease. But what causes the deposition of fatty substances in an artery with its resulting thickening and narrowing of the blood vessels? No one knows for sure. It is assumed that if no deposits or thickening occurred, the atherosclerotic process and its complications would not begin.

The possible relationship between blood lipid levels, plaque formation, and coronary heart disease has been much debated. Blood may contribute to the fatty components of plaque formation, although the exact process is unknown.

Multiple Risk Factors

Despite many unanswered questions about the specific cause(s) of atherosclerosis, a number of factors believed to increase the risk of developing this condition have been identified. They are listed below.

- Age
- Sex
- Genetic makeup
- Abnormal electrocardiogram (EKG)
- Environmental stress
- Hypertension
- Cigarette smoking
- Personality and behavior
- Lack of physical activity
- Use of alcohol (current evidence suggests that moderate drinking may reduce the risk of atherosclerosis)
- Use of drugs such as oral contraceptive pills
- High blood uric acid level
- High level of blood lipid chemicals
    Cholesterol; triglycerides; fatty acids and phospholipids; lipoproteins
- High blood insulin level
- Dietary factors
    High caloric intake
    High fat intake, especially saturated fat; insufficient polyunsaturated fat intake
    High cholesterol intake
    High sucrose intake
    High or low intake of certain minerals
    High coffee intake
    Low fiber intake
    Nutrient deficiencies
- Presence of other diseases
    Diabetes mellitus
    Gout
    Obstructive liver disease

Chapter 17
DIET AND
CARDIO-
VASCULAR
DISEASES

303

Hypothyroidism
Nephrosis
Pancreatitis

Two of the above factors are of particular significance to nutritional scientists: serum cholesterol and dietary fat.

Serum Cholesterol. High serum cholesterol is believed to be a major factor in atherosclerosis, since cholesterol is the principal lipid in plaque. Many patients with heart disease have high levels of blood cholesterol. Studies of population groups have shown that the higher the level of serum cholesterol, the higher the risk of heart disease.

Dietary Fat. Dietary fat intake appears to be related to the incidence of heart disease. If fat intake is high, the occurrence of heart disease is also high. This is particularly true of animal, or saturated fats. On the other hand, a high intake of polyunsaturated fats (mainly vegetable oil) is associated with a low serum cholesterol level and low incidence of heart disease.

The role of cholesterol and fat in the causation of heart disease is controversial. Some scientists believe they are contributory factors, whereas others do not.

Lipoproteins. In the last few years, we have learned about another group of fat-related substances in the body called **lipoproteins.** These substances, which are made up of fat and protein, are currently suspected of playing an important role in atherosclerosis.

Different forms of fat are distributed throughout the human body in the blood, fluids, fatty tissues, muscles, and organs such as the liver and kidneys. The efficient transportation of these fats from one part of the body to another requires lipoproteins, which make fat water soluble and thus easily carried by the blood.

Under normal conditions, the plasma levels of cholesterol, triglycerides, and lipoprotein exist within certain limits. In some individuals, however, a higher than normal level of these substances may occur, a condition known as **hyperlipidemia.** An excess of lipoprotein in the blood is also called **hyperlipoproteinemia.**

There are five types of hyperlipoproteinemia, which are distinguished by the lipoprotein and lipid component that is elevated in the blood. Table 17-1 summarizes this classification system. Tables 17-2 and 17-3 provide the diagnostic characteristics of hyperlipoproteinemias. In the last few years, the dietary management of hyperlipoproteinemias has received much attention. The most popular regimen was developed by the National Heart and Lung Institute of the National In-

TABLE 17-1. The Five Types of Hyperlipoproteinemia

Type	Increased Plasma Lipoprotein	Increased Plasma Lipid*	Probable Metabolic Defect
I	Chylomicrons	Triglyceride	Lipoprotein lipase fails to remove chylomicrons
IIa	Low-density lipoprotein or β-lipoprotein	Cholesterol	Low-density lipoprotein not cleared from or produced excessively in the plasma
IIb	Low-density lipoprotein (β-lipoprotein); very low density lipoprotein (pre-β-lipoprotein)	Cholesterol, triglyceride	Excessive production or decreased clearance of low-density lipoprotein and very low density lipoprotein
III	Intermediate-density lipoprotein	Triglyceride, cholesterol	Accumulation of intermediate-density lipoprotein
IV	Very low density lipoprotein or pre-β-lipoprotein	Triglyceride (cholesterol)	Overproduction or decreased clearance of the very low density lipoprotein
V	Chylomicrons; very low density lipoprotein or pre-β-lipoprotein	Triglyceride (cholesterol)	Decreased chylomicron clearance; over-production or decreased clearance of very low density lipoprotein

*Parentheses indicate minor proportion.

stitutes of Health. Even though the causes of abnormal serum lipid levels are unknown, diet therapy is designed to restore them to normal. How any dietary measure is able to achieve lower serum lipid levels is not known; the measures are employed on an empirical basis only. Table 17-4 summarizes the dietary modifications needed to achieve normolipoproteinemia.

The Prudent Diet

Although the role of diet in establishing and/or maintaining normal blood lipid levels is controversial, many clinicians agree that there is at least no harm in eliminating as many risk factors as possible from the diet. This includes eating wholesome foods with a low intake of fat and minimizing other risk factors such as inactivity, stress, and smoking.

The American Heart Association makes some specific suggestions about fat intake and diet. Obese persons should reduce to and maintain ideal body weight. Fat intake should be reduced by: (1) reducing total fat intake, (2) reducing saturated fat intake, (3) increasing polyunsaturated fat intake, and (4) reducing cholesterol intake. To achieve this modification of fat intake, the American Heart Association has developed the *fat-controlled diet* (sometimes called the fat-regulated, preventive, or prudent diet). Table 17-5 lists the foods permitted and pro-

Chapter 17
DIET AND
CARDIO-
VASCULAR
DISEASES

305

TABLE 17-2. Diagnostic Characteristics of the Five Types of Hyperlipoproteinemia

Criterion	Type I	Type IIa (endogenous)	Type IIb (exogenous)	Type III	Type IV	Type V
Designation	Hyperchylo-micronemia	Hypercholes-terolemia	Hypercholes-terolemia	Hypercholes-terolemia; hyperglyc-eridemia*	Hyperglyc-eridemia	Hyperglyc-eridemia
Chemistry						
Cholesterol (per 100 mL blood)	Normal, slightly elevated	300–600 mg	300–600 mg	350–800 mg	Normal, slightly ele-vated	250–350 mg
Triglyceride (per 100 mL blood)	5,000–10,000 mg	Normal	150–400 mg	400–800 mg	200–2,000 mg	500–5,000 mg
Plasma after storage at 4 °C	Creamy top layer, clear infranatant	Clear	Slightly turbid	Varies: clear, cloudy or milky	Clear, cloudy or milky	Creamy layer over turbid infranatant
Lipoprotein						
Chylomicrons	Increased	—	—	—	—	Increased
Very low density	—	—	Increased	—	Increased	Increased
Intermediate density	—	—	—	Increased	—	—
Low density	—	Increased	Increased	—	—	—
Age of onset	Under 10	Often during childhood	25–45	20–35	Over 20	Over 20
Frequency or etiology	Rare	Common	Environ-mental	Uncommon	Most common	Uncommon
Clinical features						
Xanthoma[1]	Yes	Yes	Yes	Yes	Yes	Yes
Hepato-splenomegaly	Yes	—	—	—	Rare	Yes
Abdominal pain	Yes	—	—	—	—	Yes
Pancreatitis	Occasionally	—	—	—	—	Yes
Lipemia retinalis	Yes	—	—	—	Yes	Yes
Paresthesia	—	—	—	—	—	Occasionally
Arcus corneae juvenilis	—	Yes	Yes	Occasionally	—	—
Other features						
Fat tolerance	Very abnormal	—	—	—	—	Abnormal
Glucose tolerance	—	—	—	Abnormal	Abnormal	Abnormal
Serum uric acid level	—	—	—	Increased	Increased	Increased
Atherosclerotic tendency	None	Very high	Very high	High risk of peripheral vascular disease	High	Unknown

Note: The symbol "—" means (1) No information is available; (2) clinical status is normal; (3) the symptom is not present.

*Hyperglyceridemia is equivalent to hypertriglyceridemia.

[1] See Table 17-3 for the types of xanthoma involved.

TABLE 17-3. Hyperlipoproteinemias and the Development of Xanthomas

Type of Hyperlipopro- teinemia	Eruptive Xanthoma	Tendon Xanthoma	Xanthelasma	Tuberous Xanthoma	Planar Xanthoma	Tuberoeruptive Xanthoma
I	Yes	—	—	—	—	—
IIa	—	Yes, some- times with polyarthritis	Yes	Yes	—	—
IIb	—	Yes, some- times with polyarthritis	Yes	Yes	—	—
III	—	Yes	Occasionally	—	Yes	Yes
IV	Occasionally	—	—	—	—	Occasionally
V	Yes	—	—	—	—	Occasionally

Note: Xanthoma is a yellow papule, nodule, or plaque in the skin due to lipid deposits; seen microscopically, the lesions show light cells with foamy protoplasm.

hibited in this dietary regimen. Table 17-6 presents the meal planning for a representative 2,000 kcal diet. The daily meal plan is low in total fat, saturated fat, and cholesterol and high in polyunsaturated fat. Caloric intake is not restricted, but if weight loss is necessary, the number of calories consumed must be reduced.

HYPERTENSION

Definition and Symptoms

Hypertension refers to an arterial blood pressure reading that is higher than normal over a period of time. An acceptable blood pressure reading is 140/90 (systolic/diastolic) mm Hg. Standard medical textbooks list the upper limits of normal blood pressure in different age groups. The clinical distinction between normal and elevated blood pressure, however, is made by the attending physician.

Usually, there are no symptoms of hypertension until complications appear that result from damage to the kidneys, heart, and circulatory system. By the time many of these complications are evident, it may be too late to help an individual. Heart attack or stroke may soon follow, often with fatal results. If symptoms of hypertension are noticeable,

Chapter 17
DIET AND
CARDIO-
VASCULAR
DISEASES

307

TABLE 17-4. Recommended Dietary Prescriptions for Different Types of Hyperlipoproteinemias

Diet Characteristics	Type I	Type IIa	Type IIb	Type III	Type IV	Type V
Nutrient(s) regulated	Fat	Fat	Protein, fat, carbo-hydrate	Protein, fat, carbo-hydrate	Protein, fat, carbo-hydrate	Protein, fat, carbohydrate
Achieve and main-tain ideal body weight	No*	No*	Yes	Yes	Yes	Yes
Protein:						
% total calories	Any	Any	20	20	15–25	15–25
Carbohydrate:						
% total calories	Any	Any	40	40	45	50
Restrictions	None	None	Sweets	Sweets	Sweets	Sweets
Fat:						
% total calories	12–20†	Any	40	40	20–35	12–30‡
Saturated fat, % total calories	Any	4–7.5	4–7.5	4–7.5	4–7.5	4–7.5
PUFA,§ % total calories	Any	8–13‖	8–13‖	8–13‖	8–13‖	8–13‖
P/S ratio˙	Any	1.5–3.0/1	1.9/1	1.2–2.4/1	1–2.4/1	0.5–1.5/1
Cholesterol per day	No limit	100–300 mg	100–300 mg	100–300 mg	300–500 mg	300–500 mg
Alcohol	Not recommended	May be used with discretion	0–2 oz hard liquor#	0–2 oz hard liquor#	0–2 oz hard liquor#	Not recommended

*No restriction on caloric intake.
†Limited to 25 to 35 g per day.
‡As low as practical.
§Polyunsaturated fatty acids.
‖High level of PUFAs is recommended.
˙PUFA/saturated fatty acids.
#Amount of liquor consumed must replace equivalent amount of carbohydrate prescribed.

they include dizziness, headaches, and/or palpitations. High blood pressure is a very important risk factor in the development of cardiovascular diseases. The higher the blood pressure, the greater the risk.

Incidence and Causes

It is estimated that there may be 25 or 30 million Americans with un-identified, untreated, or poorly controlled high blood pressure. Some important considerations in hypertension are race, age, and sex. Black

TABLE 17-5. Foods Permitted and Prohibited in a Fat-Controlled Preventive Diet

Food Group	Foods Permitted	Foods Prohibited
Beverages	Coffee: regular, decaffeinated Soft drinks: regular, low calorie Tea: weak, strong Miscellaneous: fruit juices, punches, flavored drinks, Postum Any dietetic low-calorie beverages with or without artificial sweeteners	All alcoholic beverages unless permitted by doctor; eggnog, milkshakes, malt drinks, chocolate drinks
Breads, grains, equivalents	No restriction on number of servings. Breads: Italian, raisin, white, whole wheat, Boston brown, French Vienna, cracked wheat, pumpernickel Rolls: all made with skim milk and very little saturated fat including plain pan, hard, and whole wheat Biscuits: homemade with skim milk and polyunsaturated fats Cereals: all ready-to-eat and cooked excluding those made with coconut and fat Flours: all varieties Crackers: pretzels, rusk, all others not containing butter and cheese Tortillas made with polyunsaturated oil, zwieback, bread sticks Miscellaneous products made with skim milk, permitted egg allowance, and polyunsaturated vegetable oil: English muffins, French toast, muffins, pancakes, quick breads, waffles, cornbread	Bread: made with egg and cheese Biscuits: all commercial varieties Crackers: made with butter and cheese All commercial products including doughnuts, muffins, puff pastry, popovers, sweet rolls, Danish pastry, spoon bread, unless they are homemade or special products made with skim milk and polyunsaturated fats and permitted egg allowance; all commercial mixes using saturated fats, whole milk, or dried eggs
Milk, milk products	Skim milk (fortified with vitamins A and D): fluid, powder Fermented skim milk: buttermilk, yogurt Other skim milk products: canned (evaporated), cocoa (with cocoa powder)	Fluid milk: whole, 2% low-fat Fermented whole milk: yogurt Canned whole milk: evaporated, condensed, powder Other whole milk products: regular hot chocolate, cocoa Cream: light, heavy, half and half, sour; nondairy creamers and products made from them
Cheese, cheese products	Servings must replace milk allotments. All cheeses made from partially or fully skimmed milk—e.g., uncreamed cottage; baker's, farmer, or hoop; sapsago; mozzarella, and dietetic cheese low in fat and cholesterol and high in polyunsaturated fats.	All cheeses made from cream or whole milk—e.g., brick, Camembert, American, Roquefort, blue, cream, cheddar, Gouda, Edam, Parmesan, Neufchâtel, ricotta, Swiss, processed; all cheeses not specifically permitted; any commercial products made from the above cheeses

TABLE 17-5. (continued)

Food Group	Foods Permitted	Foods Prohibited
Eggs	Three whole eggs per week maximum; no limitation on egg whites and dietetic egg substitutes; prepared in any form with permitted ingredients such as skim milk and polyunsaturated fats and oils	Eggs prepared in all other forms; egg yolk limited to 3 per week
Meats and equivalents	Maximum of 9 oz daily Chicken, turkey, veal: baked, broiled, roasted, stewed; no skin Shellfish: most varieties (shrimp is low in fat and high in cholesterol; use less than 8 oz per week) (4 oz = 1 meat equivalent) Fish: most varieties Beef, lamb, pork, ham: use less frequently; use lean cuts with visible fat trimmed, fat drippings excluded; baked, broiled, roasted, stewed Beans: baked, vegetarian, all dried forms Peas: all dried forms Nuts: all varieties except walnuts and those prohibited Peanut butter Textured vegetable protein	Goose, duck; spareribs, frankfurters, sausages, cold cuts; heavily fatty and marbled meats All forms of organ meat: chicken liver, beef liver, sweetbread, heart, kidney (If liver is eaten, use once a week. If liver is totally excluded, monitor other sources of iron.); canned pork and beans Nuts: macadamia and cashew
Desserts	All homemade cakes, pies, cookies, icings, and pie crust using permitted eggs, skim milk, and polyunsaturated oils Ice milk, fruit cobblers, imitation ice cream made with polyunsaturated oil, sherbet, water ices; gelatin, plain or fruit, fruit whips, puddings; tapioca and rice products made with skim milk, permitted eggs, and polyunsaturated oils; bread, rennet, cornstarch	Most commercial desserts such as pies, cakes, cookies, puddings, ice cream, cheesecake, eclairs, strudel, turnovers, and many others prepared with whole milk, saturated fat, cream, and eggs
Sweets	Syrups, sugars, molasses, honey; preserves, jellies, jams; hard candy, candied fruits; marshmallows, marmalades	All varieties of candy made with whole milk, saturated fat, eggs, chocolate, and chocolate sauces
Potatoes, equivalents	Number of servings not limited Potatoes: boiled, baked, mashed, creamed, scalloped with polyunsaturated fat and skim milk, salad with no egg Sweet potatoes and yams: canned, mashed, boiled, baked Bread stuffing; barley; macaroni, rice, spaghetti, noodles, bulgur, wild rice; fritters, dumplings, prepared with daily permitted egg, skim milk, and polyunsaturated fats	All potatoes and equivalents prepared with whole milk, eggs, bacon, butter, cream, cheese, meat drippings, or shortening

TABLE 17-5. (continued)

Food Group	Foods Permitted	Foods Prohibited
Fruits, vegetables	All	No restrictions except those items prepared with excluded food products
Fats	No limit on permitted fats and oils; daily servings at least 2–4 T Vegetable oils: sesame, soybean, sunflower, corn, cottonseed Margarine: made with polyunsaturated oils; if hydrogenated, must contain acceptable amount of polyunsaturated oils (recommended liquid vegetable oil listed as first ingredient, and one or more partially hydrogenated vegetable oils as additional ingredients) Gravies, sauces, salad dressings (Italian, French, mayonnaise, and similar varieties) made with skim milk, polyunsaturated oils, and other permitted ingredients	All regular butter and margarine (including completely hydrogenated items); Roquefort and blue cheese salad dressings; solid shortening, lard, bacon drippings, regular gravies, meat drippings, any dressing containing cheese Oils: olive, palm, coconut, peanut (if used, limit to small amounts)
Soups	Number of servings not limited Soups: gumbos, chowders, onion, vegetable, dehydrated, packaged, bisques, and cream Broths, consommés, bouillon cubes and powder, any clear soup with no fat Only skim milk and polyunsaturated fats permitted in both commercial and homemade soups	Any commercial soup made with whole milk and saturated fats; e.g., cream soups; any commercial soup made with bacon or ham; e.g., split pea and bean soups
Miscellaneous	Spices and seasonings: soy sauce, Worcestershire sauce, all herbs and spices, cream of tartar, baking powder, sodium bicarbonate, salt, salt substitutes, monosodium glutamate, artificial sweeteners, garlic, chutney, capers, horseradish, catsup, pickles, gelatin, popcorn Sauces: chili sauce; cranberry sauce; aspic; all barbecue, creole, sweet and sour, tomato, and cocktail sauces made with skim milk and polyunsaturated oils	Most commercial snacks such as potato chips, dips; creamed dishes; olives; frozen or packaged dinners; commercial popcorn, coffee cream substitutes; any product made with saturated oil, whole milk, and eggs not within allowance

Note: Table adapted from: (1) *The Way to a Man's Heart*. American Heart Association, 1972. By permission of the American Heart Association, Inc.; (2) *Planning Fat-Controlled Meals for 1200 and 1800 Calories*. American Heart Association, 1966. By permission of the American Heart Association, Inc.

Chapter 17
DIET AND
CARDIO-
VASCULAR
DISEASES

311

TABLE 17-6. Meal Plan for a Prudent Diet

Breakfast	Lunch	Dinner
1 serving breakfast cereal	3 oz meat or equivalent	3 oz meat or equivalent
½ c fruit or fruit juice	½ c potato or 1 serving equivalent	½ c potato or equivalent
1 sl bread or toast with 2 t margarine (vegetable oil)	½ c fruit or juice	½ c fruit or juice
Jelly or equivalent	1 serving clear broth	1 serving clear broth
½ c skim milk	½ c vegetable	½ c vegetable
Coffee or tea	1 serving salad with 1 T permitted dressing	1 serving salad with 1 T permitted dressing
1 t sugar	1 sl bread or toast or equivalent (e.g., 1 roll) with 2 t margarine (vegetable oil)	1 sl bread or equivalent (e.g., 1 roll) with 2 t margarine (vegetable oil)
Salt and pepper if needed	1 serving dessert or fruit	1 c skim milk
	Coffee or tea	1 serving dessert or fruit
	1 t sugar	Coffee or tea
	Salt and pepper if needed	1 t sugar
		Salt and pepper if needed

Note: Menu supplies 2,000 kcal, 75 to 80 g of protein, 70 to 75 g of fat, and 270 to 280 g of carbohydrate. If eggs are desired, limit to three a week.

Americans are twice as likely to have it as whites and more likely to die as a result. For unknown reasons, blood pressure increases with age, although hypertension occurs more commonly between the ages of 25 and 55. The disorder is more common in women than men.

Some of the suspected causes of hypertension are heredity, obesity, excessive salt intake, lack of physical activity, and an unwholesome lifestyle that may include excessive alcohol consumption and frequent, irregular meals. Any one of these alone may elevate blood pressure. If two or more of these factors are present, the likelihood of hypertension increases dramatically. Of all suspected causes, obesity and excessive salt intake are of the most interest to nutritionists and dietitians.

Obesity

Obesity and hypertension are related in many ways. It is more likely that an obese patient has high blood pressure, and also more likely that the same patient will die of heart disease. An obese person who does not have high blood pressure is more likely to develop hypertension than an individual of normal weight. An already hypertensive patient also has a greater tendency to gain weight than a person with normal blood pressure. This is a vicious cycle that is difficult to break.

Salt

Since the 1930s, eating too much salt throughout life has been suggested as a cause of hypertension. Some experts consider the average American salt consumption of 10 to 15 g daily to be too great. Certain other population groups (especially non-Western cultures) who have had low salt intakes since childhood also show an absence of hypertension. Restriction of salt intake can decrease blood pressure.

Treatment

There are several methods to keep hypertension under control and reduce the risk of heart disease. These include drug therapy, diet therapy, and a more wholesome lifestyle.

Drug Therapy

Drug therapy plays an important role in correcting hypertension. Diuretics and other drugs that lower blood pressure are most commonly used. By eliminating sodium, diuretics reduce the amount of fluid in the blood. Other drugs, such as hydralazine, help prevent the narrowing of the blood vessels. Drugs are most effective when used together with proper treatment of nutritional imbalances.

Diet Therapy

Dietary considerations in managing a hypertensive patient fall into two categories: (1) sodium and fluid retention, and (2) intake of calories. Because the presence of sodium causes the body to retain fluids, which is partially responsible for high blood pressure, decreasing sodium intake is important. It is now firmly established that a moderate restriction in sodium intake definitely increases the effectiveness of drug therapy for hypertension. The degree of sodium restriction is determined by: (1) the patient's clinical condition, (2) the drug therapy program, and (3) the patient's response to different treatments.

Hypertensive patients should consume enough calories to maintain an ideal weight. There are a number of special considerations for overweight patients: (1) Every effort must be made to achieve and maintain ideal body weight. (2) If dieting fails, a patient should be treated with

Chapter 17
DIET AND
CARDIO-
VASCULAR
DISEASES

313

drugs and sodium restriction. (3) A good exercise program should be established both to lower blood pressure and to reduce weight. (4) Light meals are recommended, since heavy meals cause the heart to work harder and blood pressure to fluctuate. Planning a low-sodium diet is presented below.

Everyone should follow a wholesome lifestyle, especially hypertensive individuals. This topic will be further explored at the end of this chapter.

CONGESTIVE HEART FAILURE

Symptoms

In congestive heart failure, the heart fails to pump enough blood for the body's needs. More than half of all patients with organic cardiovascular disease eventually develop congestive heart failure. Although only one side of the heart may be affected at first, the condition gradually worsens until both sides of the heart are involved. Symptoms may include: labored breathing, breathing possible only in an upright position, liver enlargement, **edema** (swelling of tissues due to excess fluid retention), and heart enlargement. In more than half of the cases of congestive heart failure, there are indentifiable causes such as pregnancy, hypertension, atherosclerosis, anemia, and excessive salt intake.

Treatment

The most common symptom of congestive heart failure is excessive retention of water and sodium, which leads to edema. The exact cause of this is unknown. Treatment goals are to increase the strength of heart muscle contractions and to reduce the retention of sodium and water. The nutritional and dietary care of patients with congestive heart failure must take into consideration the following issues: (1) the effects of particular drugs on nutritional status, (2) the control of body weight, (3) the correcting of body sodium and fluid balance, and (4) feeding routines. Drug therapy involves the use of digitalis and other drugs that increase the strength of cardiac contractions. Diuretics are used to eliminate water and sodium. All these drugs, however, can negatively affect the nutritional status of the patient.

Weight Reduction

Excessive fat hinders breathing and circulation, forces the diaphragm to rise, lowers the lung volume, and alters the position of the heart. Fat deposition around the heart can interfere with the heart muscle. Since obesity can make the heart work harder, obese patients should lose weight first. Slightly underweight persons require less oxygen and thus decrease the work the heart must perform.

Correcting Sodium and Fluid Imbalance

A liberal fluid intake can eliminate excess sodium from the body. Care must be taken to avoid combining excessive fluid intake with severe sodium restriction, however, since the result may be a dilution of body fluid rather than the desired sodium reduction. The remedy in this case is to restrict fluid intake, not to increase salt consumption.

The possible complications and side effects should always be considered when regulating body fluid and sodium. For example, sodium restriction may also result in the removal of other electrolytes from the body. Diuretics, too, have notorious side effects. One of the most common is potassium deficiency. Low blood potassium can be dangerous, since it affects the overall electrolyte balance of the body, especially if the patient is also receiving other medication. Measures to guard against excessive loss of potassium are: (1) careful prescription of diuretics and avoidance of continuous use, (2) greater use of potassium-rich foods and the use of oral potassium supplements, and (3) changing to a diuretic that does not cause excessive loss of potassium.

Feeding Routines

The routine feedings of a patient with congestive heart failure are very simple but should follow a few guidelines. Small, frequent feedings should be given to avoid fatigue and heavy breathing. The meal should be well balanced, nutritious, and light, composed mostly of easily digestible carbohydrates and a moderate amount of protein. High protein intake makes the heart work harder. Fats and vitamins should be adequate. Salt intake should be restricted according to the seriousness of the patient's condition. Finally, fiber and any food products that the patient has difficulty tolerating should not be served.

PLANNING SODIUM-CONTROLLED DIETS

A sodium-restricted diet is one in which a lower than normal amount of sodium is specified. Table 17-7 defines five types of sodium-restricted diet with five levels of sodium content. Some common descriptions for these diets are also included. For reference purposes, 23 mg sodium =

Chapter 17
DIET AND
CARDIO-
VASCULAR
DISEASES

315

TABLE 17-7. Amount of Sodium in Sodium-Controlled Diets

Diet	Approximate Sodium Content mg	Approximate Sodium Content mEq	Approximate Equivalent of Table Salt (mg NaCl)	Common Descriptive Term
1	250	11	625	Very low or rigid restriction sodium diet
2	500	22	1,250	Strict sodium restriction, severe sodium restriction, or low-sodium diet
3	1,000	43	2,500	Moderate sodium restriction diet
4	2,000	87	5,000	Mild restriction or mild sodium-regulated diet
5	≥2,000	≥87	≥5,000	Regulated diet without addition of table salt

TABLE 17-8. Approximate Nutrient Contents of the Sodium Food Exchange Lists

Sodium Food Exchange List	Food Type	Food Group	Caloric or Nutrient Level in One Exchange Sodium (mg)	kcal	Carbohydrate (g)	Fat (g)	Protein (g)
I	Milk	I-1	7	170	12	10	8
		I-2	120	170	12	10	8
II	Vegetables	II-1	9	0	0	0	0
		II-2	9	35	7	0	2
III	Fruits	III	2	40	10	0	0
IV	Bread, equivalents	IV-1	5	70	15	0	2
		IV-2	5	70	15	0	2
		IV-3	100–300	70	15	0	2
V	Meat, equivalents	V	25	75	0	5	7
VI	Fat	VI	0	45	0	5	0
VII	Alternates	VII*					

Adapted from (1) *Sodium Restricted Diet: 1000 Milligrams*, 1970; (2) *Your 500 Milligram Sodium Diet*, undated; (3) *Your Mild Sodium-Restricted Diet*, undated. American Heart Association. By permission of the American Heart Association, Inc.

*Nutrient contents vary.

TABLE 17-9. Sodium Food Exchange List I-1: Milk

Food	One Exchange	Adjustment
Low-sodium, fluid, fresh, whole milk	1 c	None
Low-sodium, reconstituted dry milk	1 c	None
Powdered low-sodium dry milk	4 T	None
Powdered low-sodium nonfat dry milk	3 T	Follow instruction on package to obtain 1 exchange. If used, must add 2 fat exchanges from List IV-1.
Reconstituted low-sodium nonfat dry milk	1 c	If used, must add 2 fat exchanges from List IV-1.
Low-sodium cocoa (low-sodium milk and cocoa powder)	⅔ c	

Foods to be avoided

1. All milk and milk products not specifically indicated.
2. All commercial milk and milk products: ice cream, sherbet, milk shakes, chocolate milk, malted milk, milk mixes, condensed milk, breakfast milk drinks, instant milk products, and others.

Note: Each exchange contains 7 mg of sodium, 170 kcal, 12 g of carbohydrate, 10 g of fat, and 8 g of protein.

Adapted from *Your 500 Milligram Sodium Diet*, undated, American Heart Association. By permission of the American Heart Association, Inc.

1 mEq sodium; mg sodium = mg sodium chloride × 0.393; and mg sodium chloride = mg sodium × 2.54.

The American Heart Association has developed Sodium Food Exchange Lists to assist in designing meal plans for such diets. Each exchange list is made up of various foods that contain approximately the same amounts of sodium, calories, protein, carbohydrate, and fat. Table 17-8 summarizes the approximate nutritional contents of these exchange lists. Tables 17-9 through 17-20 describe the specific food items permitted and prohibited within each exchange list. Table 17-21 indicates permitted and prohibited spices, condiments, gravies, and sauces for a patient on a sodium-restricted diet. Using these exchange lists, Table 17-22 presents specific meal plans (numbers of exchanges) for

Chapter 17
DIET AND
CARDIO-
VASCULAR
DISEASES

317

TABLE 17-10. Sodium Food Exchange List I-2: Milk

Food	One Exchange	Adjustment
Buttermilk, uncultured and unsalted, from whole milk	1 c	None
Buttermilk, regular, commercially cultured, from nonfat milk	½ c	If used, add 3 fat exchanges from List VI.
Chocolate milk	⅔ c	
Cocoa (powder and regular fluid milk)	⅔ c	
Ice cream	⅔ c	
Whole milk	1 c	
Whole milk dry powder	3 T	Follow instruction on package to obtain 1 exchange.
Nonfat dry milk powder	3 T	Follow instruction on package to obtain 1 exchange. If used, add 2 fat exchanges from List VI.
Reconstituted nonfat dry milk	1 c	If used, add 2 fat exchanges from List VI.
Skim milk	1 c	If used, add 2 fat exchanges from List VI.
Yogurt	1 c	

Note: Each exchange contains 120 mg of sodium, 170 kcal, 12 g of carbohydrate, 10 g of fat, and 8 g of protein.

Adapted from *Your 500 Milligram Sodium Diet*, undated, American Heart Association. By permission of the American Heart Association, Inc.

TABLE 17-11. Sodium Food Exchange List II-1: Vegetables

Food*				One Exchange
Asparagus	Cauliflower	Mushrooms	Tomatoes	½ c
Beans, green	Chicory	Okra	Turnip greens	
Beans, wax	Cucumber	Peppers, green	Watercress	
Broccoli	Eggplant	and red		
Brussels	Endive	Radishes		
sprouts	Escarole	Squash, summer		
Cabbage	Lettuce	Tomato juice,		
		canned, unsalted		
Carrots, raw				2–3 strips
Mustard greens				⅓ c
Parsley				⅓ c
Water chestnuts, raw				2–3 corms

Foods to be avoided

1. Artichokes, beet greens, celery, chard, dandelion greens, hominy, kale, sauerkraut, spinach, and white turnips.
2. Canned vegetables or vegetable juices except low-sodium dietetic products.
3. Frozen vegetables processed with salt (e.g., lima beans, frozen peas, and succotash) or with salt added during preparation.

Note: Each exchange contains 9 mg of sodium, few calories, and traces of carbohydrate, fat, and protein.

*All fresh or frozen products with no salt added or dietetic or low-sodium products.

Adapted from *Your 500 Milligram Sodium Diet*, undated, American Heart Association. By permission of the American Heart Association, Inc.

TABLE 17-12. Sodium Food Exchange List II-2: Vegetables

Food	One Exchange
Onions	½ c
Peas (fresh or low-sodium dietetic canned only)	
Pumpkin	
Rutabaga (yellow turnip)	
Squash, winter (acorn, Hubbard, etc.)	

Foods to be avoided

Same as for Sodium Food Exchange List II-1.

Note: Each exchange contains 9 mg of sodium, 35 kcal, 2 g of protein, no fat, and 7 g of carbohydrate. Two exchanges from List II-1 equals 1 exchange from List II-2.

Adapted from *Your 500 Milligram Sodium Diet*, undated, American Heart Association. By permission of the American Heart Association, Inc.

Chapter 17
DIET AND
CARDIO-
VASCULAR
DISEASES

319

TABLE 17-13. Sodium Food Exchange List III: Fruits

Food	One Exchange
Apple, small	1
Apple juice or cider	⅓ c
Applesauce	½ c
Apricot nectar	¼ c
Apricots, dried, halves	4
Apricots, fresh, medium	2
Banana, small	½
Blackberries	1 c
Blueberries	⅔ c
Cantaloupe	¼ c
Cherries, large	10
Cranberries (sweetened)	1 T
Cranberries (unsweetened)	No limit
Cranberry juice (sweetened)	⅓ c
Cranberry juice (unsweetened)	No limit
Dates	2
Fig, medium	1
Fruit cup or mixed fruits	½ c
Grapefruit, small	½
Grapefruit juice	½ c
Grape juice	¼ c
Grapes	12
Honeydew melon, medium	⅛
Lemons	No limit
Limes	No limit
Mango, small	½
Orange, small	1
Orange juice	½ c
Papaya, medium	⅓

TABLE 17-13. (continued)

Food	One Exchange
Peach, medium	1
Pear, small	1
Pineapple, small, slices	2
diced	½ c
Pineapple juice	⅓ c
Plums, medium	2
Prunes, medium	2
Prune juice	¼ c
Raisins	2 T
Raspberries	1 c
Rhubarb (sweetened)	2 T
Rhubarb (unsweetened)	No limit
Strawberries	1 c
Tangerine, large	1
Tangerine juice	½ c
Watermelon	1 c

Foods to be avoided

1. Dried fruits and all commercial products containing sodium salts or preservatives.
2. Crystallized or glazed fruit.

Note: Each exchange contains 2 mg of sodium, 40 kcal, no protein, no fat, and 10 g of carbohydrate. If sweetened fruit or fruit canned or frozen in sugar syrup is used, the caloric content may have to be adjusted.

Adapted from *Your 500 Milligram Sodium Diet*, undated, American Heart Association. By permission of the American Heart Association, Inc.

a 2,000– to 2,100–kcal diet at different sodium levels. Table 17-23 provides a sample daily menu plan for a 2,000-kcal diet with 500 mg sodium.

PREVENTING CARDIOVASCULAR DISEASE

The recent decline in the actual number of Americans suffering from heart disease confirms that public education about risk factors apparently has begun to succeed. Attitudes toward preventive health care are changing. Obviously it is to every person's advantage to adopt a lifestyle that is conducive to good health.

TABLE 17-14. Sodium Food Exchange List IV-1: Bread and Equivalents

Food	One Exchange
Bread	
White bread, sl	1
Biscuit, medium	1
Bun, hamburger	1
Corn bread, 1½-in. cube	1
Crackers, 2-in. square	5
Griddle cakes, 3 in. diam.	2
Matzo, 5-in. square	1
Muffin, medium	1
Roll, plain yeast, medium	1
Waffle, 3-in. square	1
Cereals, cooked, noninstant	
Oatmeal, rolled oats, wheat meal, farina, corn, grits, Cream of Wheat, toasted wheat germ, dried cornmeal	½ c
Cereals, dry, ready-to-eat	
Enriched Puffed Rice, Puffed Wheat, shredded wheat, Sugar Smacks, other brands (check labels)	½ c
Noodles, flours, and others	
Barley, cooked	½ c
Flour	2½ T
Macaroni, noodles, spaghetti, cooked	½ c
Popcorn	1½ c
Rice, white or brown, cooked	½ c
Tapioca, uncooked	2 T

Foods to be avoided

1. Baking powder, baking soda, and commercial mixes.
2. All instant or quick-cooking cereals and enriched products.
3. Self-rising cornmeal or flour.
4. Any dry cereals not listed.
5. Commercial graham crackers or any other crackers except low-sodium dietetic products.
6. Salted popcorn, potato chips, other chips, pretzels, other salty snack items, and salt sticks.

Note: Each exchange contains 5 mg of sodium, 70 kcal, 15 g of carbohydrate, no fat, and 2 g of protein. All items are made without salt. Where necessary sodium-free baking powder or potassium bicarbonate and low-sodium dietetic mixes are used.

Adapted from *Your 500 Milligram Sodium Diet*, undated, American Heart Association. By permission of the American Heart Association, Inc.

TABLE 17-15. Sodium Food Exchange List IV-2: Bread and Equivalents

Food (starchy vegetables)	One Exchange
Beans, baked	¼ c
Beans, cooked, navy or lima, dried or fresh	½ c
Corn	⅓ c
Lentils, cooked, dried	½ c
Parsnips	⅔ c
Peas, cooked, split, fresh or dried, green or yellow	½ c
Potato, sweet, small	½
Potato, white, mashed	½ c
Potato, white, whole, small	1

Foods to be avoided

Same as those for List IV-1.

Note: Each exchange contains 5 mg of sodium, 70 kcal, 15 g of carbohydrate, no fat, and 2 g of protein. All items are prepared without salt.

Adapted from *Your 500 Milligram Sodium Diet*, undated, American Heart Association. By permission of the American Heart Association, Inc.

TABLE 17-16. Sodium Food Exchange List IV-3: Bread and Equivalents

Food*	One Exchange	Sodium (mg)
Biscuit, medium	1	255
Bread, white, sl	1	140
Bun, hamburger	1	210
Corn bread, 1½-in. cube	1	230
Crackers, 2-in. square	5	100
Griddle cakes, 3 in. diam.	2	300
Muffin, medium	1	180
Roll, plain yeast, medium	1	140
Waffle, 3-in. square	1	180

Note: Each exchange contains 100 to 300 mg of sodium, 70 kcal, 15 g of carbohydrate, no fat, and 2 g of protein.

*Prepared with salt.

Adapted from *Your 500 Milligram Sodium Diet*, undated, American Heart Association. By permission of the American Heart Association, Inc.

TABLE 17-17. Sodium Food Exchange List V: Meat and Equivalents

Food	One Exchange
Meat, poultry, fowl*	
Beef, veal, pork, lamb; chicken, turkey, duck; quail, rabbit; tongue, chicken or pork liver; beef or calf liver[1] (all cooked)	1 oz
Seafood*	
Bass, bluefish, catfish, cod, eels, flounder, halibut, rockfish, salmon, sole, trout, tuna (low-sodium, dietetic pack) (all cooked)	1 oz
Cheese, egg, peanut butter	
Cheese, low sodium, dietetic	1 oz
Cottage cheese, unsalted	¼ c
Egg	1
Peanut butter, low sodium, dietetic	2 T

Foods to be avoided

1. Brain, kidney.
2. All processed meat products, e.g., luncheon meat, sausages, and ham.
3. All commercially processed seafood products unless dietetic.
4. Frozen seafoods containing salt, e.g., Icelandic.
5. All shellfish such as oysters, scallops, shrimp, crab, and clams.
6. Regular peanut butter.

Note: Each exchange contains 25 mg of sodium, 75 kcal, no carbohydrate, 5 g of fat, and 7 g of protein.

*Fresh unsalted, frozen unsalted, or dietetic products.

[1] 1 to 2 exchanges allowed in 2 weeks.

Adapted from *Your 500 Milligram Sodium Diet*, undated, American Heart Association. By permission of the American Heart Association, Inc.

TABLE 17-18. Sodium Food Exchange List VI-1: Fat

Food	One Exchange
Butter or margarine	1 t
Cream, heavy, sweet or sour*	1 T
Cream, light, sweet or sour*	2 T
Fat or oil, all purposes	1 t
Mayonnaise	1 t
Salad dressing	1 T
Others	
Avocado, 4 in. diam.	⅛
Nuts, small	6

Foods to be avoided

1. Bacon and bacon fat.
2. Olives.
3. Salt pork.
4. Commercial French dressing.

Note: Each exchange contains no sodium, 45 kcal, 5 g of fat, and no protein. All items are unsalted or dietetic products.

*Limited to 2 T/d.

Adapted from *Your 500 Milligram Sodium Diet*, undated, American Heart Association. By permission of the American Heart Association, Inc.

TABLE 17-19. Sodium Food Exchange List VI-2: Fat

Food	One Exchange
Butter, salted	1 t
Margarine, salted	1 t
Mayonnaise	1 t

Note: Each exchange contains 50 mg of sodium, 45 kcal, 5 g of fat, and no protein.

TABLE 17-20. Sodium Food Exchange List VII: Alternates

Food Type	Foods Permitted*	Foods Prohibited
Sugars, sweets	Low-sodium dietetic or homemade candies without salt, including hard candy, gumdrops, mints, and marshmallows; maple syrup and sugar (brown, granulated, and confectioner's)	All commercial products with salt or sodium compounds and/or butter added; molasses, corn syrup
Beverages	Coffee (instant, regular, substitute, or decaffeinated), tea, and Postum; selected carbonated beverages;† content of alcoholic beverages permitted by physician should be counted	Most commercial instant and quick drink mixes, e.g., fruit-flavored powders; fountain beverages and various brands of carbonated soft drinks
Desserts	Plain or flavored gelatin with permitted juices; pies or tapioca (pudding) made with permitted fruit and other ingredients; ices and Popsicles flavored with permitted juices and fruits; rennet dessert powder	Commercial gelatin made with sodium and other prohibited ingredients; commercial products made with salt; rennet dessert tablets
Miscellaneous	Any low-sodium dietetic products, e.g., soups, puddings; leavening agents: cream of tartar, potassium bicarbonate, sodium-free baking powder; cornmeal, tapioca, cornstarch, most spices (see text)	All forms of commercial soups (dehydrated, canned, or frozen) prepared with salt or sodium compounds

*These food items do not take into consideration the carbohydrate (quantity and quality) and caloric intake of the patient. They must be adjusted if the patient is on a weight-controlled or hyperlipoproteinemia-modified diet.

†Some beverages may be permitted depending on the degree of sodium restriction and the actual sodium content of the beverage.

Adapted from *Your 500 Milligram Sodium Diet*, undated, American Heart Association. By permission of the American Heart Association, Inc.

Chapter 17
DIET AND
CARDIO-
VASCULAR
DISEASES

323

TABLE 17-21. Spices, Condiments, Gravies, and Sauces Permitted and Prohibited in a Sodium-Regulated Diet

Products Permitted			Products Prohibited
Allspice	Horseradish, pre-	Peppermint extract	Broth, bouillon
Almond extract	pared without salt	Pimiento peppers for	Celery: seed, salt, dried or fresh leaves
Anise seed	Juniper	garnish	unless specifically indicated
Basil	Lemon juice or	Poppy seed	Horseradish prepared with salt
Bay leaf	extract	Poultry seasoning	Meat: extracts, sauces, tenderizers
Caraway seed	Mace	Purslane	MSG or sodium salt of other flavoring aids
Cardamom	Maple extract	Rosemary	Mustard, prepared
Carrots or celery (use	Marjoram	Saffron	Olives
sparingly)	Meat extract, low-	Sage	Pickles
Catsup, low-sodium	sodium dietetic	Salt substitutes (if per-	Relishes
dietetic	Meat tenderizers,	mitted by doctor)	Sugar substitute, sodium salt
Chili powder	low-sodium	Savory	Salt: regular, chili, garlic, onion
Chives	dietetic	Sesame seeds	Sauces: barbecue, soy, Worcestershire
Cinnamon	Mint	Sorrel	Wine: cooking, unless specifically
Cloves	Mustard, dry or seed	Tarragon	indicated
Cocoa (1–2 t)	Nutmeg	Thyme	
Coconut	Onion: fresh, juice,	Turmeric	
Cumin	powder	Vanilla extract	
Curry	Orange extract	Vinegar	
Dill	Oregano	Walnut extract	
Fennel	Paprika	Wine (use sparingly;	
Garlic: fresh, juice,	Parsley: fresh or	more allowed if	
powder	flakes	permitted by	
Ginger	Pepper, fresh, green,	doctor)	
	or red		
	Pepper, black, red, or		
	white		

Adapted from *Your 500 Milligram Sodium Diet*, undated, American Heart Association. By permission of the American Heart Association, Inc.

Some scientists feel that a diet of fewer saturated fats in infancy and childhood could reduce heart disease in adulthood, but this is a very controversial issue. Knowledge about the basic food groups will help in selecting an appropriate diet.

There are many things an adult can do to establish a wholesome lifestyle and thereby promote good health. It is to everyone's advantage to: (1) have regular medical checkups, (2) achieve and maintain an ideal weight, (3) eat a nutritious and well-balanced diet, (4) avoid or control high blood pressure, (5) minimize stress, (6) follow a regular exercise program, (7) drink only moderately, (8) stop smoking. Awareness and moderation are the keys to preventive health care.

TABLE 17-22. Distribution of Food Exchanges in a 2,000- to 2,100-kcal Diet at Different Sodium Levels

Sodium Food Exchange List	Food Type	Food Group	No. of Exchanges			
			250 mg sodium	500 mg sodium	1,000 mg sodium	2,000 mg sodium
I	Milk	I-1	2	—	—	—
		I-2	—	2	2	2
II	Vegetables	II-1	2	2	2	2
		II-2	2	2	2	2
III	Fruits	III	3–5	3–5	3–5	3–5
IV	Bread	IV-1* or IV-2*	6	6	3	2
		IV-3	—	—	3	4
V	Meat, equivalents	V	5	6	6	6
VI	Fat	VI-1	3–6	3–6	3–6	—
		VI-2	—	—	—	3
VII	Alternates	VII	—	—	—	1–3

*Permitted number of exchanges may be selected from one or both groups.

TABLE 17-23 Sample Menu for a 500-mg-Sodium, 2,000-kcal Diet

Breakfast	Lunch	Dinner
Juice, orange, ½ c	Mushrooms, ½ c	Mustard greens, ⅓ c
Puffed Rice, ½ c	Peas, fresh, ½ c	Margarine, unsalted, 1 t
Banana, sliced, ½	Corn bread, prepared without salt, 3-in. square, 1	Onion, ½ c
Toast, low-sodium bread, 1 sl		Muffin, prepared without salt, medium, 1
Margarine, unsalted, 1 t	Margarine, unsalted, 2 t	Margarine, unsalted, 1 t
Egg, soft cooked, 1	Chicken, unsalted, barbecued, without barbecue sauce, 2 oz	Barley, cooked, unsalted, ½ c
Milk, 1 c		Pork, roast, 3 oz
		Ice cream, ⅔ c
		Blueberries, frozen, ½ c

Note: The patient should be encouraged to use unsalted fat and alternate items (List VII) in order to achieve the caloric level of 2,000 kcal if so approved by the dietitian.

Chapter 17
DIET AND
CARDIO-
VASCULAR
DISEASES

325

STUDY QUESTIONS

1. Describe the clinical events that lead to atherosclerosis and death. What complications can result from the atherosclerotic process?
2. Describe the dietary care of a heart patient during the acute phase.
3. What are the multiple risk factors in atherosclerosis? Do some library research and discuss two non-nutritive factors in detail.
4. What correlations exist between differing levels of serum cholesterol and atherosclerosis? What is the current thinking on the relationship between ingested polyunsaturated fat and serum cholesterol level?
5. Define *lipoprotein*. What is the function of chylomicrons?
6. What are the five types of hyperlipoproteinemia? Describe their associated clinical symptoms, if any. Describe the dietary management for one type of hyperlipoproteinemia.
7. What is hypertension? What accounts for complications stemming from hypertension? What nutritional factors contribute to hypertension?
8. Name the symptoms of congestive heart failure. What is the dietary strategy in the management of congestive heart failure?
9. What preventive steps can be taken to minimize the risk of heart disease?
10. Plan a 500 mg sodium diet that provides 2,800 kcal.

REFERENCES

Alexander, S. 1980. *Running healthy: a guide to cardiovascular fitness.* Brattleboro, Vt.: The Stephen Greene Press.

American Heart Association Committee on Nutrition, Diet, and Coronary Heart Disease. 1978. *A statement for physicians and other health professionals.*

Am. J. Nurs. 1981. New concepts in understanding congestive heart failure. Part 2. How the therapeutic approaches work. 81:357.

Braunwald, E., ed. 1980. *Heart disease; a textbook of cardiovascular medicine.* Philadelphia: Saunders.

Hausman, P. 1981. *J. Sprat's legacy: the science and politics of fat and cholesterol.* New York: Richard Marek Publishers.

Hill, M. 1979. Helping the hypertensive patient control sodium intake. *Am. J. Nurs.* 79:906.

Kostas, G. 1980. A hypertension diet education program for public health nurses. *J. Amer. Dietet. Assoc.* 77:570.

———. 1980b. Evaluation and follow-up of a hypertension diet education program. *J. Amer. Dietet. Assoc.* 77:574.

Lequime, J., ed. 1980. *Prevention and treatment of coronary heart disease and its complications.* Amsterdam, Holland: Excerpta Medica.

Marsh, A. C., et al. 1980. *The sodium content of your food.* U. S. Department of Agriculture, Science and Education Administration, Home & Garden Bulletin, no. 233. Washington, D. C.

Moses, C., ed. 1980. *Sodium in medicine and health.* Baltimore: Reese Press.

National Academy of Sciences, National Research Council. 1979. *Sodium-restricted diets and the use of diuretics; rationale, complications, and practical aspects of their use.* Washington, D. C.

Chapter 17
DIET AND
CARDIO-
VASCULAR
DISEASES

327

18 DIET AND GASTROINTESTINAL DISEASES

Under normal circumstances, any food that is eaten passes through the gastrointestinal tract. Patients with intestinal disorders, therefore, must often modify their diets. Certain diet therapies are crucial to managing gastrointestinal conditions.

This chapter examines dietary considerations in treating common diseases of the stomach, small and large intestines, and the liver and the conditions of constipation and diarrhea. References will be made to: medium-chain triglycerides (MCTs), defined formula diets, oral nutrient supplements, routine progressive diets (clear liquid to full liquid to soft diets), bland diets, low- and high-residue diets, and low-fat diets. For detailed information on these topics, see other chapters as indicated in the text or refer to the index.

PROBLEMS WITH CLINICAL MANAGEMENT

Certain problems are basic to treating patients with gastrointestinal diseases. In the presence of one or more of the following difficulties, the course of recovery may be impaired: (1) unstable emotional status, such as fear, anxiety, or anger; (2) primary health problems unrelated to gastrointestinal disease (such as obesity or congestive heart failure) that nevertheless manifest symptoms of a gastrointestinal disorder; (3) abnormal nutritional status as part of a vicious cycle leading to and aggravating intestinal disease.

In addition, there is no consensus on the diagnosis and treatment of certain gastrointestinal diseases. Dietary management often varies from one clinician to another and ranges from an extremely rigid dietary regimen to a more individualized approach. However, it is generally agreed that the patient must learn healthy, lifelong dietary habits.

STOMACH

Peptic Ulcer

Refer to Figure 18-1 for names and locations of different parts of the stomach. An ulceration found in the lower end of the esophagus or any part of the stomach or duodenum is generally referred to as a **peptic ulcer.** Any acid or pepsin (an enzyme) present can further erode the ulcerated area.

Symptoms

Pain and abdominal discomfort are major symptoms of a peptic ulcer. The "midepigastric" pain—located high in the abdomen, just below the front of the chest—is often described as steady, burning, and gnawing, like a severe hunger pain. Occurring periodically, the pain lasts a few days, weeks, or months, and is usually relieved by food. Patients may lose weight or, especially in the case of complications, may experience symptoms such as nausea, vomiting, and heartburn.

Causes

Current theory holds that ulceration is related either to an excess of hydrochloric acid or to alterations of the mucosal lining that lower its resistance to acids. Protein in the diet may be prescribed to help decrease acidity, or drugs may be used to buffer or alter its secretion.

The cause of increased acid production and mucosal alteration is not known. Excess acid may be related to overactive or superfluous parietal cells; overproduction of gastrin; rapid food transit; and/or frequent consumption of alcohol, caffeine, or other stimulants.

Rapid food transit may cause continuous ulceration in patients with duodenal ulcers. Food that passes from the stomach to the duodenum, before being sufficiently digested, may cause both mechanical and chemical erosion or ulceration of the area. Such cases of ulceration tend to be more severe and prolonged.

There are several reasons why the stomach mucosa may lose resistance to secreted acid. These include: (1) local gastritis (inflammation); (2) poor nutritional status; (3) alcohol, tobacco smoke, drugs, and other local irritants; (4) such injurious conditions as infection, ischemia, and bile reflux.

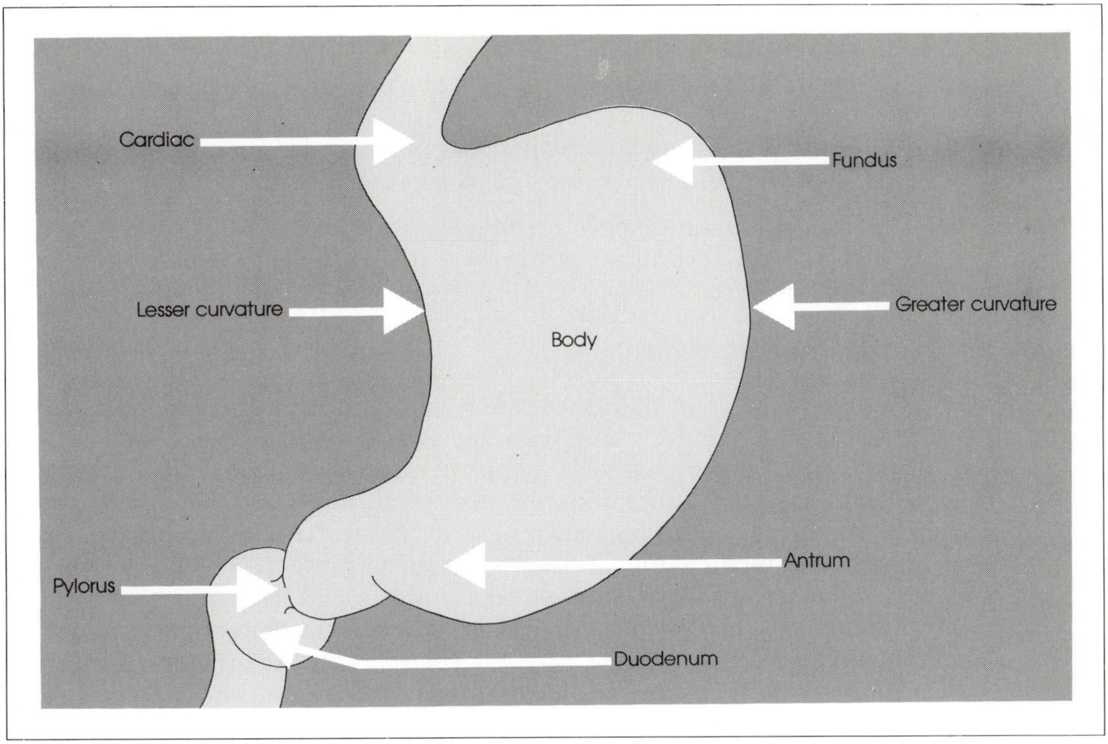

FIGURE 18-1. Parts of the stomach.

As indicated earlier, the causes of increased acid action and decreased mucosal resistance are not known. Suspected of contributing to these conditions are:

- **Heredity.** People who have parents or siblings with a history of gastric or duodenal ulcers are three times more likely to develop ulcers than those whose relatives are free of the disorder.
- **Sex differences.** More men have ulcers than women. During active reproductive years, women seem to be protected from ulcers; however, menopausal women are more susceptible to ulcer development.
- **Serum pepsinogen.** A combination of increased serum pepsinogen (an enzyme), the presence of certain pepsinogen phenotypes, and a particular psychological profile may increase the likelihood of a peptic ulcer.
- **Emotional instability.** People who are chronically anxious or depressed are definitely more prone to developing ulcers than the population in general.
- **Occupational factors.** The stress and hurry typical of certain profes-

sionals such as doctors, firefighters, and business executives predispose the individuals to ulcers.

- **Drugs and smoking.** Although many nonsmokers develop ulcers, heavy smoking is associated with an increased incidence of peptic ulcers. Drugs such as aspirin and other analgesics, alcohol, and sedatives also are implicated as a cause of peptic ulcers.

Two common types of peptic ulcers are gastric ulcers and duodenal ulcers. A list of comparisons is presented in Table 18-1.

Medical Management

The goals of ulcer therapy are to relieve pain and discomfort, to hasten healing, to prevent complications, and to avoid recurrences. An ulcer patient is encouraged to get plenty of rest, eat a modified diet, avoid irritants, and use anticholinergic drugs and antacids. If conditions warrant, surgery may be recommended. Figure 18-2 illustrates the main points of medical management of an ulcer patient.

The relationship between peptic ulcers and irritating agents in the diet has been very controversial. In the past, the dietary treatment of an ulcer patient was very stringent. The patient was ordered to consume only bland foods and to strictly avoid irritating agents. However, such conservative diet therapy is now believed to pose a number of problems. Although milk can relieve pain, it has not been proved to heal ulcers. Furthermore, the usefulness of a bland diet for an ulcer patient has been seriously questioned. At present, no known clinical or dietary method can heal an ulcer permanently. However, it is generally accepted that certain agents such as caffeine and alcohol can irritate the ulceration.

What should the dietary care be for a patient with an ulcer? The dietary strategy of most practitioners reflects two seemingly contradictory guidelines: "No acid, no ulcer" and "Let the patient enjoy his food." At present, many diet manuals use both traditional and recent diet treatments for ulcer patients. Table 18-2 indicates the different types of diet recommendations. Since antacids and drugs are usually part of clinical care, their usage is also indicated in the table. As shown in Table 18-2, during the acute phase of an ulcer, a physician will usually place a patient on a strict ulcer diet. This consists of an hourly program of 4 oz of whole milk, skim milk, or milk and cream. These feedings begin at 7 a.m. and continue until 9 p.m. The physician might also prescribe these feedings at 2-hour intervals during the night. This diet is nutritionally inadequate and should be given for only a brief period. It may be supplemented with an appropriate vitamin and mineral supplement, especially if the treatment lasts more than two or three days. In this case, the physician may prescribe other means of nutritional compensation.

TABLE 18-1. A Comparison of Gastric and Duodenal Ulcers

Criterion	Gastric Ulcer	Duodenal Ulcer
Common anatomical site	At the angulus of the stomach; adjacent to the boundary between the mucosa of the body and the antrum	Generally in the duodenal bulb or cap, i.e., the first 5 cm of the duodenum; within a centimeter of the junction between the pyloric and duodenal mucosa
Hydrochloric acid secretion	Usually normal	Usually high
Occurrence of symptoms	Usually on an empty stomach	Usually within ½ to 2 hours after a meal
Relief of symptoms	By ingesting food or antacids or vomiting	By ingesting food or antacids or vomiting
Ulcer seen by X-rays and/or endoscopy	Yes	Yes
Sex-linked factors		
Male:female incidence	2–3:1	6–12:1
Complications and mortality	Higher in men	Higher in men
Acid secretion per unit body weight	No difference between men and women	Higher in men
Female patients	More common	Less common
Percentage of total population affected	1	5–10
Annual new cases per 1,000 males at risk	1–2	3–4
Age of peak occurrence	40–60	30–50
Gastritis	Usually present, severe, and extensive	May or may not be present
Bile reflux	More frequent	Less frequent
Tendency to develop ulcer in an individual with O-type blood who lacks group AB antigen in the saliva	High	Very high

Chapter 18
DIET AND
GASTRO-
INTESTINAL
DISEASES

333

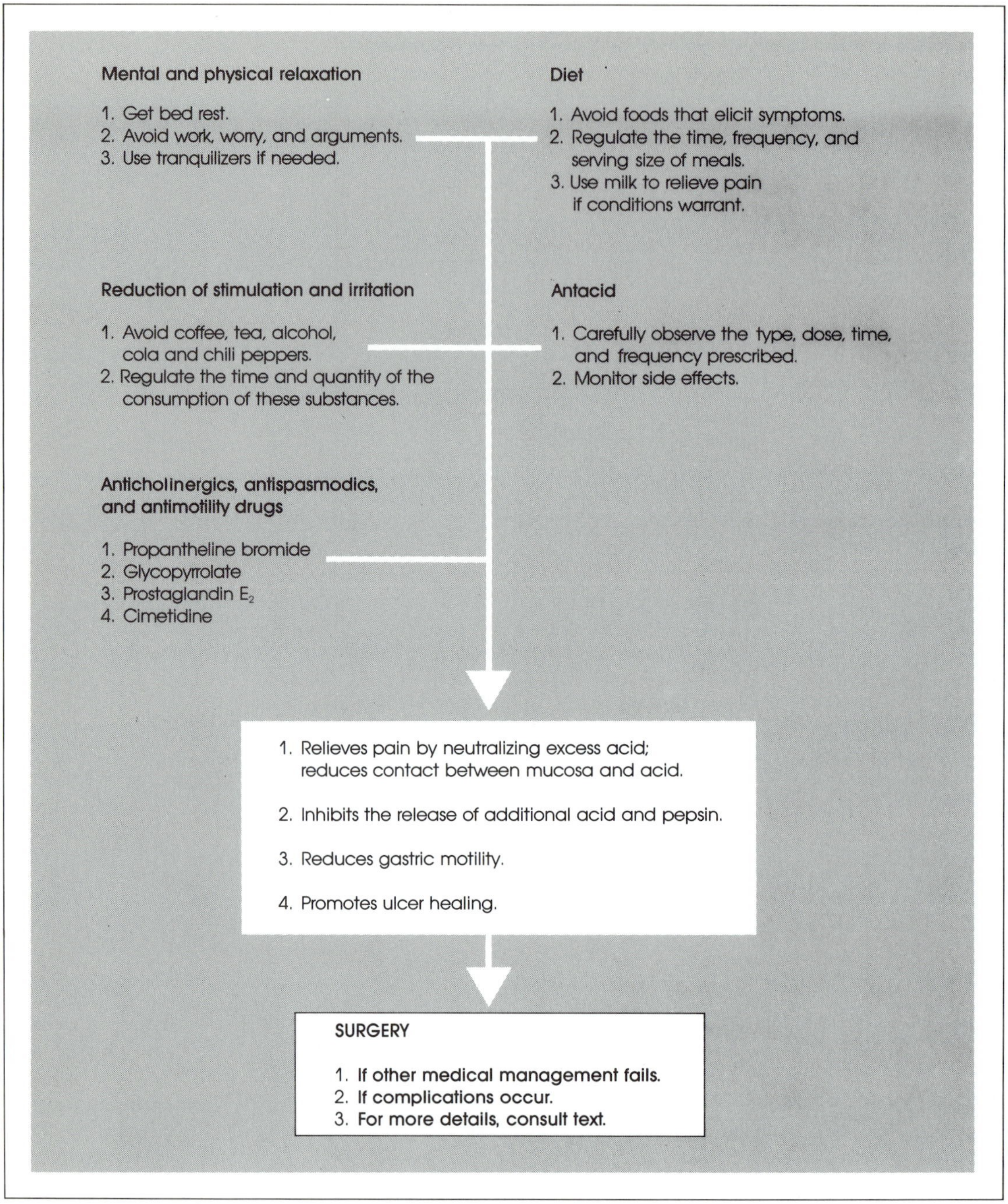

Mental and physical relaxation

1. Get bed rest.
2. Avoid work, worry, and arguments.
3. Use tranquilizers if needed.

Diet

1. Avoid foods that elicit symptoms.
2. Regulate the time, frequency, and serving size of meals.
3. Use milk to relieve pain if conditions warrant.

Reduction of stimulation and irritation

1. Avoid coffee, tea, alcohol, cola and chili peppers.
2. Regulate the time and quantity of the consumption of these substances.

Antacid

1. Carefully observe the type, dose, time, and frequency prescribed.
2. Monitor side effects.

Anticholinergics, antispasmodics, and antimotility drugs

1. Propantheline bromide
2. Glycopyrrolate
3. Prostaglandin E_2
4. Cimetidine

1. Relieves pain by neutralizing excess acid; reduces contact between mucosa and acid.

2. Inhibits the release of additional acid and pepsin.

3. Reduces gastric motility.

4. Promotes ulcer healing.

SURGERY

1. If other medical management fails.
2. If complications occur.
3. For more details, consult text.

FIGURE 18-2. Medical management of a peptic ulcer.

TABLE 18-2. Basic Types of Dietary Recommendations for Ulcer Patients with No Complications

Patient Condition	Strict Ulcer Diet	Liberalized Ulcer Diet	Individualized Ulcer Diet	Antacid*	Anticholinergic*
Acute phase with aggravating symptoms	Recommended	Optional	Optional	Hourly	Recommended
Convalescent with occasional symptoms	Optional	Optional	Optional	Hourly	Recommended
Ambulatory	Optional	Optional	Optional	Between meals and at bedtime	Discontinued
Recurring with symptoms	Optional	Optional	Optional	Hourly	May be resumed

Note: Dietitians, nurses, and physicians work together in planning any diet. Details of each diet are provided in the text.
*Prescribed by physicians.

Milk has been used to relieve ulcer pain for more than 50 years. Because of the high concentration of protein in milk, it is a very effective buffer (pH 6.7) and thus relieves ulcer pain by neutralizing excess acid. However, milk therapy has the following drawbacks:

1. The calcium in milk, when consumed in excess, can bring about hypercalcemia, and thereby a condition called milk-alkali syndrome. Hypercalcemia can also stimulate gastric acid secretion, further aggravating the ulcer.
2. A high consumption of milk can lead to weight gain. This is especially unacceptable for patients who are overweight.
3. Drinking a lot of whole milk can lead to an excessive intake of fat and cholesterol, increasing the risk of myocardial infarction and atherosclerosis.
4. The buffering capacity of milk protein is actually quite weak. Milk protein and its digested products can also eventually stimulate gastric acid secretion (acid rebound). This undesirable effect of protein in ulcer treatment is illustrated in Figure 18-3. As shown in this figure, the use of an antacid may alleviate part of the discomfort from acid rebound.

As shown in Table 18-3, a liberalized ulcer diet may also be prescribed, especially for convalescent and ambulatory patients or patients with recurring symptoms. Details of such a regimen are presented in Tables 18-4 and 18-5. The foods listed may be consumed in many small meals or in three moderate meals with three snacks interspersed. This diet eliminates substances that irritate the gastric lining or increase the

Chapter 18
DIET AND
GASTRO-
INTESTINAL
DISEASES

335

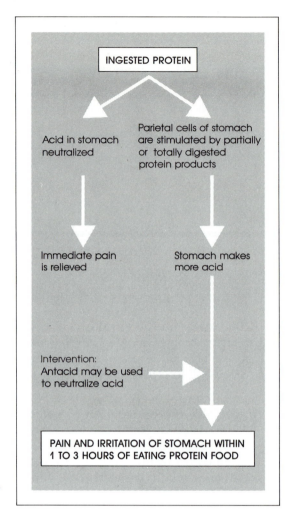

FIGURE 18-3. Contrasting effects of protein in ulcer treatment.

The diagram shows:

INGESTED PROTEIN

Acid in stomach neutralized

Parietal cells of stomach are stimulated by partially or totally digested protein products

Immediate pain is relieved

Stomach makes more acid

Intervention:
Antacid may be used to neutralize acid

PAIN AND IRRITATION OF STOMACH WITHIN 1 TO 3 HOURS OF EATING PROTEIN FOOD

flow of gastric secretions. Nutritionally, the dietary regimen is adequate if the daily food guide shown in Table 18-4 is followed.

Within the last few years, many hospitals and health practitioners have advocated an individualized diet for an ulcer patient not suffering an acute attack (see Table 18-5). Experience indicates that patients enjoy the foods on such a diet and are thus more responsive to the treatment. Table 18-5 describes the details of such a dietary regimen, which has few restrictions.

The dietary management of an ulcer patient is not yet uniform. Some physicians still prescribe the milk regimen initially and then move progressively toward the liberalized diet. Sometimes this practice

TABLE 18-3. Foods Permitted and Prohibited in a Liberalized Ulcer Diet

Food Group	Foods Permitted	Foods Prohibited
Milk, milk products	Whole milk, skim milk, plain yogurt; milkshakes; eggnog; evaporated or condensed milk; related products such as chocolate milk, low-fat milk, etc.	Any not tolerated by patient
Eggs	Any type not specifically excluded	Fried and raw* if not tolerated
Meat, poultry, fish, and cheese	Tender chicken, beef, liver, lamb, turkey (meats may be ground, chopped, or pureed if so prescribed); fish, shellfish; cottage cheese, cream cheese, mild cheeses	Meat that is tough, gristly, cured, salted, or highly spiced, such as luncheon meats, sausage, sardines, anchovies, and corned beef
Potatoes or substitute	Mashed sweet or white potato; creamed potatoes and baked without skin; rice; noodles, macaroni, spaghetti	Potato skin; any rice, pasta, or potato that is fried or highly spiced
Cereals and bread	Enriched white bread; cooked refined cereals, corn flakes, Rice Krispies, Puffed Wheat, Puffed Rice; other varieties not excluded	Cereals containing bran, whole grains, nuts, seeds, or dried fruits
Fats	Margarine, butter; sour cream; oils; mayonnaise; shortening; crisp, drained bacon	All others
Soups	Cream soups (may be strained and prepared from any permitted vegetables; use mild seasonings)	Meat broth, bouillon, consommé, other soups prepared with meat extracts; no highly seasoned soups or soups containing dried beans or peas

Chapter 18
DIET AND
GASTRO-
INTESTINAL
DISEASES

337

TABLE 18-3. (continued)

Food Group	Foods Permitted	Foods Prohibited
Fruits	Canned applesauce, apricots, cherries, peaches, pears; orange, grapefruit, tomato juice (all acidic citrus juices should be consumed in limited quantities and given when tolerated; may be diluted or sieved before serving and given during a meal; ripe bananas, oranges, grapefruit (membranes removed if not tolerated); fresh, ripe, peeled peaches and pears	Fruits not permitted, especially raw and whole fruits and those with many seeds; coconut; raisins; dried fruits
Vegetables	Canned or well-cooked peas, carrots, asparagus, summer squash, spinach; any strained vegetables	All other whole vegetables, especially if raw; other green vegetables; okra; corn; eggplant
Beverages	Milk drinks, weak tea and decaffeinated coffee, Ovaltine	Alcoholic beverages; coffee, tea; cocoa; carbonated beverages
Desserts	Plain ice cream, sherbet without fruit or nuts; cookies; wafers; custard; gelatin; angel food cake; jelly; plain puddings	Those with raisins, dried fruits, coconut, nuts, etc.
Sweets	Candies, sugar, honey, syrup, marshmallows	Chocolate candy, rich candy with nuts or fruits; preserves, jams, marmalades
Spices and dressings	Sage, paprika, thyme, mace, allspice, cinnamon; salt; cream sauces	Black pepper; chili powder; olives; mustard; nutmeg; dressings with onion, garlic, or vinegar

*Most practitioners do not recommend using raw eggs because of possible salmonella contamination.

TABLE 18-4. Daily Food Guide and Two Sample Menus for a Liberalized Ulcer Diet

Daily Food Guide		
2 cups of milk or substitute		
2 servings of meat or substitute		
4 servings of fruit and vegetables with at least 1 serving of vitamin C–rich fruit such as oranges and 1 serving of deep yellow or dark green vegetable such as spinach or squash		
4 servings of cereal or bread		

Mealtime	Menu 1	Menu 2
Breakfast	½ c orange juice 1 poached egg 1 slice toast Margarine Jelly	½ c tomato juice ½ c strained oatmeal 1 c milk Sugar
Midmorning	½ c Cream of Wheat 1 c milk Sugar	½ c plain pudding
Lunch	3 oz ground beef patty 1 baked potato (no skin) ½ c chopped spinach with cheese sauce ½ c gelatin made with fruit juice Margarine	3 oz chicken breast 1 c rice 1 t butter ½ c creamed peas ½ c orange sections (membranes removed)
Midafternoon	1 piece plain cake 1 c milk	1 c eggnog
Dinner	3 oz chicken (boiled with ingredients below) ½ c noodles ½ c mashed carrots ½ c tomato juice	3 oz chopped liver 1 c noodles ½ c asparagus tips 1 t butter ½ c gelatin dessert
Evening snack	½ c cottage cheese 4 crackers	½ c ice cream 4 plain cookies

Note: Fruit juices and other beverages may be taken halfway through each meal.

Chapter 18
DIET AND
GASTRO-
INTESTINAL
DISEASES

339

TABLE 18-5. General Principles and a Sample Menu for an Individualized Ulcer Diet

General Principles
Most foods in a regular diet are included that the individual can tolerate Highly seasoned foods or those that cause excessive gastric juice secretion are eliminated (for example, pepper, chili powder, and caffeine). Whenever possible, the patient should eat three moderate meals and snacks.

Sample Menu Plan

Breakfast	Lunch	Dinner
½ c fruit or juice	2–4 oz meat, fish, etc.	3–5 oz meat, fowl, fish,
½ c cereal	½–1 c potato or	or substitute
1–2 eggs	substitute	1 c potato or alternate
1 sl bread	½ c salad or	½ c salad or
1 t margarine	vegetable	vegetable
1 c milk	1–2 sl bread	1–2 sl bread
Weak tea or decaffeinated coffee	1 t margarine	1 t margarine
	1 c milk	Weak tea, decaffeinated coffee, or
	Weak tea or decaffeinated coffee	other beverage tolerated by patient, including milk and milk drinks

Between-meal and evening snacks: milk, ice cream, milkshakes, cookies, crackers, plain cakes, puddings, gelatins, cottage cheese (no nuts or coconut if not tolerated); amounts served as preferred by patient.

Note: Serving sizes of all meals should be according to individual need and preference.

is called "stage feeding." The patient regulates food intake, paying special attention to blandness and the size and number of servings. On the other hand, many hospitals, especially university research facilities, immediately begin the individualized diet after the acute phase of the disease has passed.

Regardless of diet, the patient should adopt the following guidelines, with which the dietitian and nurse should help the patient comply:

1. Meals should be regular, frequent, and served in small portions. Four to six feedings a day are preferable. Large meals should be avoided.
2. The timing of meals is important. Late-evening snacks should be discouraged, since the food may stimulate nocturnal acid secretion, causing pain during the night.

3. Chewing, eating, and drinking should be done slowly.
4. Stressful activity before and after each meal should be avoided. The patient should rest at these times if possible.
5. Cigarettes (or other forms of tobacco) and alcohol should be avoided before meals or on an empty stomach. Patients who insist on drinking alcoholic beverages should consume them with food.

Antacid therapy is usually combined with dietary management of an ulcer patient for the following reasons: (1) Antacids can neutralize hydrochloric acid and help to reduce ulceration. (2) Antacids prevent ulcer formation. (3) Antacids can promote healing.

Antacids vary in potency, effectiveness, and side effects. For example, tablets are less effective as a neutralizing agent and more expensive than liquid antacids. Antacids with a high sodium content are inadvisable for a patient with hypertension or heart disease.

Depending on the antacid used, possible side effects include constipation, diarrhea, and hypercalcemia. Compounds containing magnesium, for instance, may cause diarrhea. Long-term ingestion of calcium carbonate may lead to hypercalcemia, which can increase acid production.

An antacid has a very short-lasting buffering capacity when ingested on an empty stomach. The buffering effect is much longer when an antacid is taken 1 to 3 hours after a meal. Thus, during the acute phase of an ulcer, a patient is usually asked to take an antacid hourly after each meal, starting at breakfast and continuing until bedtime. However, many patients are awakened by pain at night (often at regular hours). Under these circumstances, the patient should wake up 1 hour before the expected pain and take some antacid. In most patients, this alleviates the pain.

SMALL INTESTINE

Syndromes of Intestinal Malabsorption

The **malabsorption syndrome,** which involves the failure to absorb nutrients properly, is the major clinical problem of the small intestine. Nutrient malabsorption may be due to: (1) a failure in digestion because bile salts, digestive enzymes, and/or normal peristalsis are lacking; (2) a failure in absorption because of a deficiency of mucosal enzymes and/or inflammation of the intestinal mucosa; (3) a failure in transportation because of the blockage of the lymphatic system and the portal veins (through intestinal) and/or a deficiency of a specific blood transport protein.

Physical signs of malabsorption include diarrhea, weight loss, ab-

Chapter 18
DIET AND
GASTRO-
INTESTINAL
DISEASES

341

TABLE 18-6. Common Malabsorption Diseases of the Small Intestine

Cause of Small Intestine Malabsorption	Disease Entity	Precipitating Cause(s)
Absence of digestive juice from pancreas	Cystic fibrosis Pancreatitis	Genetic Many, including alcoholism
Absence of bile	Diseases of the gallbladder and liver	Many, including liver cirrhosis and gallstones
Absence of specific disaccharidases	Deficiency of lactase, maltase, sucrase, isomaltase, or trehalase	Genetic, acquired, other causes
Overpopulation of bacteria in the upper small intestine	Blind-loop syndrome	Anatomical changes because of inflammation or surgery
Specific diseases of small intestinal walls	Crohn's disease Celiac sprue Tropical sprue Radiation enteritis Malignancy	Unknown Unknown, possibly genetic Unknown X-ray exposure Unknown
Surgical resection	Short-bowel syndrome Obesity bypass	Surgical intervention secondary to a specific intestinal disease Jejunoileal shunt or stomach stapling formed by surgical intervention to treat morbid obesity

dominal cramps, distention, and sometimes fever. Vitamin, mineral, and protein deficiencies also can result from malabsorption, with possible serious effects on the body. For example, a lack of folic acid and vitamin B_{12} can cause anemia.

Patients with malabsorption diseases also exhibit symptoms such as increased oxalic acid absorption. This increased absorption, accompanied by inflammation of the small intestine, increases the risk of developing urinary calculi (stones).

Some common malabsorption diseases of the small intestine are listed in Table 18-6. Three of these are discussed below.

Cystic Fibrosis

Cystic fibrosis, an inherited disease, is most common in infants and children but also occurs in adults. It is estimated that about 1 child per 1,500 to 3,500 live births is affected. Two major sites of this disease are the exocrine area of the pancreas and the mucous and sweat glands of the body. The mucous glands produce a tenacious and viscid mucous secretion, and an excessive amount of sodium chloride is found in the sweat.

If the affected child is not treated, overt symptoms ocurring during the first year may include any or all of the following: (1) frequent large bowel movements with foul odor, (2) substandard weight gain with good appetite, (3) abdominal bloating, (4) moderate to severe steatorrhea (fatty stool), (5) frequent and excessive crying, (6) potential sodium deficiency and circulatory collapse resulting from an excessive salt loss in sweat, and (6) frequent episodes of pneumonia. This last symptom by itself can indicate cystic fibrosis. At present, the proper diagnosis of a child with cystic fibrosis is determined from clinical symptoms, the level of sodium chloride in sweat, and x-rays of the chest.

Children with uncontrolled cystic fibrosis have a typical profile. They have a retarded body weight for their age and height, with occasional arrested growth. They are undersized, with a bloated belly and wasted arms and legs, and they appear malnourished. Early diagnosis and management can restore body size and the deposition of muscle and fat. This allows the children to regain a normal appearance, although sexual development may be delayed. However, complete recovery is possible in some cases.

Treatment

Pancreatic enzymes administered to children with cystic fibrosis definitely improve their condition. As the enzyme extracts are used (Viokase and Cotazym are the most common), the digestive problems abate. The children gain weight and their physical development improves.

Menu planning should be adapted to foods that the child finds acceptable, the clinical condition of the child, and the child's response to enzyme treatment. The diet should be high in calories and protein with a modified fat content. If fat intake is to be reduced, medium-chain triglycerides (MCTs) used in food preparation can increase energy intake, promote weight gain, and reduce fat malabsorption problems (also see Chapters 5 and 14).

Dry skim milk powder fortified with fat-soluble vitamins can be used to treat protein deficiency. This substance can be added to dishes prepared for regular meals and is an inexpensive, easy, and effective way to add calories and protein to the diet.

Lactose Intolerance

By the time ingested carbohydrates reach the small intestine, they are mainly in disaccharide form. Disaccharides, to be absorbed, must be digested, split, or hydrolyzed to monosaccharides. Special enzymes called *disaccharidases* are responsible for such hydrolysis. They are lo-

Chapter 18
DIET AND
GASTRO-
INTESTINAL
DISEASES

343

cated in the mucosa of the duodenum, jejunum, and ileum. Deficiencies in any of these disaccharidases may cause intestinal maldigestion and malabsorption.

Disaccharidase deficiency is an inborn error of carbohydrate metabolism. Some infants are born with a low activity of certain intestinal disaccharidases and, as a result, are unable to digest particular disaccharides. Lactase deficiency or lactose intolerance is probably the most common form of this disorder. Its occurrence is common among blacks, Orientals, and certain ethnic groups.

Individuals at any age with lactase deficiency may not show any overt clinical symptoms when ingesting lactose. Others exhibit such symptoms as loud bowel sounds (borborygmi), bloating, flatulence, cramps, and diarrhea if a certain amount of whole milk is ingested. The unabsorbed lactose remains in the intestine and creates a high osmotic load, drawing a large amount of water from the body fluids. In addition, action of the bacteria in the colon causes a large amount of lactic acid, carbon dioxide, butyric acid, and other volatile substances to form from the lactose.

Since milk is the major source of lactose, many of these individuals are unable to tolerate fluid milk. A child with lactose intolerance usually benefits from a lactose-restricted diet that excludes only nonfermented milk and milk products. Such a limited diet may not have adequate amounts of some or all of the following nutrients: calcium, iron, and vitamins A, D, E, K, and B_2. Particular attention must be paid to providing this child with his or her RDAs.

Celiac Disease

A patient's sensitivity to flour protein (gluten) results in **celiac disease.** As shown in Figure 18-4, flour is made up of about 10 percent protein; Table 18-7 shows the general composition of this protein. Flour protein sensitivity tends to run in families and is called gluten enteropathy, nontropical sprue, or celiac sprue.

Mucosal atrophy of the small intestine is invariably a symptom of celiac disease. Cells change from columnar in shape to squamous, or flat, and villi are also lacking (see Figure 18-5). These abnormal cells secrete only small amounts of digestive enzymes.

Other symptoms include diarrhea, steatorrhea, bulky and foamy stools with very bad odor, two to four bowel movements daily, loss of appetite and weight, and emaciation. The patient may show many of the symptoms of malnutrition, including bone pain, rough skin, and nutrient deficiencies leading to anemia. In children, a failure to thrive is characteristic.

Excluding all foods containing gluten—chiefly buckwheat, malt, oats, rye, barley, and wheat—is the basic principle of diet therapy for

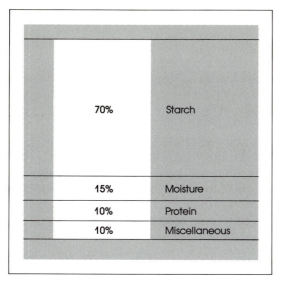

70%	Starch
15%	Moisture
10%	Protein
10%	Miscellaneous

FIGURE 18-4. Composition of wheat flour. The protein contains gliadin, a toxic substance responsible for celiac disease.

TABLE 18-7. Types of Protein in Flour Protein

Type of Protein	Substance in Which Soluble	Protein Fraction (% content)*
Gliadins	Ethanol	α-gliadin[†] (30)
		β-gliadin (30)
		γ-gliadin (30)
		ω-gliadin (10)
Glutenins	Dilute alkali	—
Albumins	Water	—
Globulins	Saline solution	—

*Obtained by starch gel electrophoresis.
[†]Currently, this is considered responsible for celiac disease.

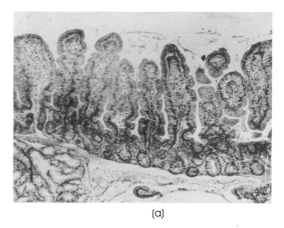

(a)

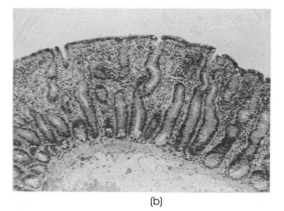

(b)

FIGURE 18-5. Mucosal surface of the small intestine of a patient with celiac sprue. (From M. R. Brown and C. B. Lillibridge, *Clinical Pediatrics* 1975; 14:76) (a) Normal duodenal mucosa with long, fingerlike villi, tall epithelial cells, short crypts in relation to total villous height, moderate cellularity of the lamina propria. (b) Specimen from a patient with gluten-sensitive enteropathy. Total flattening of mucosal surface, elongated deep crypts, short epithelial cells, and intense infiltration of lamina propria with mononuclear cells.

celiac disease. Patients respond dramatically to such a regimen. Most children show a marked improvement in 1 to 2 weeks, whereas adults take 1 to 3 months. The degree of improvement is directly related to the extent the patient adheres to the diet. Symptoms, including mucosal changes, gradually disappear. Children gain weight and begin to thrive; diarrhea and steatorrhea clear up. Although some children must continue treatment at least 5 years, others must exclude gluten from their

Chapter 18
DIET AND
GASTRO-
INTESTINAL
DISEASES

345

diet permanently. Adult patients seem to have less chance of complete recovery.

A gluten-restricted diet is difficult to follow, since foods containing gluten are used so extensively. However, patients who understand celiac disease are more likely to become aware of those products that contain gluten and to follow their prescribed diet conscientiously. Gluten-free wheat products are available, and such products as tapioca, rice, and corn flour may be substituted for those containing gluten.

If a patient is already malnourished when treatment begins, high amounts of calories, protein, vitamins, and minerals should be given as well. Treatment also should provide fluids and electrolyte compensation, especially potassium, magnesium, and calcium; MCTs; and vitamin supplements.

Patients can learn to plan meals to meet their daily RDAs with the help of food guides. Table 18-8 lists those foods that are permitted or prohibited in a gluten-restricted diet. Table 18-9 provides a sample meal plan for such a diet.

LARGE INTESTINE

Diseases and disorders (including surgery) of the large intestine include the irritable bowel syndrome, ulcerative colitis, diverticular diseases, colostomy, hemorrhoidectomy, and cancer. Table 18-10 summarizes the causes, symptoms, and dietary managements of the first three diseases (other disorders are discussed in Chapter 20).

Ulcerative Colitis

The symptoms of ulcerative colitis are recognizable, though the cause of the disease is unknown (see Table 18-10). An acute attack may require intravenous feeding, followed by the routine hospital progressive diet. Regular food should be provided as soon as the patient has recovered sufficiently.

To rest the bowel the patient should be given frequent, small feedings of a bland, low-residue diet. Table 18-11 provides a sample menu from such a diet, while Table 18-12 shows a moderately low-fiber diet. Bland diets take into consideration all forms of irritants—osmotic, chemical, thermal, and mechanical. Foods that may act as irritants include fruits, vegetables, juices, spices, alcohol, and hot and cold drinks and foods.

In general, a high-protein, high-carbohydrate, high-calorie diet with appropriate vitamin and mineral supplements is recommended. Caloric content should be about 2,000 to 3,500 kcal, while the protein contribution should be 100 to 150 g. Protein should be high-quality, such as eggs,

TABLE 18-8. Foods Permitted and Prohibited in a Gluten-Restricted Diet

Food Group	Foods Permitted	Foods Prohibited
Meat, poultry	Those prepared without prohibited grains or their flours	All products using the prohibited flours, including swiss steak, chili con carne, commercial sausages (e.g., weiners), gravies, sauces, stews, batter, stuffings, croquettes
Fish	All fish and shellfish containing no restricted grains or their flours	Any product made with the restricted grains and flours; e.g., wheat flour breaded fish sticks and shrimp
Cheese	All not specifically prohibited	Processed cheese and cheese spread prepared with gluten as a stabilizer
Eggs	All frozen and fresh eggs and egg substitutes without restricted grains or their flours	All others
Textured vegetable proteins	All those made from soy ingredients	All others
Milk, milk products	All not specifically prohibited	Milkshakes and malted milk
Fats, oils	Butter, margarine, cream and cream substitutes; bacon; olive oil, vegetable oil, salad oil; vegetable (hydrogenated) shortening; mayonnaise	Salad dressings thickened with wheat or rye products; cream, butter, white sauce made with forbidden flour
Cereals	All cereals made from rice, corn and rice; e.g., Sugar Pops, Rice Krispies, Corn Chex, cornflakes, Puffed Rice, Frosted Flakes, Cream of Rice, grits, hominy, and cornmeal	All cereals containing prohibited grains; e.g., Cream of Wheat
Bread	Muffins, pone, and cornbread prepared without wheat flour; rolls, muffins, and breads prepared with cornmeal, cornstarch, lima bean flour, and arrowroot; rice pancakes; products made with low-gluten wheat starch	All products made from prohibited grains, e.g., sweet rolls, crackers, muffins, prepared mixes, bread crumbs, commercial yeast
Vegetables, vegetable juices	All vegetables and juices; sauces made with potato flour or cornstarch may be used	Vegetables prepared with cracker crumbs, bread, or cream sauces thickened with prohibited flours or cereals
Fruits, fruit juices	All fruits and juices	Fruit sauces thickened with prohibited grains
Potatoes or substitutes	Potatoes, rice, grits, corn, sweet potatoes, dried peas and beans	Pasta
Sweets	All unless specifically prohibited	Candies and chocolate syrup with bases made from prohibited grains
Soups	Cream or vegetable soups thickened with cornstarch or potato flour; meat stock; clear broths	Milk and cream soups; bouillon cubes or powdered soups; canned soups; soups with prohibited grain products; soups thickened with wheat flour

TABLE 18-8. (continued)

Food Group	Foods Permitted	Foods Prohibited
Beverages	Coffee, tea, cocoa, chocolate, carbonated beverages, milk, Kool-aid	Ale, beer, malted milk; instant cocoa, coffee, or tea; cereal beverages; milk shakes; others including Ovaltine, Postum
Desserts	Products made with permitted grains; plain or fruit-flavored gelatin; homemade ice, ice cream, sherbet, Popsicles; cornstarch, rice and tapioca puddings; cakes, pies, and cookies, using water, sugar, and fruits	All products made with prohibited grains, e.g., pastries (cakes), desserts (ice cream cones, sherbet), prepared mixes
Miscellaneous	Herbs, pepper, olives, salt, vinegar, catsup, pickles, relishes, spices; sauces prepared from permitted grains and their flours; peanut butter, nuts, flavoring extracts, popcorn	Creamed and scalloped foods; au gratin dishes, rarebit; fritters, timbales, malt products, prepared mixes of all kinds, condiments prepared with cereal

TABLE 18-9. Sample Meal Plan for a Gluten-Restricted Diet

Breakfast	Lunch	Dinner
Juice	Meat	Meat, fish, or poultry
Cereal, hot or dry	Potato	Potato
Scrambled egg(s)	Vegetable	Vegetable
Cornbread (special)	Salad with dressing	Juice
Margarine	Fruit or dessert	Fruit or dessert
Jelly	Cornbread	Cornbread with margarine
Milk	Margarine	Milk
Coffee or tea	Milk	Beverage
Sugar	Beverage	Cream
Cream	Cream	Sugar
Salt, pepper	Sugar	Salt, pepper
	Salt, pepper	

meat, and cheese. The amount of fat is determined by the degree of steatorrhea. MCTs (see Chapters 5 and 14) may be substituted for regular fats.

Diverticular Diseases

A **diverticulum** is a blind pouch along the length of the colon. *Diverticulosis* refers to the presence of diverticula (plural of diverticulum), while *diverticulitis* is inflammation of the colon caused by a perforated

TABLE 18-10. Causes, Symptoms, and Dietary Management of Some Colon Disorders

Colon Disorder	Dietary Treatment*
Irritable bowel syndrome Also known as colon spasm and colon neurosis. Most common gastrointestinal disorder. Causes unknown. Symptoms: abdominal pain with occasional watery diarrhea. Constipation may be present.	Controversial, not used by many clinicians. If there is constipation, follow the dietary regimen for constipation discussed in text.
Ulcerative colitis Also known as idiopathic proctocolitis or inflammatory bowel disease. Causes unknown. Symptoms: diarrhea, rectal bleeding, nausea, anorexia, weight loss, loss of protein, vitamins, or minerals in the bowel, dehydration, abdominal tenderness and distention, fever and tachycardia, allergy. Symptoms sometimes absent.	All dietary procedures are supportive and nonspecific. No one diet can heal, cure, or prevent disorder. Bland or low-residue diet may be used. Food items to which patient is allergic should be identified and prohibited. Lactose intolerance corrected by eliminating dairy products. Undernourishment may be reversed. Anabolic hormones may help patients gain weight. Intravenous feeding may be indicated.
Diverticular diseases Covers a range of colon disorders. A diverticulum is a blind pouch along the colon. One disorder is diverticulitis of the colon because of a perforated diverticulum. Causes are unknown. Symptoms: pain, altered bowel habit, bleeding, infection and perforation. Symptoms sometimes absent.	Some success with a high-fiber diet, although some patients still benefit from a bland and low-residue diet.

*This is usually only a component of the overall medical management plan.

diverticulum. Diverticular disease is a term covering one or more of these diseases of the large intestine.

Most patients with diverticulosis are without symptoms. However, some develop pain, changes in bowel habits, bleeding, infection, and perforation. Patients with other symptoms also sometimes report pain in the lower abdomen. Constipation alternates with diarrhea. Some patients have blood and mucus in the stool. Massive hemorrhage may also occur with diverticulitis.

In the past, a low-residue diet was prescribed for patients with symp-

Chapter 18
DIET AND
GASTRO-
INTESTINAL
DISEASES

349

TABLE 18-11. Sample Menu for a Bland and Minimum-Fiber Diet

Breakfast	Lunch	Dinner
Orange juice, strained, ½ c	Chicken, tender, 3 oz	Beef patty, well cooked, 3 oz
Farina, ½ c	Rice, ½ c	Mashed potato, ½ c
Milk, 1 c	Vegetable juice, 1 c	White bread, 1 sl
Toast, white bread, 1 sl	White bread, 1 sl	Grapefruit juice, strained, ½ c
Margarine	Ice cream, ½ c	Custard, ½ c
Sugar	Vanilla wafers, 2	Margarine
Jelly	Milk, 1 c	Coffee or tea
Coffee or tea	Coffee or tea	
	Snacks	
	Gelatin	
	Crackers	

Note: This menu contains about 1 g of fiber. Quantities of servings should be adjusted to meet the needs of the individual.

TABLE 18-12. Sample Menu for a Moderately Low-Fiber Diet

Breakfast	Lunch	Dinner
Tomato juice, ½ c	Melted cheese sandwich:	Roast beef, tender, 3 oz
Egg, poached, 1	White bread, 2 sl	Potato, mashed, 1 c
Toast, white bread, 1 sl	Cheese, mild, 2 oz	Carrots, cooked, ½ c
Bacon, 2 sl	Green beans, ½ c	Orange juice, strained, ½ c
Margarine	Apple juice, ½ c	White bread, 1 sl
Jelly	Gelatin, 1 c	Margarine
Coffee or tea	Vanilla wafers, 2	Ice cream, ½ c
	Coffee or tea	Coffee or tea
	Snacks	
	Milk, 1 c	
	Cookies, plain, 2	

Note: This menu contains about 3 to 4 g of fiber. Quantities of servings should be adjusted to meet the needs of the individual.

toms of diverticular disease. The belief was that such a diet minimizes irritation to the intestine and inhibits formation of gas and distention of the bowel. Recently it has been suspected that diverticula could develop from the long-term consumption of low-fiber foods. Instead of a low-residue diet, a high-fiber diet now is more commonly prescribed.

Unprocessed bran is recommended to increase dietary fiber, the amount determined by individual need. An average of 2 teaspoons of unprocessed bran three times a day (the equivalent of 2 to 3 g of fiber) usually relieves the symptoms of the disease. Desired results include decreased diverticulitis, return of normal bowel habits, and a lessening of pain. Patients with diverticular diseases in the inflammatory and bleeding stages may still require a low-residue diet.

Constipation

Constipation is a symptom of an underlying condition, not a disease in itself. Caused by a lack of food, insufficient dietary roughage, and/or inadequate water intake, constipation also may result from emotional stress.

Certain intestinal diseases also affect constipation. Crohn's disease (regional enteritis), irritable bowel syndrome, tumor, obstruction, and defective electrolyte transfer may contribute to constipation. In addition, various medical conditions, such as hypothyroidism, may be causative factors.

Drugs, too, may lead to constipation. Such drugs as opiates, antihypertensives, calcium carbonate, aluminum hydroxide, and antacids should be considered.

Once any organic cause of constipation has been eliminated, the patient's habits should be reviewed. The omission of breakfast, irregular dietary habits, lack of exercise or activity, and the intake of certain drugs and laxatives all can lead to constipation, particularly in older patients.

High-fiber foods—whole grain cereals and bread, leafy vegetables, and fruit—or unprocessed bran provide necessary roughage. Prunes, rhubarb, figs, dates, bananas, and applesauce are good laxatives as well as being high in fiber and residues. A high-fiber menu plan is shown in Table 18-13. See the references for this chapter for information on the fiber content of foods.

Diarrhea

Diarrhea is the frequent passage of loose or watery unformed stools with or without mucus. Whether acute or chronic, diarrhea is a symptom and not a disease. Its causes can be psychological (nervousness), purely physical (intestinal bacteria), or the result of an intestinal dis-

Chapter 18
DIET AND
GASTRO-
INTESTINAL
DISEASES

351

TABLE 18-13. A High-Fiber Menu Plan

Breakfast	Lunch	Dinner
Dried figs, stewed, 3	Fish, baked, 3 oz	Beef stew, with vege-
Oatmeal, 1 c	Potato, baked, with	tables, 1 c
100% Bran*, 2 T	skin, 1	Cole slaw, ½ c
Toast, whole wheat, 1 sl	String beans, ½ c	Beets, buttered, ½ c
Margarine	Lettuce and tomato	Muffins, bran, 2
Jam, 2 T	salad:	Margarine
Coffee or tea	Tomato, ½	Ice cream, 1 c
	Lettuce leaves, 3	Chocolate sauce, ½ c
	Bread, whole wheat,	Coffee or tea
	1 sl	
	Margarine	
	Pudding, chocolate,	
	¾ c	
	Cookies, oatmeal and	
	raisin, 2	
	Snacks	
	Strawberries,	
	½ c	
	Ice cream, ½ c	

Note: This menu contains approximately 12 to 13 g of undigestible fiber.
*A breakfast cereal marketed by Nabisco; it contains about 7.5% fiber.

ease (such as Crohn's disease). Diarrhea also may be a symptom of non-intestinal disease, such as diabetes.

Diet therapy for diarrhea begins with clear liquids and gradually progresses to a bland, low-residue diet. Lost nutrients, such as minerals, vitamins, and protein, must be replaced. Diets should be adequate in protein, calories, and other essential nutrients.

LIVER

Essential Functions

The liver performs many important functions. The major ones are:

- Receiving and storing absorbed nutrients, including monosaccharides, amino acids, fatty acids.
- Metabolizing nutrients, thereby helping maintain blood glucose levels.
- Synthesizing and secreting bile.

- Detoxifying poisonous and waste substances in the blood.
- Storing blood. Because the liver can store 500 to 1,000 mL of blood, it is sometimes referred to as a blood reservoir.

Liver Cirrhosis

Liver (hepatic) cirrhosis is a degenerative disease characterized by chronic hepatic insufficiency. Symptoms include: (1) a reduced number of liver cells, (2) the derangement of the blood circulation system in the liver, (3) nodular regeneration throughout the remaining liver cells, and (4) death and scarring of liver cells.

Factors known to be able to produce the disease are: excessive alcohol consumption, poisoning by toxic substances, infections (e.g., hepatitis), and inborn errors in metabolism such as Wilson's disease. Severe malnutrition such as **kwashiorkor** also may lead to the development of liver cirrhosis.

Early symptoms include weakness, tiredness, weight loss and wasting, abdominal pain, and diarrhea. Skin lesions, jaundice, and nausea and vomiting may develop later.

The medical management of a cirrhotic patient consists of diet therapy, bed rest, medications, and removal of the cause of the disorder. Improvement of the patient's nutritional status is of primary importance. Aggressive nutritional measures may be needed, such as hospital or commercial high-nutrient preparations, tube feedings, and parenteral alimentation (see Chapter 14).

Patients with liver cirrhosis are susceptible to blood diseases, such as hypochromic microcytic anemia from iron deficiency. A patient with liver failure also may develop ascites (accumulation of protein fluid in the abdominal cavity), edema, or hepatic encephalopathy, which is described below.

Hepatic Encephalopathy

Hepatic or portal system encephalopathy is a disorder caused by failure of the liver to remove toxic waste. If the liver cannot function properly, ammonia accumulating in the liver will not be converted to urea. The conditions that cause hepatic encephalopathy include:

- Liver failure, as in hepatitis or cirrhosis.
- Elevated amines and ammonia in the blood.
- Drugs: sedatives, tranquilizers, and narcotics.
- Alkalosis and low blood potassium.
- Azotemia (excess urea in the blood) from misuse of diuretics or from renal failure.
- Alcoholism, infection, and some surgical procedures.

Chapter 18
DIET AND
GASTRO-
INTESTINAL
DISEASES

353

The patient manifests clinical signs: neurological and psychiatric disturbances (e.g., confusion, personality changes, and flapping tremor of the hands); intestinal bleeding; and coma (eventual development in some patients). These symptoms result from ammonia reaching the brain and gut bacteria invading the blood and organs.

The medical management of hepatic encephalopathy and coma consists of controlling the bleeding in the gastrointestinal tract, avoiding all medications containing ammonia or its salts, administering antibiotics, correcting any electrolyte imbalance, and diet therapy. The main purpose of diet therapy is to restrict the amount of nitrogenous substances, mainly ammonia, in the gastrointestinal tract and blood and to stop the catabolism of lean body mass.

If protein intake is restricted, the patient should be given good quality products such as milk, cheese, eggs, and meat, which contain high levels of essential amino acids. That is, the protein should have a high biological value. This, together with a generous amount of carbohydrate and fat, will provide an acceptable diet.

STUDY QUESTIONS

1. What are some basic problems with the clinical management of gastrointestinal diseases? How has the controversy affected treatment?
2. Define *peptic ulcer*. What are its symptoms? Etiology? What can increase stomach acid secretion in an ulcer patient? Why does this occur?
3. Discuss three factors that may predispose a person to develop a peptic ulcer.
4. How does the dietary strategy for the treatment of an ulcer revolve around two contradictory opinions? What guidelines should be uniformly followed?
5. How do antacids help an ulcer patient? What form is most effective? What precautions should be followed with different types of antacid?
6. What is the major clinical problem of the small intestine? Why does it occur? Briefly describe its symptoms, diagnosis, and treatment.
7. How does pancreatitis occur? What factors may cause it? Define *replacement therapy*.
8. What is celiac disease? Discuss the physiological abnormalities that lead to this condition. By what means can a dramatic improvement of this condition occur?

9. Define *diverticulum*. How is it related to diverticulosis? What change in the treatment of diverticulosis has taken place? Why?
10. What clinical disorders show that cystic fibrosis may be present? What special nutritional needs result from this disease? How is cystic fibrosis treated?

REFERENCES

Aman, R. A. 1980. Treating the patient, not the constipation. *Am. J. Nurs.* 80:1634.

Berk, J. E., ed. 1980. *Developments in digestive diseases.* Philadelphia: Lea & Febiger.

Grossman, M. I. 1980. New medical and surgical treatments for peptic ulcer disease. *Am. J. Med.* 69:647.

———. 1981. *Peptic ulcer: a guide for the practicing physician.* Chicago: Year Book.

Katz, A. J., and Falchuk, Z. M. 1975. Current concepts in gluten sensitive enteropathy. *Ped. Clin. N.A.* 22:767.

Kurtz, R. C., ed. 1981. *Contemporary issues in clinical nutrition.* Vol. I: Nutrition in gastrointestinal disease. New York: Churchill Livingstone.

Lebenthal, E. 1981. *Gastrointestinal disease and nutritional inadequacies.* Vol. 2. New York: Raven Press.

McCaffery, T. D. 1975. Regulating the constipated patient. *Drug Therapy* 5:41.

Page, D. M., and Bayless, T. M., eds. 1981. *Lactose digestion: clinical and nutritional implications.* Baltimore: Johns Hopkins University Press.

Winick, M., ed. 1980. Nutrition and gastroenterology. *Current concepts in nutrition.* Vol. 9. New York: Wiley.

Chapter 18
DIET AND
GASTRO-
INTESTINAL
DISEASES

355

19 DIET AND KIDNEY DISEASES

Everyone needs at least one kidney to survive. In some patients with chronic kidney disease a successful kidney transplant can make a normal life possible or at least allow the patient to live. Others require kidney dialysis, a process whereby waste products are mechanically removed from the blood. For all kidney patients, however, dietary management is an essential part of their treatment—not only to enhance life but to sustain it. We will first study the structure and functions of a normal kidney.

THE NORMAL KIDNEY

Structure

The basic structural unit of the human kidney is the nephron. Each kidney has between 1 and 1.5 million nephrons. Figure 19-1 shows a longitudinal section of a kidney, and Figure 19-2 describes the different parts of a nephron. Figure 19-3 illustrates how each nephron is bathed in a "blood bed." Blood enters the glomerule through the efferent arterioles, passing through a network of capillaries, venules, and intralobular veins. Blood leaves the kidney through the renal veins (see Figure 19-3).

Each renal capsule, composed of the glomerulus and Bowman's capsule (see Figure 19-3), filters fluid and passes it through the proximal convoluted tubule, Henle's loop, the distal convoluted loop, and finally

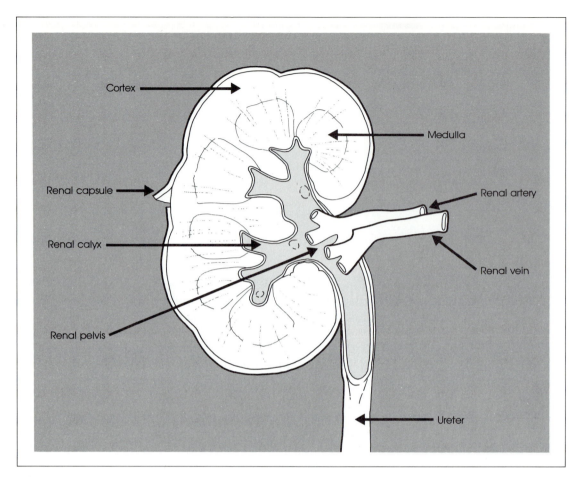

FIGURE 19-1. Section of a kidney.

the collecting tubule. This fluid drains through the ureters and enters the bladder as urine, which is normally excreted at an average rate of 1,000 to 1,500 mL daily. Each tubule can influence the final concentration of excreted urine by secreting and/or reabsorbing certain substances in response to hormonal stimulation.

Functions

There are three indicators of normal kidney function—excretory (clearance) capacity, blood analysis, and urine analysis. The clearance capacity refers to the amount of plasma completely filtered per minute. Blood analysis measures levels of certain substances, such as blood urea nitro-

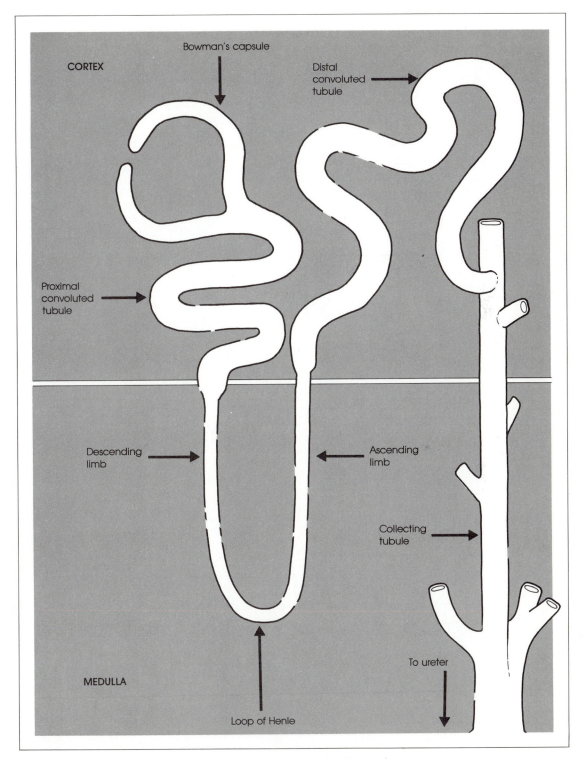

FIGURE 19-2. Parts of a nephron unit. The kidney contains 1 to 1.5 million nephrons.

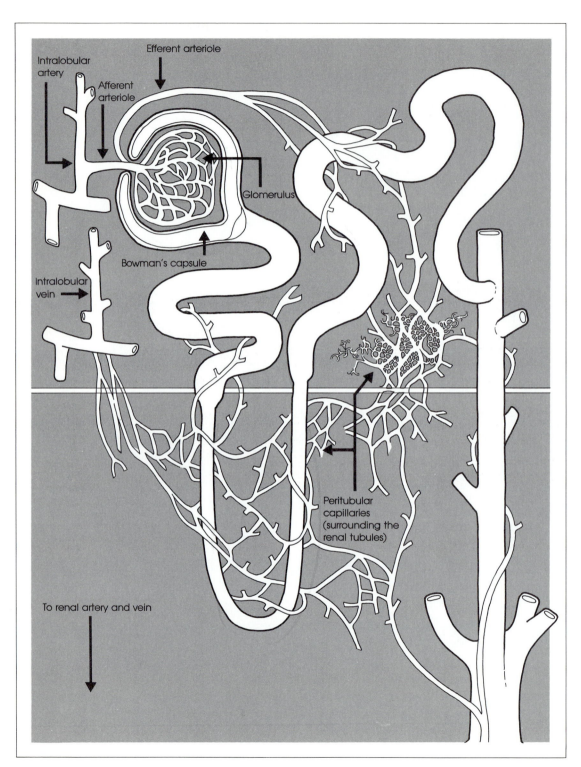

FIGURE 19-3. Blood circulation through a nephron unit.

gen (BUN) and creatinine. Urine analysis measures the amounts of fat and protein, the number and types of cells, and the amount of blood.

The kidneys perform several important functions. First, they rid the blood of waste materials, toxic substances, and excess fluid. Second, they maintain a state of neutrality within the body that is neither too acidic nor too alkaline. Third, they release and/or reabsorb electrolytes and other substances as needed and convert vitamin D into its active form. Finally, the kidneys stimulate the formation of red blood cells.

THE DISEASED KIDNEY

Although there are many forms of kidney disorders, only a few common terms are used to describe the analytical findings of the patients' blood and urine.

- **Hematuria:** blood in the urine
- **Proteinuria:** protein in the urine
- **Pyuria:** pus in the urine
- **Albuminuria:** albumin in the urine
- **Oliguria:** scanty urine
- **Azotemia:** occurrence of high levels of nitrogenous substances in the blood; e.g., urea or creatinine
- **Uremia:** presence of urinary constituents in the blood

All of the above symptoms or conditions are potentially dangerous to health. Unusually high levels of urea in the blood, for example, can poison the individual.

Figure 19-4 lists the different clinical conditions in kidney patients. Each disorder may be managed by a specific nutritional or dietary strategy. Remember that the information in Figure 19-4 is highly simplified and requires careful interpretation by a professional.

Table 19-1 summarizes the causes, symptoms, and suggested dietary treatment for different kidney malfunctions. In the following sections we provide more details for two such disorders, nephrotic syndrome and chronic renal failure. Then we will proceed to explore the implementation of dietary treatment for kidney patients.

NEPHROTIC SYNDROME AND CHRONIC RENAL FAILURE

The symptoms of nephrotic syndrome are edema, proteinuria, and body wasting. A severely restricted sodium intake, plus a diuretic in certain cases, is prescribed to control the edema. Chapter 17 discusses low-sodium diets and the proper use of diuretics. The nephrotic patient's

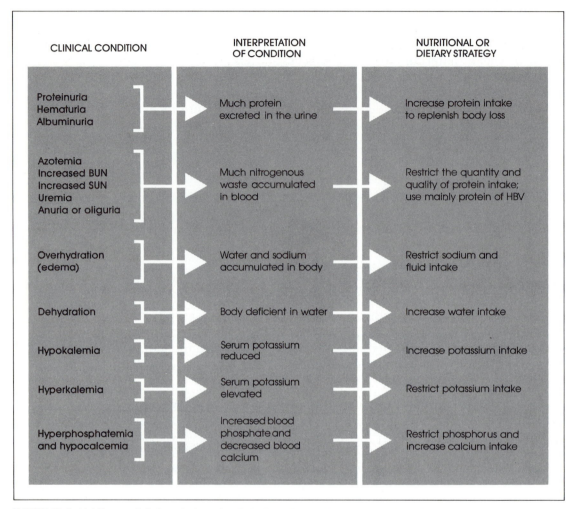

FIGURE 19-4. Nutrition and dietary strategy for clinical conditions of the kidney. HBV = high biological value.

wasted condition is corrected by a high-calorie, high-protein diet. Vitamin and mineral supplements are also recommended.

A nephrotic patient who develops hypertension may suffer kidney failure. Diet therapy for such patients must be carefully planned to avoid further accumulation of nitrogenous waste in the blood.

Certain disorders lead to the slow destruction of kidney tubules, resulting in chronic renal failure (see Table 19-1), sometimes called end-stage renal disease. Too little of a nutrient may be as harmful as too much for a patient with chronic renal failure. Nutrient intake must be carefully adjusted to the kidney's filtering capacity. Tables 19-1 and 19-3

TABLE 19-1. Causes, Symptoms, and Dietary Managements of Various Renal Disorders

Disorder	Causes and Symptoms	Dietary Management
Acute nephritic syndrome	An example of the syndrome is acute glomerulonephritis, caused by poststreptococcal infection of tonsils, pharynx, and skin. Most common in children and adolescents. Symptoms vary from mild to severe: fever, discomfort, headache, slight edema, decreased urine volume, mild hypertension, hematuria, proteinuria, and salt and water retention. Prognosis ranges from complete recovery to renal failure.	Controversial. Some clinicians prefer restriction of protein, fluid, and sodium intakes, while others do not. Diet therapy may be similar to the initial management of acute renal failure; e.g., 25 g of protein (70%–80% HBV) and 500 mg of sodium. Fluid permitted varies with the patient. See text.
Nephrotic syndrome	A group of symptoms resulting from certain kidney disorders (infection, chemical poisoning, etc.). Causes unknown in some patients. Symptoms: edema, proteinuria, and body wasting.	Restore fluid and electrolyte balance; reverse body wasting (malnutrition); correct hyperlipidemia if present. Details are given in text.
Acute renal failure	Abrupt renal malfunction because of infection, trauma, injury, chemical poisoning, pregnancy. Symptoms: nausea, lethargy, anorexia. Oliguria may be present at first, followed by diuresis. Azotemia may also be present.	Restore fluid and electrolyte balance, eliminate azotemia, implement nutritional rehabilitation. Dietary treatment similar to that for acute glomerulonephritis (one type of acute nephritic syndrome). Many patients need dialysis, especially if progressing to chronic renal failure.
Chronic renal failure	This results from a slow destruction of kidney tubules, which may be due to infection, hypertension, hereditary defect, drugs, etc. Symptoms develop as shown in Table 19-2. Nutritional complications are shown in Table 19-3.	Balance fluid and electrolytes, correct metabolic acidosis, minimize toxic effects of uremia, and implement nutritional rehabilitation. Details are in text.

should be studied with the information discussed below. Table 19-2 describes the four stages of chronic renal failure.

Sodium, Potassium, and Fluid Balance

The regulation of both sodium and water intake is essential in the treatment of chronic renal failure. A proper balance must be determined on an individual basis, however.

An elevated level of potassium is dangerous and should be controlled

TABLE 19-2. Four Stages of Chronic Renal Failure

Stage 1	Mild initial stage: hypertension, proteinuria, and hyperuricemia may be present; creatinine clearance is decreased.
Stage 2	Renal insufficiency stage: azotemia, inability to concentrate urine, nocturia, mild anemia, and creatinine clearance less than 50 mL/min for an adult.
Stage 3	Renal failure stage: creatinine clearance less than 10–15 mL/min; polyuria, hyperphosphatemia, and possibly hyperkalemia are present; calcium, chloride, and sodium blood levels are decreased; metabolic acidosis is present; hypertension may be present.
Stage 4	Terminal stage: uremias.

Characteristic symptoms
1. Classic triad: azotemia, acidosis, anemia.
2. Signs: tiredness, weakness, shortness of breath, waxy and pale complexion, abdominal pain, nausea, vomiting, diarrhea, oliguria.
3. Blood chemistry: mild to severe hyperkalemia; increased BUN, creatinine, phosphate, sulfate, chloride; decreased bicarbonate, pH (plasma).

Possible complications
1. Heart: pericardial effusion, pericarditis, and left heart failure accompanied by overt pulmonary edema.
2. Hypertension: frequently present; may produce convulsion, headache, and left heart failure.
3. Osteodystrophy: rickets and osteomalacia; may be disabling.
4. Neuropathy: incapacitated peripheral nervous system.
5. Encephalopathy: may produce convulsion.
6. Retinopathy: hemorrhage, exudate, and impairment of vision.
7. Bleeding: from mucous membranes.

either by limiting dietary intake or by medication. More information on this topic is presented later in this chapter.

Need for Protein, Calories, and Fat

Patients with chronic renal failure must limit their protein intake to avoid accumulation of nitrogen in the blood. On the other hand, adequate protein is needed for tissue maintenance and repair. Again, a proper balance must be determined on an individual basis. Such a balance reduces uremic symptoms, such as intestinal problems, nausea, and vomiting. Patients feel better and have an improved appetite.

TABLE 19-3. Nutritional Complications during Terminal Stage of Chronic Renal Failure

1. Increased nitrogenous waste products in blood
2. Water retained and not excreted
3. Potassium, phosphorus, magnesium, and acid retained and not excreted
4. Failure to adjust to sodium intake by excretion or reabsorption
5. Decreased calcium absorption
6. Vitamin deficiencies
7. Cachexia: weight loss, loss of body fat and lean body mass, retarded growth in young patients, loss of plasma protein (especially albumin)

In most patients, a caloric intake of 35 to 45 kcal/kg body weight per day is adequate. Providing enough calories is difficult, however, because of restrictions on intakes of protein, potassium, sodium, and water. Caloric consumption is automatically limited when the amount of food is small.

In general, needed calories should be derived from three sources: (1) fatty foods, (2) foods high in carbohydrate and low in protein, and (3) high-calorie nutrient supplements. Enough calories should be provided to prevent protein from becoming the major source of energy in the diet. Various methods of feeding a patient a large amount of calories are described in Chapter 14.

In the final stages of kidney failure, some patients may need measures to regulate the serum level of triglycerides, thus reducing the risk of heart disease. Chapter 17 provides more information on the role of lipids in a sound diet.

Anemia is common in patients whose kidneys are functioning at less than normal capacity. Oral supplements of iron and folic acid in progressive amounts are prescribed.

Supplements

Uremic patients usually need vitamin and mineral supplements, since without them they show low blood levels of water-soluble vitamins. Patients on a diet of less than 50 g of protein per day are especially likely to develop vitamin deficiencies and should be carefully monitored. Deficiencies of vitamins A, D, E, and K are less common.

TABLE 19-4. Hypothetical Diet Prescriptions for Treating Different Types of Renal Diseases

Type of Disorder	Protein (g)	Sodium (mEq)	Sodium (mg)	Potassium (mEq)	Potassium (mg)	Diet Specification
Acute glomerulonephritis	25	20	460	26	1,014	A
Nephrotic syndrome	100	40	920	70	2,730	B
Acute renal failure with oliguria	25	20	460	26	1,014	C
Chronic renal failure	40	40	920	40	1,560	D
with no dialysis	60	60	1,380	60	2,340	E
Renal failure with dialysis	100	50	1,150*	80	3,120†	F

Note: In general, patients should be encouraged to eat as many calories as possible. They should be taught how to achieve a high caloric intake and simultaneously comply with the diet prescriptions. Fluid, phosphorus, and calcium intakes are discussed in the text.

*If the patient's condition permits, a prescription of 2,000 to 3,000 mg of sodium is preferred, which improves compliance.

†This assumes that the patient excretes some potassium. If urinary potassium is very low, this may be lowered to 2,000 to 3,000 mg.

NUTRITIONAL AND DIETARY CARE OF KIDNEY PATIENTS

Dietary management for patients with any of the kidney diseases discussed so far (see Table 19-1) involves regulation of the intake of protein, sodium, potassium, phosphorus, calcium, and/or fluid. There are three basic considerations: (1) individualized diet prescription, (2) careful selection of foods consistent with the principles of renal dietetics, and (3) education of the patient and his or her family.

Kidney patients vary greatly in their dietary and nutritional needs. The degree to which kidneys are functioning normally, general clinical condition, and nutritional complications all play a role. It is important, therefore, that diet prescriptions be highly individualized.

Renal Food Exchange Lists

Table 19-4 lists the diet prescriptions for some hypothetical patients with various types of kidney disorders. To assist with diet planning, special food exchange lists have been designed.

Exchange lists arrange foods in groups, each of which contains foods with a similar content of protein, sodium, and potassium. By using such lists, patients may select or exchange any item within a group, thereby simplifying the entire process of diet formulation.

Currently, such lists have been developed by individuals, organizations, and clinics. Space limitation does not permit the reproduction of

TABLE 19-5. Nutrient Contents of Foods within the Renal Food Exchange Lists

Renal Food Exchange List	Food Type	Protein (g)	Sodium (mEq)	Sodium (mg)	Potassium (mEq)	Potassium (mg)
I	Milk and milk products	4	2.6	60	4.4	170
II	Vegetables II-1	1	0.4	10	3.8	150
	Vegetables II-2	2	0.4	10	3.8	150
	Vegetables II-3	1	1.1	25	6.4	250
	Vegetables II-4	2	1.1	25	6.4	250
III	Fruits III-1	0.5	0	0	2.6	100
	Fruits III-2	0.5	0	0	3.8	150
IV	Grain products IV-1	2	0.4	10	1.3	50
	Grain products IV-2	2	5.2	120	1.3	50
V	Meat and equivalents	7	1.3	30	2.8	110
VI	Fats	0	2.2	50	0	0
VII	Alternates*					

*Nutrient contents variable and usually not significant.

such lists. The references for this chapter provide many sources where such lists may be obtained. In the following, selected aspects of these lists are discussed.

Table 19-5 summarizes these lists, showing the food types in each list and their approximate amount of protein, sodium, and potassium. Table 19-6 provides examples of food items within Renal Food Exchange Lists I to VI.

Table 19-7 describes the food products included under Renal Food Exchange List VII: Alternates. This list shows the types of beverages permitted as well as a category of free foods that the patient may eat with no limitation.

Special semisynthetic, low-protein, starchy commercial products (Table 19-8) and some natural ones (arrowroot, sago, and tapioca; see Table 19-7) are used frequently. These two exchange measures provide satisfying staples without adding unwanted protein. Certain commercial nutrient solutions and supplements (Table 19-9) and the free foods in Table 19-7 help provide large amounts of calories without increasing the patient's consumption of protein and electrolytes. For extremely malnourished patients, intravenous feeding of extra calories is sometimes indicated.

TABLE 19-6. Examples of Food Items within each Renal Food Exchange List

Renal Food Exchange List	Examples of food items
I	½ c whole milk = ½ c plain yogurt
II-1	½ c fresh cooked eggplant = ½ c fresh cooked zucchini
II-2	4 large spears of asparagus = ⅓ c cooked frozen turnip greens
II-3	¼ c raw diced celery = ½ c boiled rutabaga
II-4	1 stalk fresh cooked medium broccoli = ½ c cooked frozen brussels sprouts
III-1	1 c raw cranberries = 1 whole fancy tangerine
III-2	½ c canned grape juice = 5 whole fresh Damson plums
IV-1	½ c Puffa Puffa Rice = ½ c minute brown rice
IV-2	1 raised roll = 1 pancake
V	1 oz fresh cooked fish = ¼ c low-sodium cottage cheese
VI	1 t salted regular butter = 1 t Miracle Whip

Using the information in Table 19-4, one can assign the appropriate number of exchanges to each diet prescription listed in Table 19-5. The result is shown in Table 19-10. Using the exchange lists from a professional reference source, one can translate the meal plans in Table 19-10 into sample menus. The last step is to divide the exchanges permitted the patient into three meals per day. Table 19-11 gives the sample menu complying with the hypothetical dietary prescription for patients on dialysis.

Other Dietary Considerations

A patient who needs more sodium and potassium than prescribed (Table 19-4) or contained in the meal plans and menus (e.g., Table 19-11) should be encouraged to eat more fruit. A second option is to provide the

TABLE 19-7. Renal Food Exchange List VII: Alternates

VII-1 Permitted beverages*

Colas: Coca, Pepsi, and RC	Hoffman sodas, regular, any flavor	Popsicles
Cranberry juice cocktail	Kool-aid	Root beer
Faygo sodas, regular, any flavor	Lemonade, frozen, reconstituted	Schweppes mixers, all varieties
Ginger ale	Limeade, frozen, reconstituted	7-Up
Hawaiian Punch		

VII-2 Special beverages

A. Obtain doctor's permission for drinking alcoholic beverages and include their sodium and potassium content; e.g., beer has 80 mg of potassium and 25 mg of sodium in 1 c.

B. Include the potassium content in instant coffee (100 mg of potassium and no sodium in 1 t) and tea (100 mg of potassium and no sodium in one bag used to make medium strength drink).

VII-3 Foods permitted with no limitation

Arrowroot	Gumdrops	Marshmallows
Butter and margarine, unsalted	Honey	Mints, fondant, pillow
Candy, hard, clear	Instant, N-Rich	Rich's whip topping
Coffee Rich	Jams	Sago
Cool Whip	Jellies	Shortenings and oils
Cornstarch	Jelly beans	Sugar, white
Dream Whip	Life Savers	Syrup, corn or maple
Gum, chewing	Lollipops	Tapioca, granular
		Wheat starch

*The exact fluid content must be incorporated into prescribed fluid intake if the amount is regulated.

patient with a list of foods with known sodium and potassium contents from which to select additional items.

Most of the satisfying carbohydrate foods like rice, potatoes, and spaghetti are restricted items, so that meal plans and menus tend to be monotonous and unappetizing. To improve a meal's flavor and thereby encourage patients to follow the diet therapy prescribed, low-protein starch products should be used as often as possible. Also, patients should be given commercial supplements and free foods frequently to increase caloric intake.

Fluid requirements vary from patient to patient. The approximate amount of fluid in the different *categories* (not each item) of food may be obtained from standard reference books. The amount of water in a beverage is listed on the label. The moisture level of certain special items is indicated in Table 19-12.

TABLE 19-8. Low-Protein Products for Kidney Patients

Manufacturer	Product
National distributors	
General Mills	Paygel-P Wheat Starch (dietetic), Paygel Baking Mix (dietetic), Paygel Low Protein Bread (dietetic, ready-to-serve), dp Low Protein Cookies with chocolate flavored chips. Aprotein products (from Carlo Erba, Milan, Italy): tagliatelle (flat noodles), rigatini (elbow macaroni), anellini (ring macaroni), porridge (semolino), rusk and hot cereals (ready-to-serve). All products contain: 0.1–0.9 g protein, 0.0–70 mg sodium, and 0–20 mg potassium in a 3- or 4-oz serving, except rusk, which contains about 400 mg of potassium. Check producer's literature.
Doyle Pharmaceuticals	Resource Baking Mix
Regional distributors*	
Chicago Dietetic Supply	Cellu: Lo/Protein baking mix, Lo/Protein pasta imitation macaroni, Lo/Na baking powder
Ener-G Foods (Seattle, WA)	Jolly Joan: low-protein baking mix and low-protein bread (ready-to-serve)
Vita-Wheat Baked Products (Ferndale, MI)	Low-protein, low-gluten bread; low-protein, low-gluten cookies

*Ask the companies and other local manufacturers about availability. Check company literature for contents of protein, sodium, and potassium. Consult the Kidney Foundation for new and additional products.

Patients with renal disorders have difficulty following their diets because low-protein, salt-restricted foods are often tasteless and boring. Several measures may be taken to minimize the problem of ensuring that the kidney patient eats enough of the foods prescribed. These measures include: (1) consideration for the patient's food preferences; (2) distribution of allowed protein evenly throughout the day; (3) preparation of meals that are attractive, varied, and as tasty as possible; (4) use of cookbooks, exchange lists, recipes, and menus designed specifically for kidney patients; and (5) participation in organizations for patients with renal disorders.

Patient and Family Education

Kidney patients can enjoy a better quality of life. Their lives literally depend on their willingness to accept appropriate nutrition and diet. Patient education should emphasize the following important topics:

TABLE 19-9. Chemical Nutritional Solutions (Supplements) for Patients with Kidney Diseases

Product	Characteristics	Manufacturer
Cal Power	546 kcal per 8 oz; protein- and fat-free; low in electrolytes; mixed-carbohydrate solution; ready-to-eat; 8-oz carton	General Mills
Controlyte	1,000 kcal per 7 oz; protein-free; low in electrolytes; cornstarch hydrolysate, vegetable oil; in powder form	Doyle
Hycal	295 kcal per 4 oz; protein- and fat-free; no electrolytes; glucose solution; ready-to-eat; 4-oz bottle; lemon, lime, orange, and black currant flavors, with new flavors being added	Beecham
Lipomul	600 kcal per 100 mL at normal dilution; protein- and carbohydrate-free; no electrolytes; oral fat emulsion; water miscible	Upjohn
Polycose	400 kcal per 100 mL at normal dilution; protein- and fat-free; low in electrolytes; hydrolyzed products of cornstarch; in powder form; almost tasteless	Ross

(1) normal kidney functions, kidney diseases, and the stages of disease development; (2) causes of symptoms and associated personality changes; (3) fluid and electrolyte disturbances; and (4) nutritional and dietary needs.

Patients need understanding and emotional support to adjust to kidney disease and dietary modifications. Psychological counseling may be indicated when patients find it difficult to make the necessary adjustments. Friends and family members who are willing to listen to and encourage the patient can enhance his or her sense of well-being.

As much information as possible should be provided the kidney patient regarding food purchasing and preparation. The contents of the Renal Food Exchange Lists, creative cooking methods, alternate foods (Table 19-7), special low-protein products (Table 19-8), and nutrient supplements (Table 19-9) should be familiar tools. Special occasions such as birthdays and Christmas as well as emergencies require planning. Also, such hidden sources of sodium and potassium as drinking water, tobacco, medicine, toothpaste, and mouthwash should be noted.

The restriction of sodium is discussed in Chapter 17. Potassium intake is more difficult to control, since this mineral is found in large quantities in a variety of foods—meat, milk, eggs, fruits, and vegetables.

TABLE 19-10. Meal Plans for Hypothetical Diet Prescriptions for Patients with Kidney Diseases

Food Group	Renal Food Exchange List	No. of Exchanges					
		Acute glomerulonephritis A	Nephrotic syndrome B	Acute renal failure with oliguria C	Chronic renal failure with no dialysis D	 E	Renal failure with dialysis F
Milk and milk products	I	1	3	1	1	2	3
Vegetables	II-1	2	2	2	1	1	2
	II-2	1	2	1	1	1	1
	II-3	0	0	0	1	1	1
	II-4	0	0	0	0	1	0
Fruits	III-1	0	5	2	2	2	3
	III-2	2	0	0	1	2	2
Grain products	IV-1	1	5	1	0	0	4
	IV-2	1	2	1	1	4	3
Meat and equivalents	V	2	7	2	4	5	10
Fats	VI	4	5	4	12	11	5
Alternates*	VII						

*The patient's diet is brought up to a high caloric level by means of nutrient supplements, free foods, and low-protein bakery products. See text for more information. Alternates may be taken as desired except when otherwise instructed.

Patients who must restrict fluid intake should learn how to measure and record fluid amounts accurately. The units of liquid measure such as milliliters per cubic centimeter (mL/cm^3), teaspoon, tablespoon, cup, fluid ounce, quart, and liter, should be familiar to patients.

Although kidney patients may eat in restaurants occasionally, they must still follow the prescribed diet, including fluid restrictions. Substitutions may be made if they do not exceed the allotment for specific restricted nutrients. Table 19-13 provides a sample menu for eating out, and Table 19-14 presents some suggestions for a brown bag lunch.

RENAL STONES

The symptoms of kidney stones (renal calculi) may range from none to severe back pain and ashen pallor. Pain is caused by distention of the ureter from an accumulation of urine behind the stone. Stones blocking the ureter at its junction with the bladder are most likely to cause pain.

TABLE 19-11. Sample Menu Complying with the Hypothetical Dietary Prescriptions for Patients on Dialysis

Breakfast	Lunch	Dinner
Pear nectar, 1 c	Salad:	Cauliflower, fresh,
Cream of Rice (non-	Lettuce, ½ c	cooked, ½ c
instant), ½ c	Radish, sliced, 2 T	Kale, fresh, cooked,
Margarine, 2 t	Carrots, raw, grated,	½ c
Eggs, poached, 2	¼ c	Bread, French, 1 sl
Cantaloupe, fresh, ¼ c	Mushrooms, sliced,	Margarine, 2 t
Milk, ½ c	¼ c	Chicken, fried, 4 oz
Alternates, nutrient sup-	Lemon juice, pepper	Gelatin, plain, ½ c
plement, and low-	Bread, low sodium, 1 sl	Fruit salad, canned, in
protein bread*	Bread, whole wheat,	heavy syrup, ½ c
	1 sl	Dream Whip, ¼ c
	Mayonnaise, 1 t	Milk, ½ c
	Roast beef, 4 oz	Alternates, nutrient sup-
	Fruit salad:	plement, and low-
	Honeydew, fresh,	protein bread*
	¼ c	
	Peach, fresh, sliced,	
	⅔	
	Milk, ½ c	
	Alternates, nutrient sup-	
	plement, and low-	
	protein bread*	

Note: The diet provides approximately 100 g of protein, 1,150 mg (50 mEq) of sodium, and 3,120 mg (80 mEq) of potassium. Without alternates, nutrient supplement, and low-protein bread, this menu contains about 2,000 to 2,100 kcal.

*The patient is encouraged to eat as many of the nonexcluded items as possible. See text for more information.

TABLE 19-12. Water Contents of Special Products

Food	Quantity	Approximate Water Content (mL)
Yogurt	½ c	120
Ice cream, 16% fat	⅔ c	90
Sherbet	½ c	120
Gelatin dessert	½ c	120
Lemon pudding, plain	½ c	120
Whip and Chill	½ c	120
Popsicle	1	100

TABLE 19-13. Restaurant Meal Suggestion for Patients with Kidney Diseases

	Food Groups					
	Protein foods (meat, milk, etc.)	Bread and equivalents	Fruits and vegetables	Beverage	Fat	Alternates
Breakfast	Milk Egg(s), scrambled	Toast, white bread, 1 sl Cream of Wheat, ⅓ c	Orange juice, ¼ c	Hot tea	Butter or margarine	Jelly, jam, sugar, pepper
	Food Groups					
	Protein foods (meat, milk, etc.)	Bread and equivalents	Fruits and vegetables	Dessert	Beverage	Alternates
Lunch	Chicken, fried, 1 piece	Bread, French, 1 sl	Green salad	Plain gelatin	Iced tea	Sugar, lemon wedge, oil, vinegar
	Food Groups					
	Protein foods (meat, milk, etc.)	Bread and equivalents	Fruits and vegetables	Dessert	Beverage	Alternates
Dinner	Steak, charcoal-broiled	Bread, whole wheat, 1 sl	Green salad Boiled potato	Fruit salad	Red wine Coffee	Sugar, oil, and vinegar Cream, butter, and margarine

Note: Most serving sizes and numbers are not specified. These must be determined according to diet prescriptions.

Patients identified as having renal stones should be taught how to collect stones small enough to pass through the urinary tract so that they can be analyzed. A combination of sophisticated techniques is used to identify the type of stone produced by an individual. Such information is helpful in determining the cause of the stone's formation and possible measures against further problems. Various types of stones are listed in Table 19-15. Although kidney stones can be removed surgically, other medical measures are available for their management. A relatively new technique is to use high-frequency sound waves to break up the stone.

Calcium Stones

Calcium stones are most likely when the patient is excreting a large amount of calcium in the urine. Other causes of kidney stones are listed below:

TABLE 19-14. Brown Bag Lunch Menu Suggestion for Patients with Kidney Problems

Sandwich:
 Roast beef, lean, unsalted, 1 oz
 Bread, low sodium, with unsalted
  butter, 2 sl
 Mayonnaise, unsalted, 1 t

Cole slaw, prepared without salt, ½ c

Honeydew, 1 sl

Lorna Doone (Nabisco), shortbread
 cookies, 2

Ginger ale, ½ c

Note: The contributions of protein, sodium, and potassium must be incorporated into the patient diet prescriptions.

TABLE 19-15. Types of Kidney Stones in U.S. Patients

Type of Stone	Incidence among U.S. Patients (%)
Calcium	90
Calcium oxalate	45
Calcium phosphate	5
Calcium oxalate and phosphate	40
Magnesium ammonium phosphate	2–5
Uric acid	2–5
Cystine	1–2

1. *Unknown causes* (stones are mainly made up of calcium oxalate and calcium phosphate).
2. *Excess secretions of the parathyroid glands* (mainly calcium phosphate stones).
3. *Miscellaneous causes*
 Drugs; for example, diuretics or antacids
 Diet: excessive calcium and vitamin D intake; insufficient fluid intake
 Organ disorders: kidney; small intestine
 Secondary to other diseases: Cushing's syndrome; Paget's disease
 Urinary tract infection
 Prolonged inactivity
 Excretion of excessive amounts of oxalic acid in urine
 Excessive urine alkalinity

Treatment for patients with severe symptoms emphasizes making the patient more comfortable by means of pain relievers, bed rest, and warm compresses. Patients who do not pass stones under this treatment will be assessed for possible surgery. Effort is made to identify the primary cause of the stone in patients with only minimal symptoms; however, removal of existing stones is the accepted procedure.

Some experts disagree on the use of dietary modifications as a part of the treatment for renal stones. Their reasons include: (1) predictable effectiveness; (2) questionable value of restricting a specific substance,

TABLE 19-16. Medical Management of Patients with Renal Calculi Resulting from Excess Calcium in the Urine

Treatment	Aim of Treatment	Clinical Results
Thiazide diuretics (e.g., hydrochlorothiazide)	1. Normalize urine calcium level by tubule reabsorption of calcium 2. Increase excretion of magnesium in urine (magnesium inhibits stone formation)	Urinary calcium restored to normal; overall reduction in stone formation; reduction in rate of new stone formation
Isotonic inorganic phosphates (1.5–3.0 g phosphorus per day)	1. Increase urinary pyrophosphate, which inhibits stone formation 2. Decrease urinary calcium	Reduction of stone recurrence
Oral cellulose phosphate	Inhibit calcium absorption from gut (excessive calcium absorption causes hypercalciuria)	Reduction in excretion of calcium in urine
Decreased oral calcium intake (150–350 mg/day)	Lower calcium excretion in urine	Possible reduction in stone formation
Decreased vitamin D intake (less common treatment)	Lower calcium absorption	Possible reduction in stone formation
Increased fluid intake (3–4 L/day)	Dissolve stones	Likely elimination of stones
Increased intake of acid ash foods	Acidify urine	Possible dissolution of stones

since stones are made up of different chemicals; (3) both internal and external sources of stone components. Diet therapy has, however, proved successful with some patients and is routinely prescribed.

An important practice in the treatment of calcium stones of unknown origin is the consumption of an adequate amount of fluid. The purpose of drinking plenty of fluids—at least 3 to 4 liters daily—is to dilute the urine. Since highly concentrated urine is also more alkaline, it provides an ideal environment for the precipitation of more calcium stones. Daily urine output should be 3 to 4 liters.

As shown in Table 19-16, a less alkaline condition of the urine (acidification) and a low vitamin D intake are two other diet-related methods in the treatment of calcium stones. A later discussion points up the ways in which urine may be acidified. A low vitamin D intake can be achieved by excluding all foods fortified with vitamin D, such as dairy products.

A low-calcium diet (Table 19-16) is sometimes effective in managing a patient with renal stones. Such a diet fails to provide RDAs for several nutrients, however, and is not advised for long-term use. Table 19-17 provides one example of planning a 200-mg-calcium diet. Table 19-18 provides a sample menu. To facilitate the planning of a restricted calcium diet, we can divide foods into exchange lists, each of which contains foods with approximately equal calcium contents. These exchange lists simplify the preparation of meal plans described in Tables 19-17 to 19-18. Such lists may be obtained from references for this chapter.

Calcium Phosphate Stones

Most of the management procedures in Table 19-16 also apply to kidney stones made up of calcium phosphate. A low-phosphorus, moderately low-calcium diet is sometimes used to treat such kidney stones or prevent their formation. Table 19-19 provides a sample meal for a 1,000-mg-phosphorus, 600-mg-calcium diet. Table 19-20 indicates the permitted and prohibited foods in a phosphorus-restricted diet.

Calcium Oxalate Stones

Calcium oxalate is a component of a substantial portion of kidney stones (see Table 19-15). Possible causes of excessive oxalic acid secretion include: (1) metabolic imbalances, (2) intestinal disorders, and (3) diet-related factors such as insufficient fluid intake. Treatment is as follows: (1) 3 to 4 liters of fluid daily; (2) diuretics such as thiazide; (3) oral nutrients; (4) drugs to prevent the absorption of oxalates; (5) a low-oxalate diet; (6) acidifying the patient's urine with foods and drugs.

A low-oxalate diet (see Table 19-21) in combination with other treatments may be helpful. It should be noted, however, that this diet contains inadequate amounts of a few nutrients, especially vitamin C.

Magnesium Ammonium Phosphate Stones

Magnesium ammonium phosphate stones are normally accompanied by recurring urinary tract infections. The treatment for this type of stone is prescribing antibiotics to remove infection, acidifying the urine, administering ample fluids, and removing stones surgically.

Cystine Stones

Metabolic error is responsible for the formation of cystine stones. Diagnosis of this disease, known as *cystinuria*, is important, since it recurs frequently and can cause extreme illness unless treatment is administered and/or stones are removed. Treatment includes (1) correcting the metabolic error, (2) prescribing a large intake of fluids, (3) using

TABLE 19-17. One Example of Daily Meal Planning for a 200-mg-Calcium Diet

Food Group		Approximate Calcium Content (mg)
Milk, cheese, eggs	None	0
Breads and equivalents	3 sl bread made without milk	30
Cereals, flours	1 c Puffed Rice	7
Meat, poultry, fish	3 oz chicken; 4 oz lamb; 1½ oz shad, baked	30
Vegetables	½ c beets, cooked: ½ c eggplant, cooked	30
Fruits	½ c applesauce; 2 medium nectarines; 1 medium apple	20
Fats	5–6 servings bacon fat, salad dressings, and others	5
Potatoes and equivalents	½ c noodles	15
Soup (broth of permitted meats or soups made with permitted ingredients)	No limit	0
Beverages	2–4 servings	10–20
Desserts	1 c flavored gelatin	5
Miscellaneous (sugar, nondairy creamer, sweets, etc.)	No limit	0

Note: Water used for cooking and drinking should not contain more than 35 mg of calcium per liter. Use distilled water if necessary.

TABLE 19-18. Sample Menu for a 200-mg-Calcium Diet

Breakfast	Lunch	Dinner
Juice, cranberry, ½ c	Soup, tomato, milk-free, ½ c	Fruit cocktail, canned, ½ c
Farina, ¾ c	Chicken, boneless, canned, 3 oz	Veal roast, 3 oz
Bread, made without milk, 1 sl	Mushrooms, canned, ½ c	Potato, baked, medium, 1
Margarine, 2 t	Bread, made without milk, 1 sl	Cauliflower, cooked, ½ c
Salt, pepper	Butter or margarine, 2 t	Bread, made without milk, 1 sl
Sugar	Pears, canned, ½ c	Butter or margarine, 2 t
Imitation cream, non-dairy creamer, or coffee whitener	Salt, pepper	Lemon ice, 1 c
Coffee or tea	Sugar	Imitation cream, non-dairy creamer, or coffee whitener
	Imitation cream, non-dairy creamer, or coffee whitener	Coffee or tea
	Coffee or tea	Salt, papper
		Sugar

TABLE 19-19. A Phosphorus-Restricted Diet

Breakfast	Lunch	Dinner
Juice, orange, ½ c	Roast chicken, 2 oz	Broth, chicken, 1 c
Puffed Rice, 1 c	Rice, long grain, ½ c	Roast pork, loin, 2 oz
Egg, poached, 1	Carrots, diced, cooked, ½ c	Potato, boiled, medium, 1
Toast, Italian bread, 1 sl	Green salad, 1 c	Asparagus, cooked, ½ c
Butter, 1 t	French dressing, 1 T	Fruit cocktail, ½ c
Jelly, 1 T	Bread, Italian, 2 sl	Roll, hard, 1
Milk, whole, ½ c	Butter, 2 t	Butter, 1 t
Coffee, 1 c	Milk, ½ c	Cake, angel food, 1 slice
	Gelatin, lime, ½ c	Strawberries, ½ c
		Tea

Note: This menu contains approximately 1,000 mg of phosphorus and 600 mg of calcium.

TABLE 19-20. Foods Permitted and Prohibited in a Phosphorus-Restricted Diet

Food Group	Foods Permitted	Foods Prohibited
Dairy products	1–1½ c milk daily, whole, skim, or buttermilk; 3 T dry milk; ½ oz cheddar or Swiss cheese may replace ½ c milk; one whole egg daily; no limit for egg white	Any additional servings, including cooking ingredients; all cheese and cheese spreads
Meat, fish, poultry	Beef, lamb, veal, ham, pork; turkey, chicken, duck; haddock, bluefish, cod, halibut, shad, tuna, scallops, swordfish (number of servings varies with degree of restriction)	Clams, herring, crab, lobster, mackerel, oyster, fish roe, shrimp, salmon, sardines; heart, brains, liver, kidney, sweetbread; most processed meats have added phosphate, such as cured items (check label)
Desserts	Sherbet, ices, gelatin; fruit pies, meringues (made from egg white), pudding made with permitted ingredients, fruit tapioca, fruit whip, shortbread; cookies (from white sugar), angel food cake	All forms made with milk and eggs not within daily allowance; cream-filled pies, commercial cake mixes, cakes (unless made from permitted ingredients), custard, doughnuts, rennet pudding; ice cream
Breads	Enriched commercial white bread; French or Italian bread made without milk; water rolls; soda crackers, rusks, saltines, pretzels, matzoh	Cracked wheat, brown, corn, rye, raisin, whole wheat, and any white bread made with nonfat dry milk; biscuits, pancakes, muffins, waffles, rye wafers
Beverages	Coffee, tea, fruit juices, Postum, cola, soft drinks; servings within limit since most soft drinks contain phosphate as an additive	Milk unless specifically permitted; all commercial drinks using milk powder as an ingredient; fountain beverages, cocoa, chocolate
Cereals, flours, and equivalents	Cream of Rice, Cream of Wheat, cornmeal, corn flakes, rice flakes, Puffed Rice; spaghetti, noodles, macaroni; farina, corn grits; white flour, cornstarch, tapioca	Whole-grain cereals; wheat germ, bran, corn or soy grits, bran flakes, oatmeal; shredded wheat, Puffed Wheat; flours: soybean, self-rising, whole wheat, rye
Fats, oils	Margarine, butter; French dressing; fats, lard, cooking oils, shortening	Sweet and sour cream, mayonnaise
Soups	Broth: chicken, beef, and other permitted meats; cream soups made with permitted ingredients	Cream soup made with milk and egg not within allowance; split pea, bean, lentil
Sweets	Jelly, jam, preserves; syrup; sugar, hard candy; marshmallows, clear mints (without chocolate or prohibited milk ingredients)	Molasses, brown sugar; candy made with prohibited milk or eggs; e.g., milk chocolate, fudge, caramel
Fruits	All except most commercial dried fruits (which may contain phosphate as an additive); limit consumption of commercial dates, prunes, and raisins to prescribed phosphate intake	Dried fruit unless content of phosphate specifically calculated
Vegetables	Artichokes, asparagus, brussels sprouts, cabbage, carrots, cauliflower, celery, corn, cucumber, eggplant, escarole, green and wax beans, lettuce, onions, peppers, radishes, romaine, squash, turnips; white and sweet potatoes, pumpkin	Beet greens, broccoli, chard, chick-peas, collard, dandelion greens, kale, mushrooms, okra, parsnips, peas, rutabaga, soybean sprouts, spinach, turnip greens; kidney beans, lima beans, navy beans, soybeans
Miscellaneous	Pickles, salt, seasonings, spices and condiments	Brewer's yeast, chocolate, cocoa, cream sauces, nuts, nut products, olives

TABLE 19-21. Oxalic Acid Content of Food

High Content of Oxalic Acid*

Almonds	Currants	Mustard greens	Rhubarb
Beet greens	Gooseberries	Okra	Sorrel
Beets	Grape juice	Orange juice	Soybeans
Cashews	Grapefruit	Oranges	Spinach
Chard	Grapefruit juice	Parsley	Sweet potatoes
Chocolate	Grapes	Parsnips	Tea, black
Cocoa	Green plantain	Peanut butter	Turnip greens
Collard	Kale	Peanuts	Turnips
Cranberries	Leeks	Pecans	Wax beans
Cranberry juice	Mushrooms	Prunes	Wheat germ

Moderate Content of Oxalic Acid†

Apples	Carrots	Onions (2–3 T)	Sweet potatoes
Asparagus	Celery (¼ stalk)	Peaches	Tea (some herb)
Bananas	Cereals	Pears	Tomato juice (4 oz)
Beer (12 oz)	Cherries	Pineapple	Tomatoes (½)
Blackberries	Coffee (2 c)	Plums	White potatoes
Bread (3–4 slices)	Green beans	Raspberries	
Brussels sprouts	Green peas	Soft drinks	
Cabbage	Lettuce	Strawberries	

Low Content of Oxalic Acid‡

Cauliflower, cheese, eggs, fish, margarine, meat, milk, radishes

Note: This classification applies to all items shown and any products made from them.

*These foods should be avoided by patients whenever possible (see text).

†Daily intake limited to one serving or the amount shown in parentheses.

‡There is no limit on the consumption of these foods.

chemicals to reduce the concentration of cystine in the urine, and (4) reducing the amount of cystine in the body.

Uric Acid Stones

Formation of uric acid stones may be caused by several factors: (1) the excretion of excessive uric acid, (2) high urine acidity, and (3) the presence of a primary disorder that raises the blood level of uric acid. Restricting the intake of dietary purine and chemically reducing the level of uric acid in the urine are two procedures recommended before surgery.

MODIFICATION OF URINE ACIDITY AND ALKALINITY

There are two ways to change the pH of the urine. One is to use particular drugs and the other is to consume certain foods.

Drugs

Methionine and vitamin C in the form of ascorbic acid instead of sodium ascorbate are the two drugs used most frequently to acidify urine (lower pH). From 400 to 600 mg daily of ascorbic acid or about 5 to 15 g daily of methionine are given until an acid urinary pH is obtained.

Large amounts of sodium bicarbonate or citrate will increase the urine's alkalinity. Because these substances have an unpleasant taste, they should be introduced slowly over a period of time. To avoid the formation of calcium phosphate stones, the patient must drink more fluid.

Diet

Eating certain types of food also can change the pH of a patient's urine. Some foods form an acid or alkaline residue in the body. Table 19-22 categorizes foods according to whether they produce alkaline or acidic urine. The pH of the urine can be regulated by eating more or less of the foods indicated in the table.

STUDY QUESTIONS

1. What is the basic structural unit of the kidney?
2. Define chronic renal failure. Discuss the nutritional requirements of the patient.
3. What is the reason for the high variability in the nutritional needs of kidney patients? Explain what a renal exchange list is and how it may be used. Why is the amount of LBV protein limited in the diet of a kidney patient? Obtain a complete set of exchange lists from the references provided.
4. Why is it important to educate a kidney patient in the early stages of his or her illness? What topics should be included?
5. What criticisms have been elicited by the practice of treating patients having renal stones with dietary manipulations? Which dietary treatments have met with some success?
6. Name the possible causes of excess oxalic acid excretion.

TABLE 19-22. Classification of Foods According to their Acid-Base Reactions in the Body

Alkaline-Ash-Forming or Alkaline-Urine-Producing Foods	Acid-Ash-Forming or Acid-Urine-Producing Foods	Neutral Foods
Milk and cream, all types	Meat, poultry, fish, shellfish, cheese, eggs	Butter, margarine, fats and oils (cooking), salad oil, lard
Fruits except plums, prunes, and cranberries	Plums, prunes, cranberries	Cornstarch, arrowroot, tapioca
Carbonated beverages	Corn, lentils	Sugar, honey, syrup
All vegetables except corn and lentils	Bread (especially whole wheat bread not containing baking soda or powder)	Nonchocolate candy
Chestnuts, coconut, almonds	Cereals, crackers	Coffee, tea
Molasses	Rice, noodles, macaroni, spaghetti	
Baking soda and baking powder	Peanuts, walnuts, peanut butter	
	Pastries, cakes, and cookies not containing baking soda or powder	
	Fats, bacon	

REFERENCES

Blumenkrantz, M. J., et al. 1980. Methods for assessing nutritional status of patients with renal failure. *Amer. J. Clin. Nutr.* 33:1567.

Chambers, J. K. 1981. Assessing the dialysis patient at home. *Am. J. Nurs.* 81:750.

Chantler, C., et al. 1980. Nutritional therapy in children with chronic renal failure. *Amer. J. Clin. Nutr.* 33:1682.

Gonick, H. C., ed. 1979. *Current nephrology.* Boston: Houghton Mifflin.

Greene, M. C. 1980. *Gourmet renal nutrition cookbook.* New York: Lennox Hill Hospital.

Harvey, K. B. 1980. Nutritional assessment and treatment of chronic renal failure. *Amer. J. Clin. Nutr.* 33:1586.

Hetrick, A., et al. 1979. Nutrition in renal disease: when the patient is a child. *Am. J. Nurs.* 79:2152.

Kane, T. C., et al. Undated. *Diet manual for patients with kidney disease.* Houston: Baylor College of Medicine.

Kopple, J. D. 1984. Nutritional therapy in kidney failure. In *Present knowledge in nutrition*, 5th ed. Washington, D. C.: The Nutrition Foundation.

Kopple, J. D., et al., eds. 1980. Symposium. Nutrition in renal disease. *Amer. J. Clin. Nutr.* 33:1337.

Leaf, A., and Cotran, R. S. 1980. *Renal pathophysiology.* New York: Oxford University Press.

McDonald, F. D. 1980. *Progress in clinical kidney disease and hypertension.* Vol. 1. New York: Thieme-Stratton.

Oestreich, S. J. K. 1979. Rational nursing care in chronic renal disease. *Am. J. Nurs.* 79:1096.

20 DIET, SURGERY, AND TRAUMA

Physical trauma and stress, including that from surgery, cancer and burns, requires special nutritional attention. A prolonged recovery period, possible complications, and increased human suffering otherwise may result. A successful healing process depends on aggressive dietary and nutritional support.

NUTRITIONAL SUPPORT FOR TRAUMA PATIENTS

A significant number of hospital patients are suffering from varying degrees of malnutrition. This may occur during admission or the hospital stay. Most common are vitamin and mineral deficiencies, but protein and calorie undernourishment also occur, especially among trauma patients.

Patients admitted with any form of stress or trauma often undergo a comprehensive nutritional assessment to establish: (1) nutritional status, (2) metabolic status, (3) medical conditions of the gastrointestinal system, (4) food consumption behavior, (5) nutrient needs, and (6) dietary treatment alternatives.

To initiate appropriate nutritional and dietary support for trauma patients requires an understanding of the metabolic changes that occur during surgery, burns, and body injury. There are three phases of metabolic responses to trauma—ebb, stress, and recovery. These are described in Table 20-1.

TABLE 20-1. Description of Stages of the Body in Response to Surgery and Other Forms of Trauma

Stage	Medical Term	Duration (days)	Hormonal Changes	Variations in Body Metabolites	Body Composition and Temperature Changes
1	Ebb phase, early phase	1	Not definitive	Not definitive	Decreased heat production; decreased oxygen consumption
2	Stress phase, catabolic phase, acute phase, flow phase, hypermetabolic phase	2–10	Increased blood catecholamines, glucagon, corticosteroids, thyroid hormones; decreased blood insulin	Increased blood and urine glucose and nitrogen (in the form of urea)	Muscle protein and fat breakdown, weight loss; possible body water and electrolyte loss; possible increase in body temperature and heat production; possible skin loss; loss of potassium and retention of sodium
3	Recovery phase, anabolic phase, adaptive phase	3–10	Increased blood insulin and growth hormone; decreased blood catecholamines	Increased blood ketone bodies; decreased blood glucose; slightly elevated to normal blood and urine nitrogen (in the form of urea)	Nutrient deposition; building up of body muscle

Ebb Phase

The first or *ebb phase*, is the shortest of the three, lasting only about 24 hours. The body's capacity to produce heat decreases so that the body can meet the increased demand of the environment (including the trauma), and less oxygen than normal is consumed. No significant changes in body hormones or metabolites have been observed in this first stage.

Stress Phase

The duration of the second, or *stress phase*, may vary from 2 to 10 days. Dramatic changes are taking place as the body responds to trauma. The central nervous system sends out signals via the sympathetic nervous system that trigger the release of appropriate hormones. Glands such as the adrenals, thyroid, pancreas, and pituitary respond by increasing nutrient mobilization and utilization. An important result is the breakdown of body muscle protein, increasing the output of both nitrogen and urine. This breakdown of muscle protein serves two important purposes: (1) Additional fuel is provided by the partial conversion of freed amino acids to glucose. (2) The increased nitrogen is partially converted to blood proteins and other substances that support the stresses of trauma. Because of the conversion of muscle tissue, 10 to 30 grams of protein may be lost per day during the stress phase. Also, a lack of insulin (see Table 20-1) leads to a breakdown of fat to provide more glucose for fuel.

Metabolic changes characterize the stress phase. Not only does the body use stored fat and muscle, but it mobilizes hormones called *catecholamines*, secreted by the adrenal glands, to create more heat. Together these processes result in *hypermetabolism*—a faster and more efficient use of energy. Patients lose weight and may have a mild fever. Weight loss, however, may also result from water loss. Several factors determine the degree of hypermetabolism: (1) the type and extent of injury, (2) the nutritional status of the patients, (3) the availability of fluid, (4) the extent of anesthesia.

Certain vitamins and minerals—nitrogen, potassium, phosphorus, sulfur, magnesium, zinc, and especially vitamin C—are released in the urine in increased amounts during the stress phase, indicating the loss of muscle in response to the trauma. The amount of protein and nitrogen loss depends on the type and degree of trauma. Also evident are water and potassium losses, which are usually accompanied by sodium retention.

An increase in the amount of essential nutrients and metabolites in the blood is evidence of the body's attempt to meet the additional metabolic needs caused by trauma.

Many different types of trauma may cause or exaggerate metabolic changes occurring in the stress phase. Some of the most common are: surgical stress, infection, fractures, blood loss, crush injury, burns, open wounds or tissue destruction, starvation, exposure to cold, prolonged inactivity, muscle wasting, general anesthesia, and inadequate nutritional status. If trauma is aggravated by nutrient deficiency, the patient may die from secondary malnutrition rather than from the surgery.

Recovery Phase

The last phase of response to trauma is the *recovery* or *anabolic phase.* The sympathetic nervous system begins to return to normal as the severity of the trauma decreases, triggering an increase in insulin and growth hormone in the blood. Insulin supplies glucose to cells for fuel and repair, while the growth hormone deposits nutrients throughout the body.

Most patients enter the recovery phase from 5 to 10 days after the trauma, but this period is highly variable. Transition from the stress (catabolic) to recovery (anabolic) phase depends on: (1) the type and extent of trauma, (2) body weight loss, and (3) nutrient depletion. One indicator of transition is a decrease of glucose in the blood and urine. Another is that hypermetabolism slows down. A return to normal body temperature may also be used as an indicator, though not a reliable one.

Determining the patient's transition to the recovery phase is important in providing appropriate treatment. For example, nutrients administered intravenously before the patient has entered the recovery phase may magnify and prolong hypermetabolism.

Once the patient enters the recovery phase, however, the process of protein retention begins. This retention is essential to the formation of vital body cell masses, especially in depleted abdominal organs. As the body begins to respond favorably to treatment, the danger from trauma is lessened. Both the extent of protein retention and positive nitrogen balance are determined by: (1) metabolic rate; (2) intake of amino acids and nitrogen; (3) calories available from fat, carbohydrates, and other nonprotein sources.

Nutritional treatment should begin before the patient enters the recovery phase. Determining appropriate dietary and nutritional strategy requires that three factors be considered: (1) preoperative nutritional status, (2) types of pathological abnormalities, and (3) the patient's metabolic response. When diet therapy is introduced and how the patient responds depends on: (1) the duration of the trauma stages, (2) the extent of nutrient depletion, and (3) metabolic rate. Observation of these guidelines will ensure proper patient care.

NUTRITIONAL THERAPY FOR THE SURGICAL PATIENT

Nutritional supports are important for a patient who is undergoing surgery. Preoperative dietary care prepares the patient for the operation, whereas postoperative nutritional treatment helps restore the patient to normal functioning as soon as possible. Good nutritional support contributes to the success of the entire surgical procedure.

Preoperative Diet

A preoperative diet varies according to the needs of the patient, following standards determined by the hospital. The maintenance of body fluids and electrolytes at proper levels is emphasized, sometimes requiring intravenous supplements of glucose and other nutrients.

The timing and kind of meal before surgery is also quite important. A patient should not eat for 6 to 8 hours before surgery so that food particles will not be aspirated into the lungs during recovery from anesthesia. Such an event could be fatal. For patients scheduled for morning surgery, a light evening meal with no food after midnight is recommended. If afternoon surgery is scheduled, a patient should have a breakfast of juice, toast or cereal, and coffee or tea. In emergency cases when undigested food residue is present, the patient's stomach may have to be washed out before the operation.

Gastrointestinal surgery can cause bloating ("gas") and extreme discomfort postoperatively. A preoperative liquid or low-residue diet helps avoid this complication and makes the patient's recovery period a more comfortable one.

Postoperative Diet and Nutritional Therapy

The main goal of postoperative nutritional and dietary care is for the patient to regain a normal body weight. A positive nitrogen balance is essential to subsequent muscle formation and fat deposition. First, all fluid and electrolyte imbalances should be corrected, by transfusion if necessary. The second step is to provide a carefully planned diet therapy. Finally, what the patient eats should be recorded to make sure that a proper amount and balance of nutrients is being consumed.

Major Objectives

In addition to a postoperative dietary regimen, nutritional support is needed to maintain normal body functions and tissues. Nutritional supports should also attempt to replace tissue that may have been lost during surgery, such as muscle, bone, blood, and skin. Malnourishment should be remedied, and plasma protein given to control edema and shock. Plasma protein also provides vital substances lost through bleeding and accelerates the healing process.

Inadequate nutritional supports can have dire results for the patient, including illness and even death. The return of normal body functions and the process of tissue rebuilding may be delayed. Slowing of the healing process may cause edema and muscular weakness. All of these consequences prolong convalescence and discomfort for the patient.

General Approaches

It is recommended that solid food be withheld anywhere from a few hours to 2 or 3 days after surgery. If nausea and vomiting occur, the result may be further fluid and electrolyte losses as well as discomfort. Most commonly recommended dietary supports immediately following surgery include:

1. No food by mouth.
2. Blood transfusion and intravenous feeding: fluids and electrolytes, 5% dextrose, vitamin and mineral supplements, protein-sparing solutions, combination of above.
3. Oral feeding: hospital progressive routine diet with or without supplements, liquid protein supplements with or without nonprotein calories, combination of above.
4. A combination of oral and intravenous feedings.

During this short period of food deprivation, aggressive nutritional support probably is not necessary for well-nourished individuals. Blood transfusions as well as fluid and electrolyte supplements are, however, administered when indicated.

Dextrose, usually a 5% solution in saline or water, also is sometimes prescribed. It is believed that the use of dextrose solution reduces the breakdown of protein, thereby providing needed calories. Some hospitals further recommend vitamin and mineral supplements.

When intestinal functions have stabilized—as soon as 24 hours after surgery—solid foods may be given by mouth. The feedings consist of routine hospital progressive diets over a period of 1 to 3 days. Duration depends on the patient's tolerance, strength, and type of operation.

For some patients a clear-liquid diet is best, while others are able to tolerate soft solid foods. Supplements are occasionally given, usually in the form of liquid protein, or a combination of feeding methods may also be used.

Dextrose solutions or oral liquid diets should be used with caution, since either type may be nutritionally unsound without supplements. The need for other nutritional supports such as fluids, electrolytes, protein, and calories should be carefully reviewed. Finally, a long-term dietary treatment plan should be initiated to promote a speedy recovery, as discussed below.

Postoperative Diet

A postoperative diet that provides the appropriate amount of nutrients should include: (1) 40 to 50 kcal daily per kg of body weight; (2) 12 to 15 percent of total calories as protein; (3) well-balanced intake of established RDAs; (4) carefully monitored intakes of vitamins A, K, C, B_{12}, and folic acid, plus iron and zinc.

The effective postoperative diet will be individualized. For example, a patient who has a minimal amount of tissue and blood loss, a sound preoperative nutritional status, a good appetite, and no sign of surgical complications probably requires only 35 to 40 kcal/kg per day. Serving sizes and the frequency of feedings vary, but in general postoperative patients tolerate solids best when meals are small and frequent.

Carbohydrates and fats should comprise 85 to 88 percent of the total calories in approximately equal amounts. The calories from carbohydrates and fats help correct hypermetabolism, supply energy for restoring the body to normal function, and spare protein for tissue rebuilding.

Not only should the diet for postoperative patients be well balanced and high in protein and calories, but it also should be rich in vitamins A, K, C, B_{12}, and folic acid. Vitamins A and C assist in the healing process and tissue repair. The body's ability to clot (coagulate) blood depends on vitamin K. Folic acid and vitamin B_{12} are of particular importance, since they are necessary to the production of red blood cells.

Both iron and zinc are essential to successful recovery. Iron is vital in compensating for blood loss and possible anemia, whereas zinc has an important role in wound healing. Patients must be checked for possible deficiencies of the nutrients mentioned here and given supplementation when indicated.

GASTROINTESTINAL SURGERY AND NUTRITIONAL SUPPORT

Gastrointestinal surgery introduces a number of diet management problems (see Table 20-2). These problems are discussed in the following sections for patients having undergone gastrectomy; gastric partitioning; surgery of the small intestine; and ileostomy, colostomy, and hemorrhoidectomy.

Gastrectomy

Ulcers of the stomach or duodenum may require surgery, including drainage, vagotomy (severing of the vagus nerve), repair of the pylorum, and partial or total removal of the stomach, which is called a *gastric resection* or *gastrectomy*. Some or all of the duodenum may also be removed.

The dietary plan for the management of the postgastrectomy patient (see Table 20-3) begins immediately after surgery. Depending on the patient's condition, intravenous feeding may be necessary. In this respect, postgastrectomy patients differ little from patients who undergo other surgical procedures. After this initial stage, routine hospital diets are provided. A typical meal consists of 3 or 4 oz to 8 or 10 oz of food at medium temperature. Regular food is given when the patient's bowel sounds indicate the return of a desire to eat.

TABLE 20-2. Diet Therapy for Certain Surgical Conditions of the Gastrointestinal System

Anatomical Site	Surgical Condition	Main Concern of Diet Therapy
Stomach	Gastrectomy Gastric partitioning	Dumping syndrome Multiple complications
Gallbladder	Cholecystectomy	Possible benefit from a reduced fat intake
Jejunum and ileum	Resections	Management of the short bowel syndrome and complications from obesity bypass
Colon	Ileostomy, colostomy	Support with good patient care and education
Rectum	Hemorrhoidectomy	Support and reduction of discomfort

TABLE 20-3. Dietary Management of Postgastrectomy Patients

Stage	Duration	Dietary Treatment
1	Days 1–2 or as tolerated	Nothing by mouth; possible parenteral feeding with nutritional support using amino acids or other nutrients
2	Days 2–5 or as tolerated	Clear liquid such as ice, water, clear broth, unsweetened gelatin and fruit drinks, tea; progressive diet with patient tolerance to low carbohydrate, small volume, 6–8 feedings; no sucrose; parenteral nutrition if indicated
3	Day 6 or as tolerated	Dumping syndrome prevention diet

Dumping Syndrome

A phenomenon known as **dumping syndrome** occurs when food passes from the jejunum without undergoing normal digestion and mixing by the stomach. Two types of clinical response may result. In the first, the patient experiences bloating, cramping pain, and diarrhea. The second type of response is characterized by pallor, weakness, drowsiness, warmth, fainting, palpitations, an increased pulse rate, and sweating.

In the normal digestive process, food leaves the esophagus and enters the stomach, where it is partially digested and then slowly empties into the duodenum. The small intestine receives only small amounts of food at a time. The food slowly reaches the jejunum in an orderly manner. These processes together with proper mixing and digestion produce food particles of the right size and proper dilution and prevent sudden changes of pressure in the intestine.

If part of the stomach and/or duodenum is removed, food leaves the esophagus and enters what is left of the stomach, staying only for a short time. It is then emptied into the jejunum. If a large amount of food empties into the small intestine too rapidly, the patient experiences symptoms of the dumping syndrome—bloating and pain or sweating, weakness, and palpitations. These symptoms are sometimes described collectively as the "early dumping syndrome."

The "late dumping syndrome," by contrast, is really a case of hypoglycemia. The patient experiences sweating, dizziness, and fast heartbeat from 1 to 3 hours after eating. Instead of a reaction to interference in the normal digestive process, however, these clinical manifestations are the result of the rapid depletion of blood sugar.

About 15 to 30 percent of all gastrectomy patients experience the dumping syndrome following a surgery. The symptoms are of short duration and often can be alleviated by temporarily avoiding foods or making postural changes. Eventually the weight of consumed food stretches the remaining stomach tissue to form a "mini-stomach" that holds food longer and helps prevent undigested food from reaching the jejunum.

An antidumping diet should be high in fat and protein, low in carbohydrates, and capable of maintaining body weight. Simple sugars and sweets such as candy, jams, and pastries should be avoided. Occasionally, lactose can cause diarrhea and distention; in such cases, milk and milk products should not be given.

The size and frequency of feedings and the texture and consistency of foods all are important. In general, meals should be small and frequent, including some protein and fat. Dry foods and the avoidance of excess fluids, especially with meals, produce the best results. Roughage and raw food should be given cautiously.

A 2,000 to 3,000 kcal daily intake should maintain an adequate nutritional balance in most patients. If a patient is unable to eat enough, intravenous supplements may be necessary.

Milk and milk products should be avoided only if the patient cannot tolerate them, since they provide an important source of calcium and riboflavin.

Any hypoglycemic shock experienced by the postgastrectomy patient can be temporarily relieved by consuming concentrated sugar. Reactive hypoglycemia (late dumping syndrome) can be corrected by in-

TABLE 20-4. Permitted and Prohibited Foods in an Antidumping Diet

Food Group	Foods Permitted	Foods Prohibited
Breads	All breads and crackers except those noted	Breads with nuts, jams, or dried fruits or made with bran
Fats	Margarine, butter, oil, bacon, cream, mayonnaise, French dressing	None
Cereals and equivalents	All grains, rice, spaghetti, noodles, and macaroni except those noted	Presweetened cereals
Eggs	All egg dishes	None
Meats	All tender meats, fish, poultry	Highly seasoned or smoked meats
Beverages	Tea, coffee, broth, liquid unsweetened gelatin, artificially sweetened soda (½–1 hour before and after meals)*	No milk or alcohol; carbonated beverages if not tolerated; beverages with meal unless symptoms begin to subside[†]
(The following are to be added as patient tolerance and conditions progress.)		
Vegetables	Mashed potato, all tender vegetables (peas, carrots, spinach, etc.)	None creamed; gas-forming varieties if not tolerated (cabbage, broccoli, dried beans and peas, etc.)
Fruits	Fresh or canned (unsweetened or artificially sweetened); one serving citrus fruit or juice	None canned with sugar syrup; avoid sweetened dried fruits, e.g., prunes, figs, dates
Dairy products	Milk, cheese, cottage cheese, yogurt, all in small quantities	None
Miscellaneous	Salt, catsup, mild spices, smooth peanut butter	Pickles, peppers, chili powder, nuts, olives, candy, milk gravies

Note: Check for patient tolerance and acceptability of milk and milk products.

*Some practitioners prefer 1 to 2 hours before and after meals.

[†] Some practitioners permit 4 oz of fluid with a meal.

creasing protein and fat intake while decreasing carbohydrates (see Table 20-4 for permitted and prohibited food items for an antidumping diet and Table 20-5 for sample menus).

Long-term Effects

Gastrectomy patients may suffer long-term effects from their operation. These include weight loss, failure of the body to absorb fat, and vitamin and mineral deficiencies. An appropriate diet can minimize these problems.

Weight loss following gastrectomy occurs in at least 5 percent of the

TABLE 20-5. Sample Menu Plans for an Antidumping Diet

	Soon after Surgery		Later after Surgery	
	Sample 1	Sample 2	Sample 1	Sample 2
Breakfast	Egg, poached, 1 Toast, 1 sl Butter, 1 t Banana, ½	Egg, scrambled, 1 Toast, 1 sl Butter, 1 t Peaches, ½ c	Cream of Wheat, ½ c Butter, 1 t Egg, soft-cooked, 1 Cream, 1 oz	Juice, tomato, 4 oz Oatmeal, ½ c Milk, 4 oz Bacon, crisp, 2 sl Toast, 1 sl Butter, 1 t
Snack	Gelatin, fruit-flavored, unsweetened, 1 c Cream, 1 T	Cottage cheese, 2 oz Crackers, 2	Custard, unsweetened, ½ c Crackers, 4	Milk, 1 c Crackers, 4
Lunch	Chicken breast, stewed, 3 oz Potato, mashed, ½ c Butter, 2 t	Fish, 3 oz Rice, ½ c Spinach, ½ c Butter, 2 t	Roast beef, 3 oz Rice, ½ c Peas, buttered, ½ c	Beef, patty, 3 oz Potato, ½ c Asparagus, ½ c Butter, 2 t
Snack	Cottage cheese, 2 oz Crackers, 4	Gelatin, fruit-flavored, unsweetened, 1 c	Juice, orange, ½ c Cheese, 1 oz Crackers, 2	Cottage cheese, ½ c Crackers, 4
Dinner	Meat, 3 oz Rice with grated cheese, ½ c Asparagus, tips, ½ c Margarine, 1 t	Turkey, sliced, 3 oz Potato, baked, 1 Butter, 2 t Tomato, 2 sl	Beef, 3 oz Potatoes, mashed, 1 c Carrots, ½ c Tomato, sliced, ½ Butter, 2 t	Chicken, 3 oz Noodles, 3 oz Spinach, ½ c Margarine, 1 t
Snack	Bread, 1 sl Meat, 2 oz Margarine, 1 t	Pudding, plain, un- sweetened, with whipped cream, ½ c	Pudding, un- sweetened, ¼ c	Sandwich: Bread, 2 sl Mayonnaise, 2 t Meat, 2 oz

patients and may affect up to 50 percent. Reasons for weight loss include: (1) the avoidance of food, (2) poor absorption of nutrients, and (3) hypermetabolism and attendant energy loss. Attention to dietary planning and the enhancement of the patients' appetite can encourage weight gain.

Fat malabsorption may occur because of failure of enzymes to break down fat or because of an accumulation of bacteria at the location of the surgery. As a result fatty stool is passed (steatorrhea), accompanied by diarrhea. In some cases, steatorrhea may be controlled by the use of enzyme supplements.

About 5 to 15 percent of postgastrectomy patients develop vitamin

B_{12} deficiency. Folic acid deficiency occurs in about 1 percent of the patients, resulting in anemia unless treatment is received. Other vitamin deficiencies as well as inadequate supplies of calcium and iron also may develop. All vitamin and mineral deficiencies are correctable with proper attention to food intake and periodic laboratory evaluations.

Gastric Partitioning

Procedure and Patient Selection

Gastric partitioning is performed to counteract extreme obesity. The procedure is to apply two rows of staples across the upper part of the patient's stomach, creating a pouch with a much smaller capacity than that of the stomach. Theoretically, the patient will eat less because he/she will feel full sooner.

Candidates for stomach stapling must be extremely overweight, in danger of serious obesity-related problems, and eager to lose weight. Preoperative screening and counseling should stress the necessity for family support, regular exercise, calorie counting, and behavior modification to change eating habits.

Postsurgical care

Gastric partitioning patients must be watched closely for pulmonary and cardiovascular complications. From 200 to 300 mL of fluid is given daily by tube feeding for the first 48 hours to assure proper drainage of stomach and pouch. The patient also receives electrolytes intravenously. Usually by the third day, the tube is removed and very small amounts of water and clear liquids are given, gradually progressing to pureed foods. Patients learn that they cannot tolerate too much food eaten too fast.

Patients remain on a liquid diet for 8 weeks, after which they may slowly switch to small portions of more solid foods. Vitamin supplements are always prescribed. It should be emphasized that unless eating habits are changed, the pouch will eventually stretch, and the operation will have accomplished nothing.

Surgery of the Small Intestine

Parts of the small intestine may be removed owing to pathological conditions or obesity. As much as 40 percent of the small intestine may be resected without absorption difficulties, but removing a larger portion may produce severe nutritional problems.

Short Bowel Syndrome

Short bowel syndrome occurs after the removal of a long segment of the small intestine. It is characterized by chronic diarrhea with impaired absorption of essential nutrients. The severity of absorption problems from the short bowel syndrome varies according to: (1) the length of the intestine resected, (2) the part of the intestine removed, and (3) the completeness of the resection. Substantial weight loss, anemia, and other symptoms of malnutrition can occur if no treatment is given.

Intestinal Bypass

Use of intestinal bypass to correct obesity is controversial because of the serious complications that may result. Gastric partitioning (see above discussion) is replacing the intestinal bypass, but some physicians still use the bypass procedure. Removal of a part of the digestive system reduces the patient's ability to digest and absorb food. There will be a drastic reduction in caloric intake, despite the amount of food eaten, and the patient will lose weight.

There are several possible effects from this kind of surgery, including: (1) fat malabsorption; (2) kidney stones; (3) low blood potassium, magnesium, and calcium; and (4) liver failure. A reduced capacity to absorb fat is expected—patients absorb only about 25 percent to 75 percent instead of the normal 95 percent. Other nutrients, too, are less readily absorbed. The high incidence of fatalities from liver failure is the most significant problem resulting from the intestinal bypass; the cause is unknown.

There are several desirable effects of the bypass procedure. The most important of these is substantial weight loss. Diabetic patients require less insulin and show an improved glucose tolerance. Levels of cholesterol, triglycerides, and lipoproteins are lowered in some patients. Blood pressure may also return to normal.

Postoperative medical care of patients who have had surgery of the small intestine is similar to that of other surgical patients. Once the patient is able to tolerate regular food, feedings should be small, frequent, high in protein and carbohydrates, and low in fat. Supplements of vitamins, especially vitamins A, D, K, and B_{12}, are recommended.

Ostomy and Hemorrhoidectomy

Ileostomy is a surgical procedure that creates an opening, or *stoma*, in the ileum. It is usually performed with a partial or total colectomy. By this means, patients with severe ulcerative colitis or colonic cancer are provided an alternate route to defecation.

No specific diet is prescribed for the ileostomy patient, since the digestive process is left practically intact. Good sanitary care is required to prevent infection, heal the newly formed stoma, and hasten recovery. The patient needs reassurance that a normal life is possible after the operation.

Malnourishment due to ileostomy is uncommon. Poor absorption of vitamin B_{12} as well as the loss of large quantities of fluids and electrolytes may need to be remedied, however.

Colostomy is the surgical creation of an opening in the abdominal wall. This opening serves some or all of the functions of the anus. The procedure may be temporary or permanent and may include partial or total removal of the rectum and anus and/or the colon.

A regular diet is quite possible for ostomy patients, although foods such as beer, nuts, onions, corn, lettuce, apples, and raw vegetables may cause problems. Individuals must discover for themselves what foods to avoid to prevent pain, diarrhea, and gas.

Patients need a great deal of emotional support to return to a positive self-image and a rewarding life. The care and concern of physician, family, and friends are invaluable. Membership in the ostomy self-help societies also may help the patient make the attitude adjustments necessary to living successfully with a stoma.

Hemorrhoidectomy is the surgical removal of hemorrhoids and is considered to be one of the most disagreeable of all surgical experiences. Rectal bleeding, pain, and discomfort with each bowel movement are common immediately after the operation. A low-residue diet both pre- and postoperatively may reduce these problems.

Appropriate dietary and nutritional care can play an essential role in the speedy recovery of surgical patients. Attention to the patients' nutritional needs enables them to resume an active and productive life in as short a time as possible.

STUDY QUESTIONS

1. What are the three stages of metabolic response to trauma? Describe the body's hormonal responses to stress.
2. Describe the various preoperative feeding routines for a surgical patient. What complications may result if these routines are not followed?
3. What is the goal of postoperative dietary care? How is it achieved? What are the consequences of inadequate postoperative dietary support?
4. Define the *dumping syndrome*. Why does it occur? When does it occur? How can it be alleviated?

5. What nutritional problems commonly exist in the postgastrectomy patient?
6. Differentiate between ileostomy, colostomy, and hemorrhoidectomy. Aside from nutritional therapy, what is an important role of the health professional in these situations?

REFERENCES

Alberti, K. G. M., et al. 1980. Relative role of various hormones in mediating the metabolic response to injury. *J. Parent. Ent. Nutr.* 4:141.

American College of Surgeons, Committee on Pre- and Postoperative Care. 1975. *Manual of surgical nutrition.* Philadelphia: Saunders.

Amer. J. Clin. Nutr. 1980. Symposium on surgical treatment of morbid obesity. 33:353.

Becker, H. D., and Caspary, W. F. 1980. Postgastrectomy and postvagotomy syndromes. New York: Springer.

Blackburn, G. L., and Bistrian, B. R. 1976. Nutritional care of the injured or septic patient. *Surg. Clin. N.A.* 56:1195.

Cuthbertson, D. P. 1979. The metabolic response to injury and its nutritional implications. Retrospect and prospect. *J. Parent. Ent. Nutr.* 3:108.

Deitel, M., ed. 1980. *Nutrition in clinical surgery.* Baltimore: Williams & Wilkins.

Doyle Pharmaceutical Company. N.d. *Nutrition in trauma and stress: reference manual.* Minneapolis.

Mullen, B. D., and McGinn, K. A. 1980. *The ostomy book—living comfortably with colostomies, ileostomies, and urostomies.* Palo Alto, Calif.: Bull Publishing.

Yarborough, M. F., ed. 1981. Contemporary issues in clinical nutrition. Vol. 3. In *Surgical nutrition.* New York: Churchill Livingstone.

APPENDICES
TABLES AND GLOSSARY

TABLE 1 Recommended Daily Dietary Allowance (RDA) for the United States

Age (years)	Weight (kg)	Weight (lb)	Height (cm)	Height (in)	Protein (g)	Fat-Soluble Vitamins: Vitamin A (μg RE)*	Vitamin D (μg)†	Vitamin E (mg α-TE)‡
Infants								
0.0–0.5	6	13	60	24	kg × 2.2	420	10	3
0.5–1.0	9	20	71	28	kg × 2.0	400	10	4
Children								
1–3	13	29	90	35	23	400	10	5
4–6	20	44	112	44	30	500	10	6
7–10	28	62	132	52	34	700	10	7
Males								
11–14	45	99	157	62	45	1,000	10	8
15–18	66	145	176	69	56	1,000	10	10
19–22	70	154	177	70	56	1,000	7.5	10
23–50	70	154	178	70	56	1,000	5	10
>51	70	154	178	70	56	1,000	5	10
Females								
11–14	46	101	157	62	46	800	10	8
15–18	55	120	163	64	46	800	10	8
19–22	55	120	163	64	44	800	7.5	8
23–50	55	120	163	64	44	800	5	8
>51	55	120	163	64	44	800	5	8
Pregnant						+30	+200	+5	+2
Lactating						+20	+400	+5	+3

Note: The allowances are intended to provide for individual variations among most normal persons as they live in the United States under usual environmental stresses. Diets should be based on a variety of common foods in order to provide other nutrients for which human requirements have been less well defined. See text for detailed discussion of allowances and of nutrients not tabulated.

*Retinol equivalents. 1 retinol equivalent = 1 μg of retinol or 6 μg of β-carotene.

†As cholecalciferol. 10 μg of cholecalciferol = 400 IU of vitamin D.

‡α-tocopherol equivalents. 1 mg of d-α-tocopherol = 1 α-TE.

§1 NE (niacin equivalent) is equal to 1 mg of niacin or 60 mg of dietary tryptophan.

Water-Soluble Vitamins							Minerals					
Vitamin C (mg)	Thiamin (mg)	Ribo-flavin (mg)	Niacin (mg NE)§	Vitamin B_6 (mg)	Folacin$^\|$ (μg)	Vitamin B_{12} (μg)	Calcium (mg)	Phos-phorus (mg)	Mag-nesium (mg)	Iron (mg)	Zinc (mg)	Iodine (μg)
35	0.3	0.4	6	0.3	30	0.5¶	360	240	50	10	3	40
35	0.5	0.6	8	0.6	45	1.5	540	360	70	15	5	50
45	0.7	0.8	9	0.9	100	2.0	800	800	150	15	10	70
45	0.9	1.0	11	1.3	200	2.5	800	800	200	10	10	90
45	1.2	1.4	16	1.6	300	3.0	800	800	250	10	10	120
50	1.4	1.6	18	1.8	400	3.0	1,200	1,200	350	18	15	150
60	1.4	1.7	18	2.0	400	3.0	1,200	1,200	400	18	15	150
60	1.5	1.7	19	2.2	400	3.0	800	800	350	10	15	150
60	1.4	1.6	18	2.2	400	3.0	800	800	350	10	15	150
60	1.2	1.4	16	2.2	400	3.0	800	800	350	10	15	150
50	1.1	1.3	15	1.8	400	3.0	1,200	1,200	300	18	15	150
60	1.1	1.3	14	2.0	400	3.0	1,200	1,200	300	18	15	150
60	1.1	1.3	14	2.0	400	3.0	800	800	300	18	15	150
60	1.0	1.2	13	2.0	400	3.0	800	800	300	18	15	150
60	1.0	1.2	13	2.0	400	3.0	800	800	300	10	15	150
+20	+0.4	+0.3	+2	+0.6	+400	+1.0	+400	+400	+150	#	+5	+25
+40	+0.5	+0.5	+5	+0.5	+100	+1.0	+400	+400	+150	#	+10	+50

$^\|$ The folacin allowances refer to dietary sources as determined by *Lactobacillus casei* assay after treatment with enzymes (conjugases) to make polyglutamyl forms of the vitamin available to the test organism.

¶ The recommended dietary allowance for vitamin B_{12} in infants is based on average concentration of the vitamin in human milk. The allowances after weaning are based on energy intake (as recommended by the American Academy of Pediatrics) and consideration of other factors, such as intestinal absorption.

The increased requirement during pregnancy cannot be met by the iron content of habitual American diets nor by the existing iron stores of many women; therefore the use of 30 to 60 mg of supplemental iron is recommended. Iron needs during lactation are not substantially different from those of nonpregnant women, but continued supplementation of the mother for 2 to 3 months after parturition is advisable in order to replenish stores depleted by pregnancy.

TABLE 2 Estimated Safe and Adequate Daily Intakes of Additional Selected Vitamins and Minerals for the United States

| | | Vitamins | | |
	Age (years)	Vitamin K (μg)	Biotin (μg)	Pantothenic Acid (mg)
Infants	0–0.5	12	35	2
	0.5–1	10–20	50	3
Children and adolescents	1–3	15–30	65	3
	4–6	20–40	85	3–4
	7–10	30–60	120	4–5
	>11	50–100	100–200	4–7
Adults		70–140	100–200	4–7

Source: *Recommended Dietary Allowances*, 9th ed. (Washington, D.C.: National Academy of Sciences, 1980).

Note: Because there is less information on which to base allowances, these figures are not given in the main table of the RDAs and are provided here in the form of ranges of recommended intakes.

Trace Elements*						Electrolytes		
Copper (mg)	Manganese (mg)	Fluoride (mg)	Chromium (mg)	Selenium (mg)	Molybdenum (mg)	Sodium (mg)	Potassium (mg)	Chloride (mg)
0.5–0.7	0.5–0.7	0.1–0.5	0.01–0.04	0.01–0.04	0.03–0.06	115– 350	350– 925	275– 700
0.7–1.0	0.7–1.0	0.2–1.0	0.02–0.06	0.02–0.06	0.04–0.08	250– 750	425–1,275	400–1,200
1.0–1.5	1.0–1.5	0.5–1.5	0.02–0.08	0.02–0.08	0.05–0.1	325– 975	550–1,650	500–1,500
1.5–2.0	1.5–2.0	1.0–2.5	0.03–0.12	0.03–0.12	0.06–0.15	450–1,350	775–2,325	700–2,100
2.0–2.5	2.0–3.0	1.5–2.5	0.05–0.2	0.05–0.2	0.1 –0.3	600–1,800	1,000–3,000	925–2,775
2.0–3.0	2.5–5.0	1.5–2.5	0.05–0.2	0.05–0.2	0.15–0.5	900–2,700	1,525–4,575	1,400–4,200
2.0–3.0	2.5–5.0	1.5–4.0	0.05–0.2	0.05–0.2	0.15–0.5	1,100–3,300	1,875–5,625	1,700–5,100

*Since the toxic levels for many trace elements may be only several times usual intakes, the upper levels for the trace elements given in this table should not be habitually exceeded.

TABLE 3   Mean Heights and Weights and Recommended Energy Intakes for the United States

Category	Age (years)	Weight (kg)	Weight (lb)	Height (cm)	Height (in.)	Energy Needs (with range) (kcal)	Energy Needs (with range) (MJ)
Infants	0.0–0.5	6	13	60	24	kg × 115 (95–145)	kg × .48
	0.5–1.0	9	20	71	28	kg × 105 (80–135)	kg × .44
Children	1– 3	13	29	90	35	1,300 (900–1,800)	5.5
	4– 6	20	44	112	44	1,700 (1,300–2,300)	7.1
	7–10	28	62	132	52	2,400 (1,650–3,300)	10.1
Males	11–14	45	99	157	62	2,700 (2,000–3,700)	11.3
	15–18	66	145	176	69	2,800 (2,100–3,900)	11.8
	19–22	70	154	177	70	2,900 (2,500–3,300)	12.2
	23–50	70	154	178	70	2,700 (2,300–3,100)	11.3
	51–75	70	154	178	70	2,400 (2,000–2,800)	10.1
	>76	70	154	178	70	2,050 (1,650–2,450)	8.6
Females	11–14	46	101	157	62	2,200 (1,500–3,000)	9.2
	15–18	55	120	163	64	2,100 (1,200–3,000)	8.8
	19–22	55	120	163	64	2,100 (1,700–2,500)	8.8
	23–50	55	120	163	64	2,000 (1,600–2,400)	8.4
	51–75	55	120	163	64	1,800 (1,400–2,200)	7.6
	>76	55	120	163	64	1,600 (1,200–2,000)	6.7
Pregnancy						+300	
Lactation						+500	

Source: Recommended Dietary Allowances, 9th ed. (Washington, D.C.: National Academy of Sciences, 1980).

Notes: The data in this table have been assembled from the observed median heights and weights of children together with desirable weights for adults for the mean heights of men (70 in.) and women (64 in.) between the ages of 18 and 34 years as surveyed in the U.S. population (Health, Education and Welfare/National Center for Health Statistics data).

The energy allowances for the young adults are for men and women doing light work. The allowances for the two older age groups represent mean energy needs over these age spans, allowing for a 2% decrease in basal (resting) metabolic rate per decade and a reduction in activity of 200 kcal/d for men and women between 51 and 75 years, 500 kcal for men over 75 years, and 400 kcal for women over 75. The customary range of daily energy output is shown for adults in parentheses, and is based on a variation in energy needs of ±400 kcal at any one age emphasizing the wide range of energy intakes appropriate for any group of people.

Energy allowances for children through age 18 are based on median energy intakes of children these ages followed in longitudinal growth studies. The values in parentheses are 10th and 90th percentiles of energy intake, to indicate the range of energy consumption among children of these ages.

TABLE 4   U.S. Recommended Daily Allowance (U.S. RDA)

Nutrient	Adults and Children (4 years or older)	Infants (Birth to 1 year)	Children (Under 4 years)	Pregnant or Lactating Women
Required				
Protein (g)	45 or 65*	18 or 25*	20 or 28*	45 or 65*
Vitamin A (IU)	5,000	1,500	2,500	8,000
Vitamin C (mg)	60	35	40	60
Thiamin (mg)	1.5	0.5	0.7	1.7
Riboflavin (mg)	1.7	0.6	0.8	2.0
Niacin (mg)	20	8	9	20
Calcium (mg)	1,000	600	800	1,300
Iron (mg)	18	15	10	18
Optional				
Vitamin D (IU)	400	400	400	400
Vitamin E (IU)	30	5	10	30
Vitamin B_6 (mg)	2.0	0.4	0.7	2.5
Folic acid (mg)	0.4	0.1	0.2	0.8
Vitamin B_{12} (μg)	6	2	3	8
Phosphorus (mg)	1,000	500	800	1,300
Iodine (μg)	150	45	70	150
Magnesium (mg)	400	70	200	450
Zinc (mg)	15	5	8	15
Copper (mg)	2	0.6	1	2
Biotin (mg)	0.3	0.05	0.15	0.3
Pantothenic acid (mg)	10	3	5	10

*Lower value if protein efficiency ratio is equal to or greater than that of casein; higher value if protein efficiency ratio is less than that of casein, but greater than 20%.

NUTRITIVE VALUES OF THE EDIBLE PART OF FOODS

Table 5 shows the food values in 730 common foods. Foods are grouped under the following headings: dairy products; eggs; fats and oils; fish, shellfish, meat, and poultry; fruits and fruit products; grain products; legumes (dry), nuts, and seeds; sugars and sweets; vegetables and vegetable products; and miscellaneous items.

Most of the foods listed are in ready-to-eat form. Some are basic products widely used in food preparation, such as flour, fat, and corn-meal. The weight in grams for an approximate measure of each food is shown. A footnote indicates if inedible parts are included in the description and the weight. All table notes appear on pages A58–A59.

The values for food energy (kcal) and nu-trients shown are the amounts present in the edible part of the item, that is, that portion customarily eaten—corn without the cob, meat without bone, potatoes without skins, and European-type grapes without seeds. If additional parts are eaten —the potato skin, for example—the amounts obtained of some nutrients will be somewhat greater than those shown.

Values for thiamin, riboflavin, and niacin in white flours and white bread and rolls are based on the increased enrichment levels put into effect for those products by the Food and Drug Administration in 1974. Iron values for those products and the values for enriched corn-meal, pasta, farina, and rice (except the value of riboflavin) represent the minimum levels of enrichment promulgated under the Federal Food, Drug, and Cosmetic Act of 1955. Riboflavin values of rice are for unenriched rice, as the levels

TABLE 5 Nutritive Values of the Edible Part of Foods

Food	Approximate Measures, Units, or Weight (edible part unless footnotes indicate otherwise)	Weight (g)	Water (%)	Food Energy (kcal)	Protein (g)	Fat (g)
Dairy Products (Cheese, Cream, Imitation Cream, Milk; Related Products)						
Butter. See Fats, oils; related products.						
Cheese:						
Natural:						
Blue	1 oz	28	42	100	6	8
Camembert (3 wedges per 4-oz container)	1 wedge	38	52	115	8	9
Cheddar:						
Cut pieces	1 oz	28	37	115	7	9
	1 cu. in.	17.2	37	70	4	6
Shredded	1 c	113	37	455	28	37
Cottage (curd not pressed down):						
Creamed (cottage cheese, 4% fat):						
Large curd	1 c	225	79	235	28	10
Small curd	1 c	210	79	220	26	9
Low fat (2%)	1 c	226	79	205	31	4
Low fat (1%)	1 c	226	82	165	28	2
Uncreamed (dry curd, less than ½% fat)	1 c	145	80	125	25	1
Cream	1 oz	28	54	100	2	10
Mozzarella, made with—						
Whole milk	1 oz	28	48	90	6	7
Part skim milk	1 oz	28	49	80	8	5

Dashes (—) denote lack of reliable data for a constituent believed to be present in measurable amount for added riboflavin have not been approved. Thiamin, riboflavin, and niacin values for products prepared with white flour represent the use of flour enriched at the 1974 levels; values for iron for such products represent the use of flour enriched at the 1955 level.

Niacin values are for preformed niacin occurring naturally in foods. The values do not include additional niacin that the body may form from tryptophan, an essential amino acid in the protein of most foods. Among the better sources of tryptophan are milk, meats, eggs, legumes, and nuts.

Values have been calculated from the ingredients called for in typical recipes for many of the prepared items, such as biscuits, corn muffins, macaroni and cheese, custard, and many desserts. Values for toast and cooked vegetables are without fat added, either during preparation or at the table. Some vitamins, especially ascorbic acid, may be destroyed when vegetables are cut or shredded. Since such losses vary, no deduction has been made. For meat, values are for meat cooked and drained of the drippings.

A variety of manufactured items—some of the milk products, ready-to-eat breakfast cereals, imitation cream products, fruit drinks, and various mixes—are included. Frequently those foods are fortified with one or more nutrients. If nutrients are added, this information is on the label. Values shown here for those foods are usually based on products from several manufacturers and may differ somewhat from the values provided by any one source.

Table 5 has been adapted from Table 2 of Science and Education Administration, U.S. Department of Agriculture, *Nutritive Value of Foods*, Home and Garden Bulletin no. 72, rev. (Washington, D.C., April 1981).

Nutrients in Indicated Quantity													
	Fatty Acids												
Saturated (total) (g)	**Unsaturated**		**Carbohydrate (g)**	**Calcium (mg)**	**Phosphorus (mg)**	**Iron (mg)**	**Potassium (mg)**	**Vitamin A Value (IU)**	**Thiamin (mg)**	**Riboflavin (mg)**	**Niacin (mg)**	**Ascorbic Acid (mg)**
	Oleic (g)	**Linoleic (g)**										
5.3	1.9	0.2	1	150	110	0.1	73	200	0.01	0.11	0.3	0
5.8	2.2	0.2	Trace	147	132	0.1	71	350	0.01	0.19	0.2	0
6.1	2.1	0.2	Trace	204	145	0.2	28	300	0.01	0.11	Trace	0
3.7	1.3	0.1	Trace	124	88	0.1	17	180	Trace	0.06	Trace	0
24.2	8.5	0.7	1	815	579	0.8	111	1,200	0.03	0.42	0.1	0
6.4	2.4	0.2	6	135	297	0.3	190	370	0.05	0.37	0.3	Trace
6.0	2.2	0.2	6	126	277	0.3	177	340	0.04	0.34	0.3	Trace
2.8	1.0	0.1	8	155	340	0.4	217	160	0.05	0.42	0.3	Trace
1.5	0.5	0.1	6	138	302	0.3	193	80	0.05	0.37	0.3	Trace
0.4	0.1	Trace	3	46	151	0.3	47	40	0.04	0.21	0.2	0
6.2	2.4	0.2	1	23	30	0.3	34	400	Trace	0.06	Trace	0
4.4	1.7	0.2	1	163	117	0.1	21	260	Trace	0.08	Trace	0
3.1	1.2	0.1	1	207	149	0.1	27	180	0.01	0.10	Trace	0

TABLE 5   (continued)

Food	Approximate Measures, Units, or Weight (edible part unless footnotes indicate otherwise)	Weight (g)	Water (%)	Food Energy (kcal)	Protein (g)	Fat (g)
Parmesan, grated						
Cup, not pressed down	1 c	100	18	455	42	30
Tablespoon	1 T	5	18	25	2	2
Ounce	1 oz	28	18	130	12	9
Provolone	1 oz	28	41	100	7	8
Ricotta, made with—						
Whole milk	1 c	246	72	430	28	32
Part skim milk	1 c	246	74	340	28	19
Romano	1 oz	28	31	110	9	8
Swiss	1 oz	28	37	105	8	8
Pasteurized process cheese:						
American	1 oz	28	39	105	6	9
Swiss	1 oz	28	42	95	7	7
Pasteurized process cheese food, American	1 oz	28	43	95	6	7
Pasteurized process cheese spread, American	1 oz	28	48	80	5	6
Cream, sour	1 c	230	71	495	7	48
	1 T	12	71	25	Trace	3
Cream, sweet:						
Half-and-half (cream and milk)	1 c	242	81	315	7	28
	1 T	15	81	20	Trace	2
Light, coffee, or table	1 c	240	74	470	6	46
	1 T	15	74	30	Trace	3
Whipped topping (pressurized)	1 c	60	61	155	2	13
	1 T	3	61	10	Trace	1
Whipping, unwhipped (volume about double when whipped):						
Heavy	1 c	238	58	820	5	88
	1 T	15	58	80	Trace	6
Light	1 c	239	64	700	5	74
	1 T	15	64	45	Trace	5
Cream products, imitation (made with vegetable fat):						
Sour dressing (imitation sour cream) made with nonfat dry milk	1 c	235	75	415	8	39
	1 T	12	75	20	Trace	2
Sweet:						
Creamers:						
Liquid (frozen)	1 c	245	77	335	2	24
	1 T	15	77	20	Trace	1
Powdered	1 c	94	2	515	5	33
	1 t	2	2	10	Trace	1
Whipped topping:						
Frozen	1 c	75	50	240	1	19
	1 T	4	50	15	Trace	1
Powdered, made with whole milk	1 c	80	67	150	3	10
	1 T	4	67	10	Trace	Trace
Pressurized	1 c	70	60	185	1	16
	1 T	4	60	10	Trace	1

Saturated (total) (g)	Fatty Acids Unsaturated Oleic (g)	Linoleic (g)	Carbohydrate (g)	Calcium (mg)	Phosphorus (mg)	Iron (mg)	Potassium (mg)	Vitamin A Value (IU)	Thiamin (mg)	Riboflavin (mg)	Niacin (mg)	Ascorbic Acid (mg)
19.1	7.7	0.3	4	1,376	807	1.0	107	700	0.05	0.39	0.3	0
1.0	0.4	Trace	Trace	69	40	Trace	5	40	Trace	0.02	Trace	0
5.4	2.2	0.1	1	390	229	0.3	30	200	0.01	0.11	0.1	0
4.8	1.7	0.1	1	214	141	0.1	39	230	0.01	0.09	Trace	0
20.4	7.1	0.7	7	509	389	0.9	257	1,210	0.03	0.48	0.3	0
12.1	4.7	0.5	13	669	449	1.1	308	1,060	0.05	0.46	0.2	0
—	—	—	1	302	215	—	—	160	—	0.11	Trace	0
5.0	1.7	0.2	1	272	171	Trace	31	240	0.01	0.10	Trace	0
5.6	2.1	0.2	Trace	174	211	0.1	46	340	0.01	0.10	Trace	0
4.5	1.7	0.1	1	219	216	0.2	61	230	Trace	0.08	Trace	0
4.4	1.7	0.1	2	163	130	0.2	79	260	0.01	0.13	Trace	0
3.8	1.5	0.1	2	159	202	0.1	69	220	0.01	0.12	Trace	0
30.0	12.1	1.1	10	268	195	0.1	331	1,820	0.08	0.34	0.2	2
1.6	0.6	0.1	1	14	10	Trace	17	90	Trace	0.02	Trace	Trace
17.3	7.0	0.6	10	254	230	0.2	314	260	0.08	0.36	0.2	2
1.1	0.4	Trace	1	16	14	Trace	19	20	0.01	0.02	Trace	Trace
28.8	11.7	1.0	9	231	192	0.1	292	1,730	0.08	0.36	0.1	2
1.8	0.7	0.1	1	14	12	Trace	18	110	Trace	0.02	Trace	Trace
8.3	3.4	0.3	7	61	54	Trace	88	550	0.02	0.04	Trace	0
0.4	0.2	Trace	Trace	3	3	Trace	4	30	Trace	Trace	Trace	0
54.8	22.2	2.0	7	154	149	0.1	179	3,500	0.05	0.26	0.1	1
3.5	1.4	0.1	Trace	10	9	Trace	11	220	Trace	0.02	Trace	Trace
46.2	18.3	1.5	7	166	146	0.1	231	2,690	0.06	0.30	0.1	1
2.9	1.1	0.1	Trace	10	9	Trace	15	170	Trace	0.02	Trace	Trace
31.2	4.4	1.1	11	266	205	0.1	380	20[1]	0.09	0.38	0.2	2
1.6	0.2	0.1	1	14	10	Trace	19	Trace[1]	0.01	0.02	Trace	Trace
22.8	0.3	Trace	28	23	157	0.1	467	220[1]	0	0	0	0
1.4	Trace	0	2	1	10	Trace	29	10[1]	0	0	0	0
30.6	0.9	Trace	52	21	397	0.1	763	190[1]	0	0.16[1]	0	0
0.7	Trace	0	1	Trace	8	Trace	16	Trace[1]	0	Trace[1]	0	0
16.3	1.0	0.2	17	5	6	0.1	14	650[1]	0	0	0	0
0.9	0.1	Trace	1	Trace	Trace	Trace	1	30[1]	0	0	0	0
8.5	0.6	0.1	13	72	69	Trace	121	290[1]	0.02	0.09	Trace	1
0.4	Trace	Trace	1	4	3	Trace	6	10[1]	Trace	Trace	Trace	Trace
13.2	1.4	0.2	11	4	13	Trace	13	330[1]	0	0	0	0
0.8	0.1	Trace	1	Trace	1	Trace	1	20[1]	0	0	0	0

TABLE 5 (continued)

Food	Approximate Measures, Units, or Weight (edible part unless footnotes indicate otherwise)	Weight (g)	Water (%)	Food Energy (kcal)	Protein (g)	Fat (g)
Ice cream. See Milk desserts, frozen.						
Ice milk. See Milk desserts, frozen.						
Milk:						
Fluid:						
Whole (3.3% fat)	1 c	244	88	150	8	8
Lowfat (2%):						
No milk solids added	1 c	244	89	120	8	5
Milk solids added:						
Label claim less than 10 g of protein per cup	1 c	245	89	125	9	5
Label claim 10 or more grams of protein per cup (protein fortified)	1 c	246	88	135	10	5
Lowfat (1%):						
Milk solids added:						
Label claim less than 10 g of protein per cup	1 c	245	90	105	9	2
Label claim 10 or more grams of protein per cup (protein fortified)	1 c	246	89	120	10	3
No milk solids added	1 c	244	90	100	8	3
Nonfat (skim):						
Milk solids added:						
Label claim less than 10 g of protein per cup	1 c	245	90	90	9	1
Label claim 10 or more grams of protein per cup (protein fortified)	1 c	246	89	100	10	1
No milk solids added	1 c	245	91	85	8	Trace
Buttermilk	1 c	245	90	100	8	2
Canned:						
Evaporated, unsweetened:						
Whole milk	1 c	252	74	340	17	19
Skim milk	1 c	255	79	200	19	1
Sweetened, condensed	1 c	306	27	980	24	27
Dried:						
Buttermilk	1 c	120	3	465	41	7
Nonfat instant:						
Envelope[5]	3.2 oz (net weight)	91	4	325	32	1
Cup	1 c	68[7]	4	245	24	Trace
Milk beverages:						
Chocolate milk (commercial):						
Regular	1 c	250	82	210	8	8
Lowfat (2%)	1 c	250	84	180	8	5
Lowfat (1%)	1 c	250	85	160	8	3
Eggnog (commercial)	1 c	254	74	340	10	19
Malted milk, home-prepared with 1 c of whole milk and 2 to 3 heaping teaspoons of malted milk powder (about ¾ oz)						
Chocolate	1 c of milk plus ¾ oz of powder	265	81	235	9	9

| | Fatty Acids | | | | | | | Vitamin A | | | | Ascorbic |
Saturated (total) (g)	Unsaturated Oleic (g)	Linoleic (g)	Carbo-hydrate (g)	Calcium (mg)	Phos-phorus (mg)	Iron (mg)	Potassium (mg)	Value (IU)	Thiamin (mg)	Riboflavin (mg)	Niacin (mg)	Acid (mg)
5.1	2.1	0.2	11	291	228	0.1	370	310[2]	0.09	0.40	0.2	2
2.9	1.2	0.1	12	297	232	0.1	377	500	0.10	0.40	0.2	2
2.9	1.2	0.1	12	313	245	0.1	397	500	0.10	0.42	0.2	2
3.0	1.2	0.1	14	352	276	0.1	447	500	0.11	0.48	0.2	3
1.5	0.6	0.1	12	313	245	0.1	397	500	0.10	0.42	0.2	2
1.8	0.7	0.1	14	349	273	0.1	444	500	0.11	0.47	0.2	3
1.6	0.7	0.1	12	300	235	0.1	381	500	0.10	0.41	0.2	2
0.4	0.1	Trace	12	316	255	0.1	418	500	0.10	0.43	0.2	2
0.4	0.1	Trace	14	352	275	0.1	446	500	0.11	0.48	0.2	3
0.3	0.1	Trace	12	302	247	0.1	406	500	0.09	0.34	0.2	2
1.3	0.5	Trace	12	285	219	0.1	371	80[3]	0.08	0.38	0.1	2
11.6	5.3	0.4	25	657	510	0.5	764	610[3]	0.12	0.80	0.5	5
0.3	0.1	Trace	29	738	497	0.7	845	1,000[3]	0.11	0.79	0.4	3
16.8	6.7	0.7	166	868	775	0.6	1,136	1,000[3]	0.28	1.27	0.6	8
4.3	1.7	0.2	59	1,421	1,119	0.4	1,910	260[3]	0.47	1.90	1.1	7
0.4	0.1	Trace	47	1,120	896	0.3	1,552	2,160[6]	0.38	1.59	0.8	5
0.3	0.1	Trace	35	837	670	0.2	1,160	1,610[6]	0.28	1.19	0.6	4
5.3	2.2	0.2	26	280	251	0.6	417	300[3]	0.09	0.41	0.3	2
3.1	1.3	0.1	26	284	254	0.6	422	500	0.10	0.42	0.3	2
1.5	0.7	0.1	26	287	257	0.6	426	500	0.10	0.40	0.2	2
11.3	5.0	0.6	34	330	278	0.5	420	890	0.09	0.48	0.3	4
5.5	—	—	29	304	265	0.5	500	330	0.14	0.43	0.7	2

Nutrients in Indicated Quantity

TABLE 5 (continued)

Food	Approximate Measures, Units, or Weight (edible part unless footnotes indicate otherwise)	Weight (g)	Water (%)	Food Energy (kcal)	Protein (g)	Fat (g)
Natural	1 c of milk plus ¾ oz of powder	265	81	235	11	10
Shakes, thick:[8]						
Chocolate, container	10.6 oz	300	72	355	9	8
Vanilla, container	11 oz	313	74	350	12	9
Milk desserts, frozen:						
Ice cream:						
Regular (about 11% fat):						
Hardened	½ gal	1,064	61	2,155	38	115
	1 c	133	61	270	5	14
	3-fl-oz container	50	61	100	2	5
Soft serve (frozen custard)	1 c	173	60	375	7	23
Rich (about 16% fat), hardened	½ gal	1,188	59	2,805	33	190
	1 c	148	59	350	4	24
Ice milk:						
Hardened (about 4.3% fat)	½ gal	1,048	69	1,470	41	45
	1 c	131	69	185	5	6
Soft serve (about 2.6% fat)	1 c	175	70	225	8	5
Sherbet (about 2% fat)	½ gal	1,542	66	2,160	17	31
	1 c	193	66	270	2	4
Milk desserts, other:						
Custard, baked	1 c	265	77	305	14	15
Puddings:						
From home recipe:						
Starch base:						
Chocolate	1 c	260	66	385	8	12
Vanilla (blancmange)	1 c	255	76	285	9	10
Tapioca cream	1 c	165	72	220	8	8
From mix (chocolate) and milk:						
Regular (cooked)	1 c	260	70	320	9	8
Instant	1 c	260	69	325	8	7
Yogurt:						
With added milk solids:						
Made with lowfat milk:						
Fruit-flavored[9]	8 oz	227	75	230	10	3
Plain	8 oz	227	85	145	12	4
Made with nonfat milk	8 oz	227	85	125	13	Trace
Without added milk solids:						
Made with whole milk	8 oz	227	88	140	8	7
Eggs						
Eggs, large (24 oz per dozen):						
Raw:						
Whole, without shell	1	50	75	80	6	6
White	1	33	88	15	3	Trace
Yolk	1	17	49	65	3	6
Cooked, whole:						
Fried in butter	1	46	72	85	5	6
Hard-cooked, shell removed	1	50	75	80	6	6
Poached	1	50	74	80	6	6

Saturated (total) (g)	Unsaturated Oleic (g)	Linoleic (g)	Carbohydrate (g)	Calcium (mg)	Phosphorus (mg)	Iron (mg)	Potassium (mg)	Vitamin A Value (IU)	Thiamin (mg)	Riboflavin (mg)	Niacin (mg)	Ascorbic Acid (mg)
6.0	—	—	27	347	307	0.3	529	380	0.20	0.54	1.3	2
5.0	2.0	0.2	63	396	378	0.9	672	260	0.14	0.67	0.4	0
5.9	2.4	0.2	56	457	361	0.3	572	360	0.09	0.61	0.5	0
71.3	28.8	2.6	254	1,406	1,075	1.0	2,052	4,340	0.42	2.63	1.1	6
8.9	3.6	0.3	32	176	134	0.1	257	540	0.05	0.33	0.1	1
3.4	1.4	0.1	12	66	51	Trace	96	200	0.02	0.12	0.1	Trace
13.5	5.9	0.6	38	236	199	0.4	338	790	0.08	0.45	0.2	1
118.3	47.8	4.3	256	1,213	927	0.8	1,771	7,200	0.36	2.27	0.9	5
14.7	6.0	0.5	32	151	115	0.1	221	900	0.04	0.28	0.1	1
28.1	11.3	1.0	232	1,409	1,035	1.5	2,117	1,710	0.61	2.78	0.9	6
3.5	1.4	0.1	29	176	129	0.1	265	210	0.08	0.35	0.1	1
2.9	1.2	0.1	38	274	202	0.3	412	180	0.12	0.54	0.2	1
19.0	7.7	0.7	469	827	594	2.5	1,585	1,480	0.26	0.71	1.0	31
2.4	1.0	0.1	59	103	74	0.3	198	190	0.03	0.09	0.1	4
6.8	5.4	0.7	29	297	310	1.1	387	930	0.11	0.50	0.3	1
7.6	3.3	0.3	67	250	255	1.3	445	390	0.05	0.36	0.3	1
6.2	2.5	0.2	41	298	232	Trace	352	410	0.08	0.41	0.3	2
4.1	2.5	0.5	28	173	180	0.7	223	480	0.07	0.30	0.2	2
4.3	2.6	0.2	59	265	247	0.8	354	340	0.05	0.39	0.3	2
3.6	2.2	0.3	63	374	237	1.3	335	340	0.08	0.39	0.3	2
1.8	0.6	0.1	42	343	269	0.2	439	120[10]	0.08	0.40	0.2	1
2.3	0.8	0.1	16	415	326	0.2	531	150[10]	0.10	0.49	0.3	2
0.3	0.1	Trace	17	452	355	0.2	579	20[10]	0.11	0.53	0.3	2
4.8	1.7	0.1	11	274	215	0.1	351	280	0.07	0.32	0.2	1
1.7	2.0	0.6	1	28	90	1.0	65	260	0.04	0.15	Trace	0
0	0	0	Trace	4	4	Trace	45	0	Trace	0.09	Trace	0
1.7	2.1	0.6	Trace	26	86	0.9	15	310	0.04	0.07	Trace	0
2.4	2.2	0.6	1	26	80	0.9	58	290	0.03	0.13	Trace	0
1.7	2.0	0.6	1	28	90	1.0	65	260	0.04	0.14	Trace	0
1.7	2.0	0.6	1	28	90	1.0	65	260	0.04	0.13	Trace	0

TABLE 5   (continued)

Food	Approximate Measures, Units, or Weight (edible part unless footnotes indicate otherwise)	Weight (g)	Water (%)	Food Energy (kcal)	Protein (g)	Fat (g)
Scrambled (milk added) in butter (also omelet)	1	64	76	95	6	7
Fats, Oils; Related Products						
Butter:						
Regular (1 brick or 4 sticks per pound)						
Stick (½ c)	1 stick	113	16	815	1	92
Tablespoon (about ⅛ stick)	1 T	14	16	100	Trace	12
Pat (1-in. square, ⅓ in. high; 90 per pound)	1 pat	5	16	35	Trace	4
Whipped (6 sticks or two 8-oz containers per pound)						
Stick (½ c)	1 stick	76	16	540	1	61
Tablespoon (about ⅛ stick)	1 T	9	16	65	Trace	8
Pat (1¼-in. square, ⅓ in. high; 120 per pound)	1 pat	4	16	25	Trace	3
Fats, cooking (vegetable shortenings)	1 c	200	0	1,770	0	200
	1 T	13	0	110	0	13
Lard	1 c	205	0	1,850	0	205
	1 T	13	0	115	0	13
Margarine:						
Regular (1 brick or 4 sticks per pound):						
Stick (½ c)	1 stick	113	16	815	1	92
Tablespoon (about ⅛ stick)	1 T	14	16	100	Trace	12
Pat (1-in. square, ⅓ in. high; 90 per pound)	1 pat	5	16	35	Trace	4
Soft, two 8-oz containers per pound	8 oz	227	16	1,635	1	184
	1 T	14	16	100	Trace	12
Whipped (6 sticks per pound):						
Stick (½ c)	1 stick	76	16	545	Trace	61
Tablespoon (about ⅛ stick)	1 T	9	16	70	Trace	8
Oils, salad or cooking:						
Corn	1 c	218	0	1,925	0	218
	1 T	14	0	120	0	14
Olive	1 c	216	0	1,910	0	216
	1 T	14	0	120	0	14
Peanut	1 c	216	0	1,910	0	216
	1 T	14	0	120	0	14
Safflower	1 c	218	0	1,925	0	218
	1 T	14	0	120	0	14
Soybean oil, hydrogenated (partially hardened)	1 c	218	0	1,925	0	218
	1 T	14	0	120	0	14
Soybean-cottonseed oil blend, hydrogenated	1 c	218	0	1,925	0	218
	1 T	14	0	120	0	14
Salad dressings:						
Commercial:						
Blue cheese:						
Regular	1 T	15	32	75	1	8
Low calorie (5 kcal per teaspoon)	1 T	16	84	10	Trace	1
French:						
Regular	1 T	16	39	65	Trace	6
Low calorie (5 kcal per teaspoon)	1 T	16	77	15	Trace	1

| | Fatty Acids | | | | | | | Vitamin A | | | | |
| Saturated (total) (g) | Unsaturated | | Carbo-hydrate (g) | Calcium (mg) | Phos-phorus (mg) | Iron (mg) | Potassium (mg) | Value (IU) | Thiamin (mg) | Riboflavin (mg) | Niacin (mg) | Ascorbic Acid (mg) |
	Oleic (g)	Linoleic (g)										
2.8	2.3	0.6	1	47	97	0.9	85	310	0.04	0.16	Trace	0
57.3	23.1	2.1	Trace	27	26	0.2	29	3,470[11]	0.01	0.04	Trace	0
7.2	2.9	0.3	Trace	3	3	Trace	4	430[11]	Trace	Trace	Trace	0
2.5	1.0	0.1	Trace	1	1	Trace	1	150[11]	Trace	Trace	Trace	0
38.2	15.4	1.4	Trace	18	17	0.1	20	2,310[11]	Trace	0.03	Trace	0
4.7	1.9	0.2	Trace	2	2	Trace	2	290[11]	Trace	Trace	Trace	0
1.9	0.8	0.1	Trace	1	1	Trace	1	120[11]	0	Trace	Trace	0
48.8	88.2	48.4	0	0	0	0	0	—	0	0	0	0
3.2	5.7	3.1	0	0	0	0	0	—	0	0	0	0
81.0	83.8	20.5	0	0	0	0	0	0	0	0	0	0
5.1	5.3	1.3	0	0	0	0	0	0	0	0	0	0
16.7	42.9	24.9	Trace	27	26	0.2	29	3,750[12]	0.01	0.04	Trace	0
2.1	5.3	3.1	Trace	3	3	Trace	4	470[12]	Trace	Trace	Trace	0
0.7	1.9	1.1	Trace	1	1	Trace	1	170[12]	Trace	Trace	Trace	0
32.5	71.5	65.4	Trace	53	52	0.4	59	7,500[12]	0.01	0.08	0.1	0
2.0	4.5	4.1	Trace	3	3	Trace	4	470[12]	Trace	Trace	Trace	0
11.2	28.7	16.7	Trace	18	17	0.1	20	2,500[12]	Trace	0.03	Trace	0
1.4	3.6	2.1	Trace	2	2	Trace	2	310[12]	Trace	Trace	Trace	0
27.7	53.6	125.1	0	0	0	0	0	—	0	0	0	0
1.7	3.3	7.8	0	0	0	0	0	—	0	0	0	0
30.7	154.4	17.7	0	0	0	0	0	—	0	0	0	0
1.9	9.7	1.1	0	0	0	0	0	—	0	0	0	0
37.4	98.5	67.0	0	0	0	0	0	—	0	0	0	0
2.3	6.2	4.2	0	0	0	0	0	—	0	0	0	0
20.5	25.9	159.8	0	0	0	0	0	—	0	0	0	0
1.3	1.6	10.0	0	0	0	0	0	—	0	0	0	0
31.8	93.1	75.6	0	0	0	0	0	—	0	0	0	0
2.0	5.8	4.7	0	0	0	0	0	—	0	0	0	0
38.2	63.0	99.6	0	0	0	0	0	—	0	0	0	0
2.4	3.9	6.2	0	0	0	0	0	—	0	0	0	0
1.6	1.7	3.8	1	12	11	Trace	6	30	Trace	0.02	Trace	Trace
0.5	0.3	Trace	1	10	8	Trace	5	30	Trace	0.01	Trace	Trace
1.1	1.3	3.2	3	2	2	0.1	13	—	—	—	—	—
0.1	0.1	0.4	2	2	2	0.1	13	—	—	—	—	—

Nutrients in Indicated Quantity

TABLE 5 (continued)

Food	Approximate Measures, Units, or Weight (edible part unless footnotes indicate otherwise)	Weight (g)	Water (%)	Food Energy (kcal)	Protein (g)	Fat (g)
Italian:						
Regular	1 T	15	28	85	Trace	9
Low calorie (2 kcal per teaspoon)	1 T	15	90	10	Trace	1
Mayonnaise	1 T	14	15	100	Trace	11
Mayonnaise type:						
Regular	1 T	15	41	65	Trace	6
Low calorie (8 kcal per teaspoon)	1 T	16	81	20	Trace	2
Tartar sauce, regular	1 T	14	34	75	Trace	8
Thousand Island:						
Regular	1 T	16	32	80	Trace	8
Low calorie (10 kcal per teaspoon)	1 T	15	68	25	Trace	2
Homemade:						
Cooked type [13]	1 T	16	68	25	1	2
Fish, Shellfish, Meat, Poultry; Related Products						
Fish and shellfish:						
Bluefish, baked with butter or margarine	3 oz	85	68	135	22	4
Clams:						
Raw, meat only	3 oz	85	82	65	11	1
Canned, solids and liquid	3 oz	85	86	45	7	1
Crabmeat (white or king), canned, not pressed down	1 c	135	77	135	24	3
Fish stick, breaded, cooked, frozen (4 × 1 × ½ in.)	1 fish stick or 1 oz	28	66	50	5	3
Haddock, breaded, fried [14]	3 oz	85	66	140	17	5
Ocean perch, breaded, fried [14]	1 fillet	85	59	195	16	11
Oysters, raw, meat only (13–19 medium selects)	1 c	240	85	160	20	4
Salmon, pink, canned, solids and liquid	3 oz	85	71	120	17	5
Sardines, Atlantic, canned in oil, drained solids	3 oz	85	62	175	20	9
Scallops, frozen, breaded, fried, reheated	6	90	60	175	16	8
Shad, baked with butter or margarine and bacon	3 oz	85	64	170	20	10
Shrimp:						
Canned meat	3 oz	85	70	100	21	1
French fried [16]	3 oz	85	57	190	17	9
Tuna, canned in oil, drained solids	3 oz	85	61	170	24	7
Tuna salad [17]	1 c	205	70	350	30	22
Meat and meat products:						
Bacon (20 slices per pound, raw), broiled or fried, crisp	2 slices	15	8	85	4	8
Beef, canned:						
Corned beef	3 oz	85	59	185	22	10
Corned beef hash	1 c	220	67	400	19	25
Beef,[18] cooked:						
Cuts braised, simmered, or pot-roasted:						
Lean and fat (piece, 2½ × 2½ × ¾ in.)	3 oz	85	53	245	23	16
Lean only	2.5 oz	72	62	140	22	5
Ground beef, broiled:						
Lean with 10% fat patty	3 oz	85	60	185	23	10
Lean with 21% fat patty	2.9 oz	82	54	235	20	17

| | Fatty Acids | | | | | | | | | | | |
| Saturated (total) (g) | Unsaturated | | Carbo-hydrate (g) | Calcium (mg) | Phos-phorus (mg) | Iron (mg) | Potassium (mg) | Vitamin A Value (IU) | Thiamin (mg) | Riboflavin (mg) | Niacin (mg) | Ascorbic Acid (mg) |
	Oleic (g)	Linoleic (g)										
1.6	1.9	4.7	1	2	1	Trace	2	Trace	Trace	Trace	Trace	—
0.1	0.1	0.4	Trace	Trace	1	Trace	2	Trace	Trace	Trace	Trace	—
2.0	2.4	5.6	Trace	3	4	0.1	5	40	Trace	0.01	Trace	—
1.1	1.4	3.2	2	2	4	Trace	1	30	Trace	Trace	Trace	—
0.4	0.4	1.0	2	3	4	Trace	1	40	Trace	Trace	Trace	—
1.5	1.8	4.1	1	3	4	0.1	11	30	Trace	Trace	Trace	Trace
1.4	1.7	4.0	2	2	3	0.1	18	50	Trace	Trace	Trace	Trace
0.4	0.4	1.0	2	2	3	0.1	17	50	Trace	Trace	Trace	Trace
0.5	0.6	0.3	2	14	15	0.1	19	80	0.01	0.03	Trace	Trace
—	—	—	0	25	244	0.6	—	40	0.09	0.08	1.6	—
—	—	—	2	59	138	5.2	154	90	0.08	0.15	1.1	8
0.2	Trace	Trace	2	47	116	3.5	119	—	0.01	0.09	0.9	—
0.6	0.4	0.1	1	61	246	1.1	149	—	0.11	0.11	2.6	—
—	—	—	2	3	47	0.1	—	0	0.01	0.02	0.5	—
1.4	2.2	1.2	5	34	210	1.0	296	—	0.03	0.06	2.7	2
2.7	4.4	2.3	6	28	192	1.1	242	—	0.10	0.10	1.6	—
1.3	0.2	0.1	8	226	343	13.2	290	740	0.34	0.43	6.0	—
0.9	0.8	0.1	0	167[15]	243	0.7	307	60	0.03	0.16	6.8	—
3.0	2.5	0.5	0	372	424	2.5	502	190	0.02	0.17	4.6	—
—	—	—	9	—	—	—	—	—	—	—	—	—
—	—	—	0	20	266	0.5	320	30	0.11	0.22	7.3	—
0.1	0.1	Trace	1	98	224	2.6	104	50	0.01	0.03	1.5	—
2.3	3.7	2.0	9	61	162	1.7	195	—	0.03	0.07	2.3	—
1.7	1.7	0.7	0	7	199	1.6	—	70	0.04	0.10	10.1	—
4.3	6.3	6.7	7	41	291	2.7	—	590	0.08	0.23	10.3	2
2.5	3.7	0.7	Trace	2	34	0.5	35	0	0.08	0.05	0.8	—
4.9	4.5	0.2	0	17	90	3.7	—	—	0.01	0.20	2.9	—
11.9	10.9	0.5	24	29	147	4.4	440	—	0.02	0.20	4.6	—
6.8	6.5	0.4	0	10	114	2.9	184	30	0.04	0.18	3.6	—
2.1	1.8	0.2	0	10	108	2.7	176	10	0.04	0.17	3.3	—
4.0	3.9	0.3	0	10	196	3.0	261	20	0.08	0.20	5.1	—
7.0	6.7	0.4	0	9	159	2.6	221	30	0.07	0.17	4.4	—

Nutrients in Indicated Quantity

TABLE 5   (continued)

Food	Approximate Measures, Units, or Weight (edible part unless footnotes indicate otherwise)	Weight (g)	Water (%)	Food Energy (kcal)	Protein (g)	Fat (g)
Roast, oven-cooked, no liquid added:						
Relatively fat, such as rib:						
Lean and fat (2 pieces, 4⅛ × 2¼ ×						
¼ in.)	3 oz	85	40	375	17	33
Lean only	1.8 oz	51	57	125	14	7
Relatively lean, such as heel of round:						
Lean and fat (2 pieces, 4⅛ × 2¼ ×						
¼ in.)	3 oz	85	62	165	25	7
Lean only from item 168	2.8 oz	78	65	125	24	3
Steak:						
Relatively fat, such as sirloin, broiled:						
Lean and fat (piece, 2½ × 2½ ×						
¾ in.)	3 oz	85	44	330	20	27
Lean only	2.0 oz	56	59	115	18	4
Relatively lean, such as round, braised:						
Lean and fat (piece, 4⅛ × 2¼ ×						
½ in.)	3 oz	85	55	220	24	13
Lean only	2.4 oz	68	61	130	21	4
Beef, dried, chipped	2½-oz	71	48	145	24	4
Beef and vegetable stew	1 c	245	82	220	16	11
Beef potpie (homemade), baked[19] (piece, ⅓ of 9-in.-diam. pie)	1 piece	210	55	515	21	30
Chili con carne with beans, canned	1 c	255	72	340	19	16
Chop suey with beef and pork (homemade)	1 c	250	75	300	26	17
Heart, beef, lean, braised	3 oz	85	61	160	27	5
Lamb, cooked:						
Chop, rib (cut 3 per pound with bone), broiled:						
Lean and fat	3.1 oz	89	43	360	18	32
Lean only	2 oz	57	60	120	16	6
Leg, roasted:						
Lean and fat (2 pieces, 4⅛ × 2¼ ×						
¼ in.)	3 oz	85	54	235	22	16
Lean only	2.5 oz	71	62	130	20	5
Shoulder, roasted:						
Lean and fat (3 pieces, 2½ × 2½ ×						
¼ in.)	3 oz	85	50	285	18	23
Lean only	2.3 oz	64	61	130	17	6
Liver, beef, fried[20] (slice, 6½ × 2⅜ × ⅜ in.)	3 oz	85	56	195	22	9
Pork, cured, cooked:						
Ham, light cure, lean and fat, roasted (2 pieces, 4⅛ × 2¼ × ¼ in.)[22]	3 oz	85	54	245	18	19
Luncheon meat:						
Boiled ham, slice	1 oz	28	59	65	5	5
Canned, spiced or unspiced:						
Slice, 3 × 2 × ½ in.	1 slice	60	55	175	9	15

Nutrients in Indicated Quantity												
Fatty Acids												
Saturated (total) (g)	Unsaturated		Carbo-hydrate (g)	Calcium (mg)	Phos-phorus (mg)	Iron (mg)	Potassium (mg)	Vitamin A Value (IU)	Thiamin (mg)	Riboflavin (mg)	Niacin (mg)	Ascorbic Acid (mg)
	Oleic (g)	Linoleic (g)										
14.0	13.6	0.8	0	8	158	2.2	189	70	0.05	0.13	3.1	—
3.0	2.5	0.3	0	6	131	1.8	161	10	0.04	0.11	2.6	—
2.8	2.7	0.2	0	11	208	3.2	279	10	0.06	0.19	4.5	—
1.2	1.0	0.1	0	10	199	3.0	268	Trace	0.06	0.18	4.3	—
11.3	11.1	0.6	0	9	162	2.5	220	50	0.05	0.15	4.0	—
1.8	1.6	0.2	0	7	146	2.2	202	10	0.05	0.14	3.6	
5.5	5.2	0.4	0	10	213	3.0	272	20	0.07	0.19	4.8	—
1.7	1.5	0.2	0	9	182	2.5	238	10	0.05	0.16	4.1	—
2.1	2.0	0.1	0	14	287	3.6	142	—	0.05	0.23	2.7	0
4.9	4.5	0.2	15	29	184	2.9	613	2,400	0.15	0.17	4.7	17
7.9	12.8	6.7	39	29	149	3.8	334	1,720	0.30	0.30	5.5	6
7.5	6.8	0.3	31	82	321	4.3	594	150	0.08	0.18	3.3	—
8.5	6.2	0.7	13	60	248	4.8	425	600	0.28	0.38	5.0	33
1.5	1.1	0.6	1	5	154	5.0	197	20	0.21	1.04	6.5	1
14.8	12.1	1.2	0	8	139	1.0	200	—	0.11	0.19	4.1	—
2.5	2.1	0.2	0	6	121	1.1	174	—	0.09	0.15	3.4	—
7.3	6.0	0.6	0	9	177	1.4	241	—	0.13	0.23	4.7	—
2.1	1.8	0.2	0	9	169	1.4	227	—	0.12	0.21	4.4	—
10.8	8.8	0.9	0	9	146	1.0	206	—	0.11	0.20	4.0	—
3.6	2.3	0.2	0	8	140	1.0	193	—	0.10	0.18	3.7	—
2.5	3.5	0.9	5	9	405	7.5	323	45,390[21]	0.22	3.56	14.0	23
6.8	7.9	1.7	0	8	146	2.2	199	0	0.40	0.15	3.1	—
1.7	2.0	0.4	0	3	47	0.8	—	0	0.12	0.04	0.7	—
5.4	6.7	1.0	1	5	65	1.3	133	0	0.19	0.13	1.8	—

TABLE 5 (continued)

Food	Approximate Measures, Units, or Weight (edible part unless footnotes indicate otherwise)	Weight (g)	Water (%)	Food Energy (kcal)	Protein (g)	Fat (g)
Pork, fresh, cooked: [18]						
Chop, loin (cut 3 per pound with bone), broiled:						
Lean and fat	2.7 oz	78	42	305	19	25
Lean only	2 oz	56	53	150	17	9
Roast, oven-cooked, no liquid added:						
Lean and fat (piece, 2½ × 2½ × ¾ in.)	3 oz	85	46	310	21	24
Lean only	2.4 oz	68	55	175	20	10
Shoulder cut, simmered:						
Lean and fat (3 pieces, 2½ × 2½ × ¼ in.)	3 oz	85	46	320	20	26
Lean only	2.2 oz	63	60	135	18	6
Sausages (see also Luncheon meat):						
Bologna, slice	1 oz	28	56	85	3	8
Braunschweiger, slice	1 oz	28	53	90	4	8
Brown-and-serve (10 to 11 per 8-oz package), browned	1 link	17	40	70	3	6
Deviled ham, canned	1 T	13	51	45	2	4
Frankfurter (8 per 1-lb package), cooked (reheated)	1	56	57	170	7	15
Meat, potted (beef, chicken, turkey), canned	1 T	13	61	30	2	2
Pork link (16 per 1-lb package), cooked	1 link	13	35	60	2	6
Salami:						
Dry type, slice (12 per 4-oz package)	1 slice	10	30	45	2	4
Cooked type, slice (8 per 8-oz package)	1 slice	28	51	90	5	7
Vienna sausage (7 per 4-oz can)	1	16	63	40	2	3
Veal, medium fat, cooked, bone removed:						
Cutlet (4⅛ × 2¼ × ½ in.), braised or broiled	3 oz	85	60	185	23	9
Rib (2 pieces, 4⅛ × 2¼ × ¼ in.), roasted	3 oz	85	55	230	23	14
Poultry and poultry products:						
Chicken, cooked:						
Breast, fried,[23] bones removed, ½ breast (3.3 oz with bones)	2.8 oz	79	58	160	26	5
Drumstick, fried,[23] bones removed (2 oz with bones)	1.3 oz	38	55	90	12	4
Half broiler, broiled, bones removed (10.4 oz with bones)	6.2 oz	176	71	240	42	7
Chicken, canned, boneless	3 oz	85	65	170	18	10
Chicken a la king, cooked (homemade)	1 c	245	68	470	27	34
Chicken and noodles, cooked (homemade)	1 c	240	71	365	22	18
Chicken chow mein:						
Canned	1 c	250	89	95	7	Trace
Homemade	1 c	250	78	255	31	10
Chicken potpie (homemade), baked,[19] piece (⅓ of 9-in.-diam. pie)	1 piece	232	57	545	23	31
Turkey, roasted, flesh without skin:						
Dark meat, piece, 2½ × 1⅝ × ¼ in.	4 pieces	85	61	175	26	7

Saturated (total) (g)	Fatty Acids — Unsaturated Oleic (g)	Linoleic (g)	Carbo-hydrate (g)	Calcium (mg)	Phos-phorus (mg)	Iron (mg)	Potassium (mg)	Vitamin A Value (IU)	Thiamin (mg)	Riboflavin (mg)	Niacin (mg)	Ascorbic Acid (mg)
8.9	10.4	2.2	0	9	209	2.7	216	0	0.75	0.22	4.5	—
3.1	3.6	0.8	0	7	181	2.2	192	0	0.63	0.18	3.8	—
8.7	10.2	2.2	0	9	218	2.7	233	0	0.78	0.22	4.8	—
3.5	4.1	0.8	0	9	211	2.6	224	0	0.73	0.21	4.4	—
9.3	10.9	2.3	0	9	118	2.6	158	0	0.46	0.21	4.1	—
2.2	2.6	0.6	0	8	111	2.3	146	0	0.42	0.19	3.7	—
3.0	3.4	0.5	Trace	2	36	0.5	65	—	0.05	0.06	0.7	—
2.6	3.4	0.8	1	3	69	1.7	—	1,850	0.05	0.41	2.3	—
2.3	2.8	0.7	Trace	—	—	—	—	—	—	—	—	—
1.5	1.8	0.4	0	1	12	0.3	—	0	0.02	0.01	0.2	—
5.6	6.5	1.2	1	3	57	0.8	—	—	0.08	0.11	1.4	—
—	—	—	0	—	—	—	—	—	Trace	0.03	0.2	—
2.1	2.4	0.5	Trace	1	21	0.3	35	0	0.10	0.04	0.5	—
1.6	1.6	0.1	Trace	1	28	0.4	—	—	0.04	0.03	0.5	—
3.1	3.0	0.2	Trace	3	57	0.7	—	—	0.07	0.07	1.2	—
1.2	1.4	0.2	Trace	1	24	0.3	—	—	0.01	0.02	0.4	—
4.0	3.4	0.4	0	9	196	2.7	258	—	0.06	0.21	4.6	—
6.1	5.1	0.6	0	10	211	2.9	259	—	0.11	0.26	6.6	—
1.4	1.8	1.1	1	9	218	1.3	—	70	0.04	0.17	11.6	—
1.1	1.3	0.9	Trace	6	89	0.9	—	50	0.03	0.15	2.7	—
2.2	2.5	1.3	0	16	355	3.0	483	160	0.09	0.34	15.5	—
3.2	3.8	2.0	0	18	210	1.3	117	200	0.03	0.11	3.7	3
12.7	14.3	3.3	12	127	358	2.5	404	1,130	0.10	0.42	5.4	12
5.9	7.1	3.5	26	26	247	2.2	149	430	0.05	0.17	4.3	Trace
—	—	—	18	45	35	1.3	418	150	0.05	0.10	1.0	13
2.4	3.4	3.1	10	58	293	2.5	473	280	0.08	0.23	4.3	10
11.3	10.9	5.6	42	70	232	3.0	343	3,090	0.34	0.31	5.5	5
2.1	1.5	1.5	0	—	—	2.0	338	—	0.03	0.20	3.6	—

TABLE 5 (continued)

Food	Approximate Measures, Units, or Weight (edible part unless footnotes indicate otherwise)	Weight (g)	Water (%)	Food Energy (kcal)	Protein (g)	Fat (g)
Light and dark meat:						
Chopped or diced	1 c	140	61	265	44	9
Pieces (1 slice white meat, 4 × 2 × ¼ in., and 2 slices dark meat, 2½ × 1⅝ × ¼ in.)	3 pieces	85	61	160	27	5
Light meat, piece, 4 × 2 × ¼ in.	2 pieces	85	62	150	28	3
Fruits and Fruit Products						
Apples, raw, unpeeled, without cores:						
2¾-in. diam. (about 3 per pound with cores)	1	138	84	80	Trace	1
3¼-in. diam. (about 2 per pound with cores)	1	212	84	125	Trace	1
Apple juice, bottled or canned[24]	1 c	248	88	120	Trace	Trace
Applesauce, canned:						
Sweetened	1 c	255	76	230	1	Trace
Unsweetened	1 c	244	89	100	Trace	Trace
Apricots:						
Raw, without pits (about 12 per pound with pits)	3	107	85	55	1	Trace
Canned in heavy syrup (halves and syrup)	1 c	258	77	220	2	Trace
Dried:						
Uncooked (28 large or 37 medium halves per cup)	1 c	130	25	340	7	1
Cooked, unsweetened, fruit and liquid	1 c	250	76	215	4	1
Apricot nectar, canned	1 c	251	85	145	1	Trace
Avocados, raw, whole, without skins and seeds:						
California, mid- and late-winter (with skin and seed, 3⅛-in. diam.; 10 oz)	1	216	74	370	5	37
Florida, late summer and fall (with skin and seed, 3⅝-in. diam.; 1 lb)	1	304	78	390	4	33
Banana, without peel (about 2.6 per pound with peel)	1	119	76	100	1	Trace
Banana flakes	1 T	6	3	20	Trace	Trace
Blackberries, raw	1 c	144	85	85	2	1
Blueberries, raw	1 c	145	83	90	1	1
Cantaloupe. See Muskmelons.						
Cherries:						
Sour (tart), red, pitted, canned, water pack	1 c	244	88	105	2	Trace
Sweet, raw, without pits and stems	10	68	80	45	1	Trace
Cranberry juice cocktail, bottled, sweetened	1 c	253	83	165	Trace	Trace
Cranberry sauce, sweetened, canned, strained	1 c	277	62	405	Trace	1
Dates:						
Whole, without pits	10	80	23	220	2	Trace
Chopped	1 c	178	23	490	4	1
Fruit cocktail, canned, in heavy syrup	1 c	255	80	195	1	Trace
Grapefruit:						
Raw, medium, 3¾-in. diam. (about 1 lb 1 oz):						
Pink or red, with peel	½	241[28]	89	50	1	Trace
White, with peel	½	241[28]	89	45	1	Trace
Canned, sections with syrup	1 c	254	81	180	2	Trace

| Fatty Acids | | | | | | | | | | | | |
| Saturated (total) (g) | Unsaturated | | Carbohydrate (g) | Calcium (mg) | Phosphorus (mg) | Iron (mg) | Potassium (mg) | Vitamin A Value (IU) | Thiamin (mg) | Riboflavin (mg) | Niacin (mg) | Ascorbic Acid (mg) |
	Oleic (g)	Linoleic (g)										
2.5	1.7	1.8	0	11	351	2.5	514	—	0.07	0.25	10.8	—
1.5	1.0	1.1	0	7	213	1.5	312	—	0.04	0.15	6.5	—
0.9	0.6	0.7	0	—	—	1.0	349	—	0.04	0.12	9.4	—
—	—	—	20	10	14	0.4	152	120	0.04	0.03	0.1	6
—	—	—	31	15	21	0.6	233	190	0.06	0.04	0.2	8
—	—	—	30	15	22	1.5	250	—	0.02	0.05	0.2	2[25]
—	—	—	61	10	13	1.3	166	100	0.05	0.03	0.1	3[25]
—	—	—	26	10	12	1.2	190	100	0.05	0.02	0.1	2[25]
—	—	—	14	18	25	0.5	301	2,890	0.03	0.04	0.6	11
—	—	—	57	28	39	0.8	604	4,490	0.05	0.05	1.0	10
—	—	—	86	87	140	7.2	1,273	14,170	0.01	0.21	4.3	16
—	—	—	54	55	88	4.5	795	7,500	0.01	0.13	2.5	8
—	—	—	37	23	30	0.5	379	2,380	0.03	0.03	0.5	36[26]
5.5	22.0	3.7	13	22	91	1.3	1,303	630	0.24	0.43	3.5	30
6.7	15.7	5.3	27	30	128	1.8	1,836	880	0.33	0.61	4.9	43
—	—	—	26	10	31	0.8	440	230	0.06	0.07	0.8	12
—	—	—	5	2	6	0.2	92	50	0.01	0.01	0.2	Trace
—	—	—	19	46	27	1.3	245	290	0.04	0.06	0.6	30
—	—	—	22	22	19	1.5	117	150	0.04	0.09	0.7	20
—	—	—	26	37	32	0.7	317	1,660	0.07	0.05	0.5	12
—	—	—	12	15	13	0.3	129	70	0.03	0.04	0.3	7
—	—	—	42	13	8	0.8	25	Trace	0.03	0.03	0.1	81[27]
—	—	—	104	17	11	0.6	83	60	0.03	0.03	0.1	6
—	—	—	58	47	50	2.4	518	40	0.07	0.08	1.8	0
—	—	—	130	105	112	5.3	1,153	90	0.16	0.18	3.9	0
—	—	—	50	23	31	1.0	411	360	0.05	0.03	1.0	5
—	—	—	13	20	20	0.5	166	540	0.05	0.02	0.2	44
—	—	—	12	19	19	0.5	159	10	0.05	0.02	0.2	44
—	—	—	45	33	36	0.8	343	30	0.08	0.05	0.5	76

Nutrients in Indicated Quantity

TABLE 5 (continued)

Food	Approximate Measures, Units, or Weight (edible part unless footnotes indicate otherwise)	Weight (g)	Water (%)	Food Energy (kcal)	Protein (g)	Fat (g)
Grapefruit juice:						
Raw, pink, red, or white	1 c	246	90	95	1	Trace
Canned, white:						
Unsweetened	1 c	247	89	100	1	Trace
Sweetened	1 c	250	86	135	1	Trace
Frozen, concentrate, unsweetened:						
Undiluted	6 fl oz	207	62	300	4	1
Diluted with 3 parts water by volume	1 c	247	89	100	1	Trace
Dehydrated crystals, prepared with water						
(1 lb yields about 1 gal)	1 c	247	90	100	1	Trace
Grapes, European type (adherent skin), raw:						
Thompson seedless	10	50	81	35	Trace	Trace
Tokay and Emperor (seeded)	10	60[30]	81	40	Trace	Trace
Grape juice:						
Canned or bottled	1 c	253	83	165	1	Trace
Frozen concentrate, sweetened:						
Undiluted	6 fl oz	216	53	395	1	Trace
Diluted with 3 parts water by volume	1 c	250	86	135	1	Trace
Grape drink, canned	1 c	250	86	135	Trace	Trace
Lemon, raw, size 165, without peel and seeds						
(about 4 per pound with peels and seeds)	1	74	90	20	1	Trace
Lemonade concentrate, frozen:						
Undiluted	6 fl oz	219	49	425	Trace	Trace
Diluted with 4⅓ parts water by volume	1 c	248	89	105	Trace	Trace
Lemon juice:						
Raw	1 c	244	91	60	1	Trace
Canned or bottled, unsweetened	1 c	244	92	55	1	Trace
Frozen, single strength, unsweetened	6 oz	183	92	40	1	Trace
Limeade concentrate, frozen:						
Undiluted	6 fl oz	218	50	410	Trace	Trace
Diluted with 4⅓ parts water by volume	1 c	247	89	100	Trace	Trace
Lime juice:						
Raw	1 c	246	90	65	1	Trace
Canned, unsweetened	1 c	246	90	65	1	Trace
Muskmelons, raw, with rind, without seed cavity:						
Cantaloupe, orange-fleshed (with rind and						
seed cavity, 5-in. diam., 2⅓ lb), with rind	½	477[33]	91	80	2	Trace
Honeydew (with rind and seed cavity, 6½-in.						
diam., 5¼ lb), with rind	1/10	226[33]	91	50	1	Trace
Oranges, all commercial varieties, raw:						
Whole, 2⅝-in. diam., without peel and seeds						
(about 2½ per pound with peel and						
seeds)	1	131	86	65	1	Trace
Sections without membranes	1 c	180	86	90	2	Trace
Orange juice:						
Raw, all varieties	1 c	248	88	110	2	Trace
Canned, unsweetened	1 c	249	87	120	2	Trace

Saturated (total) (g)	Unsaturated Oleic (g)	Unsaturated Linoleic (g)	Carbo-hydrate (g)	Calcium (mg)	Phos-phorus (mg)	Iron (mg)	Potassium (mg)	Vitamin A Value (IU)	Thiamin (mg)	Riboflavin (mg)	Niacin (mg)	Ascorbic Acid (mg)
—	—	—	23	22	37	0.5	399	[29]	0.10	0.05	0.5	93
—	—	—	24	20	35	1.0	400	20	0.07	0.05	0.5	84
—	—	—	32	20	35	1.0	405	30	0.08	0.05	0.5	78
—	—	—	72	70	124	0.8	1,250	60	0.29	0.12	1.4	286
—	—	—	24	25	42	0.2	420	20	0.10	0.04	0.5	96
—	—	—	24	22	40	0.2	412	20	0.10	0.05	0.5	91
—	—	—	9	6	10	0.2	87	50	0.03	0.02	0.2	2
—	—	—	10	7	11	0.2	99	60	0.03	0.02	0.2	2
—	—	—	42	28	30	0.8	293	—	0.10	0.05	0.5	Trace[25]
—	—	—	100	22	32	0.9	255	40	0.13	0.22	1.5	32[31]
—	—	—	33	8	10	0.3	85	10	0.05	0.08	0.5	10[31]
—	—	—	35	8	10	0.3	88	—	0.03[32]	0.03[32]	0.3	[32]
—	—	—	6	19	12	0.4	102	10	0.03	0.01	0.1	39
—	—	—	112	9	13	0.4	153	40	0.05	0.06	0.7	66
—	—	—	28	2	3	0.1	40	10	0.01	0.02	0.2	17
—	—	—	20	17	24	0.5	344	50	0.07	0.02	0.2	112
—	—	—	19	17	24	0.5	344	50	0.07	0.02	0.2	102
—	—	—	13	13	16	0.5	258	40	0.05	0.02	0.2	81
—	—	—	108	11	13	0.2	129	Trace	0.02	0.02	0.2	26
—	—	—	27	3	3	Trace	32	Trace	Trace	Trace	Trace	6
—	—	—	22	22	27	0.5	256	20	0.05	0.02	0.2	79
—	—	—	22	22	27	0.5	256	20	0.05	0.02	0.2	52
—	—	—	20	38	44	1.1	682	9,240	0.11	0.08	1.6	90
—	—	—	11	21	24	0.6	374	60	0.06	0.04	0.9	34
—	—	—	16	54	26	0.5	263	260	0.13	0.05	0.5	66
—	—	—	22	74	36	0.7	360	360	0.18	0.07	0.7	90
—	—	—	26	27	42	0.5	496	500	0.22	0.07	1.0	124
—	—	—	28	25	45	1.0	496	500	0.17	0.05	0.7	100

TABLE 5 (continued)

Food	Approximate Measures, Units, or Weight (edible part unless footnotes indicate otherwise)	Weight (g)	Water (%)	Food Energy (kcal)	Protein (g)	Fat (g)
Frozen concentrate:						
Undiluted	6 fl oz	213	55	360	5	Trace
Diluted with 3 parts water by volume	1 c	249	87	120	2	Trace
Dehydrated crystals, prepared with water						
(1 lb yields about 1 gal)	1 c	248	88	115	1	Trace
Orange and grapefruit juice:						
Frozen concentrate:						
Undiluted	6 fl oz	210	59	330	4	1
Diluted with 3 parts water by volume	1 c	248	88	110	1	Trace
Papayas, raw, ½-in. cubes	1 c	140	89	55	1	Trace
Peaches:						
Raw:						
Whole, 2½-in. diam., peeled, pitted (about						
4 per pound with peels and pits)	1	100	89	40	1	Trace
Sliced	1 c	170	89	65	1	Trace
Canned, yellow-fleshed, solids and liquid						
(halves or slices):						
Syrup pack	1 c	256	79	200	1	Trace
Water pack	1 c	244	91	75	1	Trace
Dried:						
Uncooked	1 c	160	25	420	5	1
Cooked, unsweetened, halves and juice	1 c	250	77	205	3	1
Frozen, sliced, sweetened:						
10-oz container	1 container	284	77	250	1	Trace
Cup	1 c	250	77	220	1	Trace
Pears:						
Raw, with skin, cored:						
Anjou, 3-in. diam. (about 2 per pound with						
cores and stems)	1	200	83	120	1	1
Bartlett, 2½-in. diam. (about 2½ per pound						
with cores and stems)	1	164	83	100	1	1
Bosc, 2½-in. diam. (about 3 per pound with						
cores and stems)	1	141	83	85	1	1
Canned, solids and liquid, syrup pack, heavy						
(halves or slices)	1 c	255	80	195	1	1
Pineapple:						
Raw, diced	1 c	155	85	80	1	Trace
Canned, heavy syrup pack, solids and liquid:						
Crushed, chunks, tidbits	1 c	255	80	190	1	Trace
Slices and liquid:						
Large	1 slice; 2¼ T liquid	105	80	80	Trace	Trace
Medium	1 slice; 1¼ T liquid	58	80	45	Trace	Trace
Pineapple juice, unsweetened, canned	1 c	250	86	140	1	Trace
Plums:						
Raw, without pits:						
Japanese and hybrid (2⅛-in. diam., about						
6½ per pound with pits)	1	66	87	30	Trace	Trace
Prune-type (1½-in. diam., about 15 per						
pound with pits)	1	28	79	20	Trace	Trace

Saturated (total) (g)	Oleic (g)	Linoleic (g)	Carbohydrate (g)	Calcium (mg)	Phosphorus (mg)	Iron (mg)	Potassium (mg)	Vitamin A Value (IU)	Thiamin (mg)	Riboflavin (mg)	Niacin (mg)	Ascorbic Acid (mg)
—	—	—	87	75	126	0.9	1,500	1,620	0.68	0.11	2.8	360
—	—	—	29	25	42	0.2	503	540	0.23	0.03	0.9	120
—	—	—	27	25	40	0.5	518	500	0.20	0.07	1.0	109
—	—	—	78	61	99	0.8	1,308	800	0.48	0.06	2.3	302
—	—	—	26	20	32	0.2	439	270	0.15	0.02	0.7	102
—	—	—	14	28	22	0.4	328	2,450	0.06	0.06	0.4	78
—	—	—	10	9	19	0.5	202	1,330[34]	0.02	0.05	1.0	7
—	—	—	16	15	32	0.9	343	2,260[34]	0.03	0.09	1.7	12
—	—	—	51	10	31	0.8	333	1,100	0.03	0.05	1.5	8
—	—	—	20	10	32	0.7	334	1,100	0.02	0.07	1.5	7
—	—	—	109	77	187	9.6	1,520	6,240	0.02	0.30	8.5	29
—	—	—	54	38	93	4.8	743	3,050	0.01	0.15	3.8	5
—	—	—	64	11	37	1.4	352	1,850	0.03	0.11	2.0	116[35]
—	—	—	57	10	33	1.3	310	1,630	0.03	0.10	1.8	103[35]
—	—	—	31	16	22	0.6	260	40	0.04	0.08	0.2	8
—	—	—	25	13	18	0.5	213	30	0.03	0.07	0.2	7
—	—	—	22	11	16	0.4	83	30	0.03	0.06	0.1	6
—	—	—	50	13	18	0.5	214	10	0.03	0.05	0.3	3
—	—	—	21	26	12	0.8	226	110	0.14	0.05	0.3	26
—	—	—	49	28	13	0.8	245	130	0.20	0.05	0.5	18
—	—	—	20	12	5	0.3	101	50	0.08	0.02	0.2	7
—	—	—	11	6	3	0.2	56	30	0.05	0.01	0.1	4
—	—	—	34	38	23	0.8	373	130	0.13	0.05	0.5	80[27]
—	—	—	8	8	12	0.3	112	160	0.02	0.02	0.3	4
—	—	—	6	3	5	0.1	48	80	0.01	0.01	0.1	1

TABLE 5 (continued)

Food	Approximate Measures, Units, or Weight (edible part unless footnotes indicate otherwise)	Weight (g)	Water (%)	Food Energy (kcal)	Protein (g)	Fat (g)
Canned, heavy syrup pack (Italian prunes), with pits and liquid:						
Cup	1 c[36]	272	77	215	1	Trace
Portion	3; 2¾ T liquid[36]	140	77	110	1	Trace
Prunes, dried, "softenized," with pits:						
Uncooked	4 extra large or 5 large	49[36]	28	110	1	Trace
Cooked, unsweetened, all sizes, fruit and liquid	1 c	250[36]	66	255	2	1
Prune juice, canned or bottles	1 c	256	80	195	1	Trace
Raisins, seedless:						
Cup, not pressed down	1 c	145	18	420	4	Trace
Packet, ½ oz (1½ T)	1 packet	14	18	40	Trace	Trace
Raspberries, red:						
Raw, capped, whole	1 c	123	84	70	1	1
Frozen, sweetened	10 oz	284	74	280	2	1
Rhubarb, cooked, added sugar:						
From raw	1 c	270	63	380	1	Trace
From frozen, sweetened	1 c	270	63	385	1	1
Strawberries:						
Raw, whole berries, capped	1 c	149	90	55	1	1
Frozen, sweetened:						
Sliced	10 oz	284	71	310	1	1
Whole	1 lb (about 1¾ c)	454	76	415	2	1
Tangerine, raw, 2⅜-in. diam., size 176, without peel (about 4 per pound with peels and seeds)	1	86	87	40	1	Trace
Tangerine juice, canned, sweetened	1 c	249	87	125	1	Trace
Watermelon, raw, 4 × 8 in. wedge with rind and seeds (1/16 of 32⅔-lb melon, 10 × 16 in.),	1	926[37]	93	110	2	1
Grain Products						
Bagel, 3-in. diam.:						
Egg	1	55	32	165	6	2
Water	1	55	29	165	6	1
Barley, pearled, light, uncooked	1 c	200	11	700	16	2
Biscuits, baking powder, 2-in. diam. (enriched flour, vegetable shortening):						
Homemade	1	28	27	105	2	5
From mix	1	28	29	90	2	3
Bread crumbs (enriched):[38]						
Dry, grated	1 c	100	7	390	13	5
Soft. See Bread, White.						
Bread:						
Boston brown bread, canned, slice, 3¼ × ½ in.[38]	1 sl	45	45	95	2	1
Cracked wheat (¾ enriched wheat flour, ¼ cracked wheat):[38]						
Loaf	1 lb	454	35	1,195	39	10
Slice (18 per loaf)	1 sl	25	35	65	2	1

Nutrients in Indicated Quantity												
Fatty Acids												
Saturated	Unsaturated		Carbo-		Phos-			Vitamin A				Ascorbic
(total)	Oleic	Linoleic	hydrate	Calcium	phorus	Iron	Potassium	Value	Thiamin	Riboflavin	Niacin	Acid
(g)	(g)	(g)	(g)	(mg)	(mg)	(mg)	(mg)	(IU)	(mg)	(mg)	(mg)	(mg)
—	—	—	56	23	26	2.3	367	3,130	0.05	0.05	1.0	5
—	—	—	29	12	13	1.2	189	1,610	0.03	0.03	0.5	3
—	—	—	29	22	34	1.7	298	690	0.04	0.07	0.7	1
—	—	—	67	51	79	3.8	695	1,590	0.07	0.15	1.5	2
—	—	—	49	36	51	1.8	602	—	0.03	0.03	1.0	5
—	—	—	112	90	146	5.1	1,106	30	0.16	0.12	0.7	1
—	—	—	11	9	14	0.5	107	Trace	0.02	0.01	0.1	Trace
—	—	—	17	27	27	1.1	207	160	0.04	0.11	1.1	31
—	—	—	70	37	48	1.7	284	200	0.06	0.17	1.7	60
—	—	—	97	211	41	1.6	548	220	0.05	0.14	0.8	16
—	—	—	98	211	32	1.9	475	190	0.05	0.11	0.5	16
—	—	—	13	31	31	1.5	244	90	0.04	0.10	0.9	88
—	—	—	79	40	48	2.0	318	90	0.06	0.17	1.4	151
—	—	—	107	59	73	2.7	472	140	0.09	0.27	2.3	249
—	—	—	10	34	15	0.3	108	360	0.05	0.02	0.1	27
—	—	—	30	44	35	0.5	440	1,040	0.15	0.05	0.2	54
—	—	—	27	30	43	2.1	426	2,510	0.13	0.13	0.9	30
0.5	0.9	0.8	28	9	43	1.2	41	30	0.14	0.10	1.2	0
0.2	0.4	0.6	30	8	41	1.2	42	0	0.15	0.11	1.4	0
0.3	0.2	0.8	158	32	378	4.0	320	0	0.24	0.10	6.2	0
1.2	2.0	1.2	13	34	49	0.4	33	Trace	0.08	0.08	0.7	Trace
0.6	1.1	0.7	15	19	65	0.6	32	Trace	0.09	0.08	0.8	Trace
1.0	1.6	1.4	73	122	141	3.6	152	Trace	0.35	0.35	4.8	Trace
0.1	0.2	0.2	21	41	72	0.9	131	0[39]	0.06	0.04	0.7	0
2.2	3.0	3.9	236	399	581	9.5	608	Trace	1.52	1.13	14.4	Trace
0.1	0.2	0.2	13	22	32	0.5	34	Trace	0.08	0.06	0.8	Trace

TABLE 5 (continued)

Food	Approximate Measures, Units, or Weight (edible part unless footnotes indicate otherwise)	Weight (g)	Water (%)	Food Energy (kcal)	Protein (g)	Fat (g)
French or Vienna, enriched: [38]						
Loaf	1 lb	454	31	1,315	41	14
Slice:						
French (5 × 2½ × 1 in.)	1 sl	35	31	100	3	1
Vienna (4¾ × 4 × ½ in.)	1 sl	25	31	75	2	1
Italian, enriched:						
Loaf	1 lb	454	32	1,250	41	4
Slice, 4½ × 3¼ × ¾ in.	1 sl	30	32	85	3	Trace
Raisin, enriched: [38]						
Loaf	1 lb	454	35	1,190	30	13
Slice (18 per loaf)	1 sl	25	35	65	2	1
Rye:						
American, light (⅔ enriched wheat flour, ⅓ rye flour):						
Loaf	1 lb	454	36	1,100	41	5
Slice (4¾ × 3¾ × 7/16 in.)	1 sl	25	36	60	2	Trace
Pumpernickel (⅔ rye flour, ⅓ enriched wheat flour):						
Loaf	1 lb	454	34	1,115	41	5
Slice (5 × 4 × ⅜ in.)	1 sl	32	34	80	3	Trace
White, enriched: [38]						
Soft-crumb type:						
Loaf	1 lb	454	36	1,225	39	15
Slice (18 per loaf)	1 sl	25	36	70	2	1
Toast	1 sl	22	25	70	2	1
Slice (22 per loaf)	1 sl	20	36	55	2	1
Toast	1 sl	17	25	55	2	1
Loaf	1½ lb	680	36	1,835	59	22
Slice (24 per loaf)	1 sl	28	36	75	2	1
Toast	1 sl	24	25	75	2	1
Slice (28 per loaf)	1 sl	24	36	65	2	1
Toast	1 sl	21	25	65	2	1
Crumbs	1 c	45	36	120	4	1
Cubes	1 c	30	36	80	3	1
Firm-crumb type:						
Loaf	1 lb	454	35	1,245	41	17
Slice (20 per loaf)	1 sl	23	35	65	2	1
Toast	1 sl	20	24	65	2	1
Loaf	2 lb	907	35	2,495	82	34
Slice (34 per loaf)	1 sl	27	35	75	2	1
Toast	1 sl	23	24	75	2	1
Whole wheat:						
Soft-crumb type: [38]						
Loaf	1 lb	454	36	1,095	41	12
Slice (16 per loaf)	1 sl	28	36	65	3	1
Toast	1 sl	24	24	65	3	1
Firm-crumb type: [38]						
Loaf	1 lb	454	36	1,100	48	14

| | Fatty Acids | | | | | | | | | | | |
Saturated (total) (g)	Unsaturated Oleic (g)	Unsaturated Linoleic (g)	Carbo-hydrate (g)	Calcium (mg)	Phos-phorus (mg)	Iron (mg)	Potassium (mg)	Vitamin A Value (IU)	Thiamin (mg)	Riboflavin (mg)	Niacin (mg)	Ascorbic Acid (mg)
3.2	4.7	4.6	251	195	386	10.0	408	Trace	1.80	1.10	15.0	Trace
0.2	0.4	0.4	19	15	30	0.8	32	Trace	0.14	0.08	1.2	Trace
0.2	0.3	0.3	14	11	21	0.6	23	Trace	0.10	0.06	0.8	Trace
0.6	0.3	1.5	256	77	349	10.0	336	0	1.80	1.10	15.0	0
Trace	Trace	0.1	17	5	23	0.7	22	0	0.12	0.07	1.0	0
3.0	4.7	3.9	243	322	395	10.0	1,057	Trace	1.70	1.07	10.7	Trace
0.2	0.3	0.2	13	18	22	0.6	58	Trace	0.09	0.06	0.6	Trace
0.7	0.5	2.2	236	340	667	9.1	658	0	1.35	0.98	12.9	0
Trace	Trace	0.1	13	19	37	0.5	36	0	0.07	0.05	0.7	0
0.7	0.5	2.4	241	381	1,039	11.8	2,059	0	1.30	0.93	8.5	0
0.1	Trace	0.2	17	27	73	0.8	145	0	0.09	0.07	0.6	0
3.4	5.3	4.6	229	381	440	11.3	476	Trace	1.80	1.10	15.0	Trace
0.2	0.3	0.3	13	21	24	0.6	26	Trace	0.10	0.06	0.8	Trace
0.2	0.3	0.3	13	21	24	0.6	26	Trace	0.08	0.06	0.8	Trace
0.2	0.2	0.2	10	17	19	0.5	21	Trace	0.08	0.05	0.7	Trace
0.2	0.2	0.2	10	17	19	0.5	21	Trace	0.06	0.05	0.7	Trace
5.2	7.9	6.9	343	571	660	17.0	714	Trace	2.70	1.65	22.5	Trace
0.2	0.3	0.3	14	24	27	0.7	29	Trace	0.11	0.07	0.9	Trace
0.2	0.3	0.3	14	24	27	0.7	29	Trace	0.09	0.07	0.9	Trace
0.2	0.3	0.2	12	20	23	0.6	25	Trace	0.10	0.06	0.8	Trace
0.2	0.3	0.2	12	20	23	0.6	25	Trace	0.08	0.06	0.8	Trace
0.3	0.5	0.5	23	38	44	1.1	47	Trace	0.18	0.11	1.5	Trace
0.2	0.3	0.3	15	25	29	0.8	32	Trace	0.12	0.07	1.0	Trace
3.9	5.9	5.2	228	435	463	11.3	549	Trace	1.80	1.10	15.0	Trace
0.2	0.3	0.3	12	22	23	0.6	28	Trace	0.09	0.06	0.8	Trace
0.2	0.3	0.3	12	22	23	0.6	28	Trace	0.07	0.06	0.8	Trace
7.7	11.8	10.4	455	871	925	22.7	1,097	Trace	3.60	2.20	30.0	Trace
0.2	0.3	0.3	14	26	28	0.7	33	Trace	0.11	0.06	0.9	Trace
0.2	0.3	0.3	14	26	28	0.7	33	Trace	0.09	0.06	0.9	Trace
2.2	2.9	4.2	224	381	1,152	13.6	1,161	Trace	1.37	0.45	12.7	Trace
0.1	0.2	0.2	14	24	71	0.8	72	Trace	0.09	0.03	0.8	Trace
0.1	0.2	0.2	14	24	71	0.8	72	Trace	0.07	0.03	0.8	Trace
2.5	3.3	4.9	216	449	1,034	13.6	1,238	Trace	1.17	0.54	12.7	Trace

TABLE 5 (continued)

Food	Approximate Measures, Units, or Weight (edible part unless footnotes indicate otherwise)	Weight (g)	Water (%)	Food Energy (kcal)	Protein (g)	Fat (g)
Slice (18 per loaf)	1 sl	25	36	60	3	1
Toast	1 sl	21	24	60	3	1
Breakfast cereals:						
Hot type, cooked:						
Corn (hominy) grits, degermed:						
Enriched	1 c	245	87	125	3	Trace
Unenriched	1 c	245	87	125	3	Trace
Farina, quick-cooking, enriched	1 c	245	89	105	3	Trace
Oatmeal or rolled oats	1 c	240	87	130	5	2
Wheat, rolled	1 c	240	80	180	5	1
Wheat, whole meal	1 c	245	88	110	4	1
Ready-to-eat:						
Bran flakes (40% bran), added sugar, salt, iron, vitamins	1 c	35	3	105	4	1
Bran flakes with raisins, added sugar, salt, iron, vitamins	1 c	50	7	145	4	1
Corn flakes:						
Plain, added sugar, salt, iron, vitamins	1 c	25	4	95	2	Trace
Sugar-coated, added salt, iron, vitamins	1 c	40	2	155	2	Trace
Corn, oat flour, puffed, added sugar, salt, iron, vitamins	1 c	20	4	80	2	1
Corn, shredded, added sugar, salt, iron, thiamin, niacin	1 c	25	3	95	2	Trace
Oats, puffed, added sugar, salt, minerals, vitamins	1 c	25	3	100	3	1
Rice, puffed:						
Plain, added iron, thiamin, niacin	1 c	15	4	60	1	Trace
Presweetened, added salt, iron, vitamins	1 c	28	3	115	1	0
Wheat flakes, added sugar, salt, iron, vitamins	1 c	30	4	105	3	Trace
Wheat, puffed:						
Plain, added iron, thiamin, niacin	1 c	15	3	55	2	Trace
Presweetened, added salt, iron, vitamins	1 c	38	3	140	3	Trace
Wheat, shredded, plain	1 oblong biscuit or ½ c spoon-size biscuits	25	7	90	2	1
Wheat germ, without salt and sugar, toasted	1 T	6	4	25	2	1
Buckwheat flour, light, sifted	1 c	98	12	340	6	1
Bulgur, canned, seasoned	1 c	135	56	245	8	4
Cake icings. See Sugars and Sweets.						
Cakes made from cake mixes with enriched flour:[46]						
Angel food:						
Whole cake (9¾-in. diam. tube cake)	1	635	34	1,645	36	1
Piece, 1/12 of cake	1	53	34	135	3	Trace
Coffee cake:						
Whole cake (7¾ × 5⅝ × 1¼ in.)	1	430	30	1,385	27	41
Piece, ⅙ of cake	1	72	30	230	5	7
Cupcake, made with egg, milk, 2½-in. diam.:						
Without icing	1	25	26	90	1	3
With chocolate icing	1	36	22	130	2	5

Nutrients in Indicated Quantity												
Fatty Acids												
Saturated (total) (g)	Unsaturated		Carbo-hydrate (g)	Calcium (mg)	Phos-phorus (mg)	Iron (mg)	Potassium (mg)	Vitamin A Value (IU)	Thiamin (mg)	Riboflavin (mg)	Niacin (mg)	Ascorbic Acid (mg)
	Oleic (g)	Linoleic (g)										
0.1	0.2	0.3	12	25	57	0.8	68	Trace	0.06	0.03	0.7	Trace
0.1	0.2	0.3	12	25	57	0.8	68	Trace	0.05	0.03	0.7	Trace
Trace	Trace	0.1	27	2	25	0.7	27	Trace[40]	0.10	0.07	1.0	0
Trace	Trace	0.1	27	2	25	0.2	27	Trace[40]	0.05	0.02	0.5	0
Trace	Trace	0.1	22	147	113[41]	[42]	25	0	0.12	0.07	1.0	0
0.4	0.8	0.9	23	22	137	1.4	146	0	0.19	0.05	0.2	0
—	—	—	41	19	182	1.7	202	0	0.17	0.07	2.2	0
—	—	—	23	17	127	1.2	118	0	0.15	0.05	1.5	0
—	—	—	28	19	125	5.6	137	1,540	0.46	0.52	6.2	0
—	—	—	40	28	146	7.9	154	2,200[43]	[44]	[44]	[44]	0
—	—	—	21	[44]	9	[44]	30	[44]	[44]	[44]	[44]	13[45]
—	—	—	37	1	10	[44]	27	1,760	0.53	0.60	7.1	21[45]
—	—	—	16	4	18	5.7	—	880	0.26	0.30	3.5	11
—	—	—	22	1	10	0.6	—	0	0.33	0.05	4.4	13
—	—	—	19	44	102	4.0	—	1,100	0.33	0.38	4.4	13
—	—	—	13	3	14	0.3	15	0	0.07	0.01	0.7	0
—	—	—	26	3	14	[44]	43	1,240[45]	[44]	[44]	[44]	15[45]
—	—	—	24	12	83	4.8	81	1,320	0.40	0.45	5.3	16
—	—	—	12	4	48	0.6	51	0	0.08	0.03	1.2	0
—	—	—	33	7	52	[44]	63	1,680	0.50	0.57	6.7	20[45]
—	—	—	20	11	97	0.9	87	0	0.06	0.03	1.1	0
—	—	—	3	3	70	0.5	57	10	0.11	0.05	0.3	1
0.2	0.4	0.4	78	11	86	1.0	314	0	0.08	0.04	0.4	0
—	—	—	44	27	263	1.9	151	0	0.08	0.05	4.1	0
—	—	—	377	603	756	2.5	381	0	0.37	0.95	3.6	0
—	—	—	32	50	63	0.2	32	0	0.03	0.08	0.3	0
11.7	16.3	8.8	225	262	748	6.9	469	690	0.82	0.91	7.7	1
2.0	2.7	1.5	38	44	125	1.2	78	120	0.14	0.15	1.3	Trace
0.8	1.2	0.7	14	40	59	0.3	21	40	0.05	0.05	0.4	Trace
2.0	1.6	0.6	21	47	71	0.4	42	60	0.05	0.06	0.4	Trace

TABLE 5 (continued)

Food	Approximate Measures, Units, or Weight (edible part unless footnotes indicate otherwise)	Weight (g)	Water (%)	Food Energy (kcal)	Protein (g)	Fat (g)
Devil's food with chocolate icing:						
Whole, 2-layer cake (8- or 9-in. diam.)	1	1,107	24	3,755	49	136
Piece, 1/16 of cake	1	69	24	235	3	8
Cupcake, 2½-in. diam.	1	35	24	120	2	4
Gingerbread:						
Whole cake (8-in. square)	1	570	37	1,575	18	39
Piece, 1/9 of cake	1	63	37	175	2	4
White, 2-layer with chocolate icing:						
Whole cake (8- or 9-in. diam.)	1	1,140	21	4,000	44	122
Piece, 1/16 of cake	1	71	21	250	3	8
Yellow, 2-layer with chocolate icing:						
Whole cake (8- or 9-in. diam.)	1	1,108	26	3,735	45	125
Piece, 1/16 of cake	1	69	26	235	3	8
Cakes made from home recipies using enriched flour:[47]						
Boston cream pie with custard filling:						
Whole cake (8-in. diam.)	1	825	35	2,490	41	78
Piece, 1/12 of cake	1	69	35	210	3	6
Fruitcake, dark:						
Loaf, 1 lb (7½ × 2 × 1½ in.)	1 lb	454	18	1,720	22	69
Slice, 1/30 of loaf	1 slice	15	18	55	1	2
Plain, sheet cake:						
Without icing:						
Whole cake (9-in. square)	1	777	25	2,830	35	108
Piece, 1/9 of cake	1	86	25	315	4	12
With uncooked white icing:						
Whole cake (9-in. square)	1	1,096	21	4,020	37	129
Piece, 1/9 of cake	1	121	21	445	4	14
Pound:[49]						
Loaf, 8½ × 3½ × 3¼ in.	1	565	16	2,725	31	170
Slice, 1/17 of loaf	1	33	16	160	2	10
Sponge cake:						
Whole cake (9¾-in. diam. tube cake)	1	790	32	2,345	60	45
Piece, 1/12 of cake	1	66	32	195	5	4
Cookies made with enriched flour:[50] [51]						
Brownie with nuts:						
Homemade, 1¾ × 1¾ × 7/8 in.:						
From home recipe	1	20	10	95	1	6
From commercial recipe	1	20	11	85	1	4
Frozen, with chocolate icing,[52] 1½ × 1¾ × 7/8 in.	1	25	13	105	1	5
Chocolate chip:						
Commercial, 2¼-in. diam., 3/8 in. thick	4	42	3	200	2	9
Homemade, 2⅓-in. diam.	4	40	3	205	2	12
Fig bars, square (15/8 × 15/8 × 3/8 in.) or rectangular (1½ × 1¾ × ½ in.)	4	56	14	200	2	3
Gingersnaps, 2-in. diam., ¼ in. thick	4	28	3	90	2	2
Macaroons, 2¾-in. diam., ¼ in. thick	2	38	4	180	2	9

| | Fatty Acids | | | | | | | | | | | |
| Saturated (total) (g) | Unsaturated | | Carbo-hydrate (g) | Calcium (mg) | Phos-phorus (mg) | Iron (mg) | Potassium (mg) | Vitamin A Value (IU) | Thiamin (mg) | Riboflavin (mg) | Niacin (mg) | Ascorbic Acid (mg) |
	Oleic (g)	Linoleic (g)										
50.0	44.9	17.0	645	653	1,162	16.6	1,439	1,660	1.06	1.65	10.1	1
3.1	2.8	1.1	40	41	72	1.0	90	100	0.07	0.10	0.6	Trace
1.6	1.4	0.5	20	21	37	0.5	46	50	0.03	0.05	0.3	Trace
9.7	16.6	10.0	291	513	570	8.6	1,562	Trace	0.84	1.00	7.4	Trace
1.1	1.8	1.1	32	57	63	0.9	173	Trace	0.09	0.11	0.8	Trace
48.2	46.4	20.0	716	1,129	2,041	11.4	1,322	680	1.50	1.77	12.5	2
3.0	2.9	1.2	45	70	127	0.7	82	40	0.09	0.11	0.8	Trace
47.8	47.8	20.3	638	1,008	2,017	12.2	1,208	1,550	1.24	1.67	10.6	2
3.0	3.0	1.3	40	63	126	0.8	75	100	0.08	0.10	0.7	Trace
23.0	30.1	15.2	412	553	833	8.2	734[48]	1,730	1.04	1.27	9.6	2
1.9	2.5	1.3	34	46	70	0.7	61[48]	140	0.09	0.11	0.8	Trace
14.4	33.5	14.8	271	327	513	11.8	2,250	540	0.72	0.73	4.9	2
0.5	1.1	0.5	9	11	17	0.4	74	20	0.02	0.02	0.2	Trace
29.5	44.4	23.9	434	497	793	8.5	614[48]	1,320	1.21	1.40	10.2	2
3.3	4.9	2.6	48	55	88	0.9	68[48]	150	0.13	0.15	1.1	Trace
42.2	49.5	24.4	694	548	822	8.2	669[48]	2,190	1.22	1.47	10.2	2
4.7	5.5	2.7	77	61	91	0.8	74[48]	240	0.14	0.16	1.1	Trace
42.9	73.1	39.6	273	107	418	7.9	345	1,410	0.90	0.99	7.3	0
2.5	4.3	2.3	16	6	24	0.5	20	80	0.05	0.06	0.4	0
13.1	15.8	5.7	427	237	885	13.4	687	3,560	1.10	1.64	7.4	Trace
1.1	1.3	0.5	36	20	74	1.1	57	300	0.09	0.14	0.6	Trace
1.5	3.0	1.2	10	8	30	0.4	38	40	0.04	0.03	0.2	Trace
0.9	1.4	1.3	13	9	27	0.4	34	20	0.03	0.02	0.2	Trace
2.0	2.2	0.7	15	10	31	0.4	44	50	0.03	0.03	0.2	Trace
2.8	2.9	2.2	29	16	48	1.0	56	50	0.10	0.17	0.9	Trace
3.5	4.5	2.9	24	14	40	0.8	47	40	0.06	0.06	0.5	Trace
0.8	1.2	0.7	42	44	34	1.0	111	60	0.04	0.14	0.9	Trace
0.7	1.0	0.6	22	20	13	0.7	129	20	0.08	0.06	0.7	0
—	—	—	25	10	32	0.3	176	0	0.02	0.06	0.2	0

TABLE 5 (continued)

Food	Approximate Measures, Units, or Weight (edible part unless footnotes indicate otherwise)	Weight (g)	Water (%)	Food Energy (kcal)	Protein (g)	Fat (g)
Oatmeal with raisins, 2⅝-in. diam., ¼ in. thick	4	52	3	235	3	8
Plain, prepared from commercial chilled dough, 2½-in. diam., ¼ in. thick	4	48	5	240	2	12
Sandwich type (chocolate or vanilla), 1¾-in. diam., ⅜ in. thick	4	40	2	200	2	9
Vanilla wafers, 1¾-in. diam., ¼ in. thick	10	40	3	185	2	6
Cornmeal:						
Whole-grain, unbolted, dry form	1 c	122	12	435	11	5
Bolted (nearly whole grain), dry form	1 c	122	12	440	11	4
Degermed, enriched:						
Dry form	1 c	138	12	500	11	2
Cooked	1 c	240	88	120	3	Trace
Degermed, unenriched:						
Dry form	1 c	138	12	500	11	2
Cooked	1 c	240	88	120	3	Trace
Crackers: [38]						
Graham, plain, 2½-in. square	2	14	6	55	1	1
Rye wafers, whole grain, 1⅞ × 3½ in.	2	13	6	45	2	Trace
Saltines, made with enriched flour	4 crackers	11	4	50	1	1
Danish pastry (enriched flour), plain without fruit or nuts: [54]						
Ounce	1 oz	28	22	120	2	7
Packaged ring, 12 oz	1	340	22	1,435	25	80
Round piece, about 4¼-in. diam. × 1 in.	1 pastry	65	22	275	5	15
Doughnut, made with enriched flour: [38]						
Cake type, plain, 2½-in. diam., 1 in. high	1	25	24	100	1	5
Yeast-leavened, glazed, 3¾-in. diam., 1¼ in. high	1	50	26	205	3	11
Macaroni, enriched, cooked (cut lengths, elbows, shells):						
Firm stage (hot)	1 c	130	64	190	7	1
Tender stage:						
Cold	1 c	105	73	115	4	Trace
Hot	1 c	140	73	155	5	1
Macaroni (enriched) and cheese:						
Canned [55]	1 c	240	80	230	9	10
Homemade (served hot) [56]	1 c	200	58	430	17	22
Muffin made with enriched flour: [38]						
Homemade:						
Blueberry, 2⅜-in. diam., 1½ in. high	1	40	39	110	3	4
Bran	1	40	35	105	3	4
Corn (enriched, degermed cornmeal and flour), 2⅜-in. diam., 1½ in. high	1	40	33	125	3	4
Plain, 3-in. diam., 1½ in. high	1	40	38	120	3	4
From mix, egg, milk:						
Corn, 2⅜-in. diam., 1½ in. high [58]	1	40	30	130	3	4
Noodles, chow mein, canned	1 c	45	1	220	6	11
Noodles (egg noodles), enriched, cooked	1 c	160	71	200	7	2

| Fatty Acids | | | | | | | | | | | | |
| Saturated (total) (g) | Unsaturated | | Carbo-hydrate (g) | Calcium (mg) | Phos-phorus (mg) | Iron (mg) | Potassium (mg) | Vitamin A Value (IU) | Thiamin (mg) | Riboflavin (mg) | Niacin (mg) | Ascorbic Acid (mg) |
	Oleic (g)	Linoleic (g)										
2.0	3.3	2.0	38	11	53	1.4	192	30	0.15	0.10	1.0	Trace
3.0	5.2	2.9	31	17	35	0.6	23	30	0.10	0.08	0.9	0
2.2	3.9	2.2	28	10	96	0.7	15	0	0.06	0.10	0.7	0
—	—	—	30	16	25	0.6	29	50	0.10	0.09	0.8	0
0.5	1.0	2.5	90	24	312	2.9	346	620[53]	0.46	0.13	2.4	0
0.5	0.9	2.1	91	21	272	2.2	303	590[53]	0.37	0.10	2.3	0
0.2	0.4	0.9	108	8	137	4.0	166	610[53]	0.61	0.36	4.8	0
Trace	0.1	0.2	26	2	34	1.0	38	140[53]	0.14	0.10	1.2	0
0.2	0.4	0.9	108	8	137	1.5	166	610[53]	0.19	0.07	1.4	0
Trace	0.1	0.2	26	2	34	0.5	38	140[53]	0.05	0.02	0.2	0
0.3	0.5	0.3	10	6	21	0.5	55	0	0.02	0.08	0.5	0
—	—	—	10	7	50	0.5	78	0	0.04	0.03	0.2	0
0.3	0.5	0.4	8	2	10	0.5	13	0	0.05	0.05	0.4	0
2.0	2.7	1.4	13	14	31	0.5	32	90	0.08	0.08	0.7	Trace
24.3	31.7	16.5	155	170	371	6.1	381	1,050	0.97	1.01	8.6	Trace
4.7	6.1	3.2	30	33	71	1.2	73	200	0.18	0.19	1.7	Trace
1.2	2.0	1.1	13	10	48	0.4	23	20	0.05	0.05	0.4	Trace
3.3	5.8	3.3	22	16	33	0.6	34	25	0.10	0.10	0.8	0
—	—	—	39	14	85	1.4	103	0	0.23	0.13	1.8	0
—	—	—	24	8	53	0.9	64	0	0.15	0.08	1.2	0
—	—	—	32	11	70	1.3	85	0	0.20	0.11	1.5	0
4.2	3.1	1.4	26	199	182	1.0	139	260	0.12	0.24	1.0	Trace
8.9	8.8	2.9	40	362	322	1.8	240	860	0.20	0.40	1.8	Trace
1.1	1.4	0.7	17	34	53	0.6	46	90	0.09	0.10	0.7	Trace
1.2	1.4	0.8	17	57	162	1.5	172	90	0.07	0.10	1.7	Trace
1.2	1.6	0.9	19	42	68	0.7	54	120[57]	0.10	0.10	0.7	Trace
1.0	1.7	1.0	17	42	60	0.6	50	40	0.09	0.12	0.9	Trace
1.2	1.7	0.9	20	96	152	0.6	44	100[57]	0.08	0.09	0.7	Trace
—	—	—	26	—	—	—	—	—	—	—	—	—
—	—	—	37	16	94	1.4	70	110	0.22	0.13	1.9	0

TABLE 5   (continued)

Food	Approximate Measures, Units, or Weight (edible part unless footnotes indicate otherwise)	Weight (g)	Water (%)	Food Energy (kcal)	Protein (g)	Fat (g)
Pancakes, (4-in. diam.):[38]						
Buckwheat, made from mix (with buckwheat and enriched flours), egg and milk added	1 cake	27	58	55	2	2
Plain:						
Homemade with enriched flour	1 cake	27	50	60	2	2
Made from mix with enriched flour; egg and milk added	1 cake	27	51	60	2	2
Pies, piecrust made with enriched flour and vegetable shortening (9-in. diam.):						
Apple:						
Whole	1 pie	945	48	2,420	21	105
Sector, ⅟₇ of pie	1 sector	135	48	345	3	15
Banana cream:						
Whole	1 pie	910	54	2,010	41	85
Sector, ⅟₇ of pie	1 sector	130	54	285	6	12
Blueberry:						
Whole	1 pie	945	51	2,285	23	102
Sector, ⅟₇ of pie	1 sector	135	51	325	3	15
Cherry:						
Whole	1 pie	945	47	2,465	25	107
Sector, ⅟₇ of pie	1 sector	135	47	350	4	15
Custard:						
Whole	1 pie	910	58	1,985	56	101
Sector, ⅟₇ of pie	1 sector	130	58	285	8	14
Lemon meringue:						
Whole	1 pie	840	47	2,140	31	86
Sector, ⅟₇ of pie	1 sector	120	47	305	4	12
Mince:						
Whole	1 pie	945	43	2,560	24	109
Sector, ⅟₇ of pie	1 sector	135	43	365	3	16
Peach:						
Whole	1 pie	945	48	2,410	24	101
Sector, ⅟₇ of pie	1 sector	135	48	345	3	14
Pecan:						
Whole	1 pie	825	20	3,450	42	189
Sector, ⅟₇ of pie	1 sector	118	20	495	6	27
Pumpkin:						
Whole	1 pie	910	59	1,920	36	102
Sector, ⅟₇ of pie	1 sector	130	59	275	5	15
Piecrust (homemade) made with enriched flour and vegetable shortening, baked, 9-in. diam.	1 shell	180	15	900	11	60
Piecrust mix with enriched flour and vegetable shortening, 10-oz. package prepared and baked, 9-in. diam.	1 shell (2-crust pie)	320	19	1,485	20	93
Pizza (cheese) baked, 4¾-in. sector; ⅛ of 12-in.-diam. pie[19]	1 sector	60	45	145	6	4
Popcorn, popped:						
Plain, large kernel	1 c	6	4	25	1	Trace

| | Fatty Acids | | | | | | | Vitamin A | | | | Ascorbic |
| Saturated (total) (g) | Unsaturated | | Carbo-hydrate (g) | Calcium (mg) | Phos-phorus (mg) | Iron (mg) | Potassium (mg) | Value (IU) | Thiamin (mg) | Riboflavin (mg) | Niacin (mg) | Acid (mg) |
	Oleic (g)	Linoleic (g)										
0.8	0.9	0.4	6	59	91	0.4	66	60	0.04	0.05	0.2	Trace
0.5	0.8	0.5	9	27	38	0.4	33	30	0.06	0.07	0.5	Trace
0.7	0.7	0.3	9	58	70	0.3	42	70	0.04	0.06	0.2	Trace
27.0	44.5	25.2	360	76	208	6.6	756	280	1.06	0.79	9.3	9
3.9	6.4	3.6	51	11	30	0.9	108	40	0.15	0.11	1.3	2
26.7	33.2	16.2	279	601	746	7.3	1,847	2,280	0.77	1.51	7.0	9
3.8	4.7	2.3	40	86	107	1.0	264	330	0.11	0.22	1.0	1
24.8	43.7	25.1	330	104	217	9.5	614	280	1.03	0.80	10.0	28
3.5	6.2	3.6	47	15	31	1.4	88	40	0.15	0.11	1.4	4
28.2	45.0	25.3	363	132	236	6.6	992	4,160	1.09	0.84	9.8	Trace
4.0	6.4	3.6	52	19	34	0.9	142	590	0.16	0.12	1.4	Trace
33.9	38.5	17.5	213	874	1,028	8.2	1,247	2,090	0.79	1.92	5.6	0
4.8	5.5	2.5	30	125	147	1.2	178	300	0.11	0.27	0.8	0
26.1	33.8	16.4	317	118	412	6.7	420	1,430	0.61	0.84	5.2	25
3.7	4.8	2.3	45	17	59	1.0	60	200	0.09	0.12	0.7	4
28.0	45.9	25.2	389	265	359	13.3	1,682	20	0.96	0.86	9.8	9
4.0	6.6	3.6	56	38	51	1.9	240	Trace	0.14	0.12	1.4	1
24.8	43.7	25.1	361	95	274	8.5	1,408	6,900	1.04	0.97	14.0	28
3.5	6.2	3.6	52	14	39	1.2	201	990	0.15	0.14	2.0	4
27.8	101.0	44.2	423	388	850	25.6	1,015	1,320	1.80	0.95	6.9	Trace
4.0	14.4	6.3	61	55	122	3.7	145	190	0.26	0.14	1.0	Trace
37.4	37.5	16.6	223	464	628	7.3	1,456	22,480	0.78	1.27	7.0	Trace
5.4	5.4	2.4	32	66	90	1.0	208	3,210	0.11	0.18	1.0	Trace
14.8	26.1	14.9	79	25	90	3.1	89	0	0.47	0.40	5.0	0
22.7	39.7	23.4	141	131	272	6.1	179	0	1.07	0.79	9.9	0
1.7	1.5	0.6	22	86	89	1.1	67	230	0.16	0.18	1.6	4
Trace	0.1	0.2	5	1	17	0.2	—	—	—	0.01	0.1	0

Nutrients in Indicated Quantity

TABLE 5   (continued)

Food	Approximate Measures, Units, or Weight (edible part unless footnotes indicate otherwise)	Weight (g)	Water (%)	Food Energy (kcal)	Protein (g)	Fat (g)
With oil (coconut) and salt added, large kernel	1 c	9	3	40	1	2
Sugar coated	1 c	35	4	135	2	1
Pretzels, made with enriched flour:						
Dutch, twisted, 2¾ × 2⅝ in.	1	16	5	60	2	1
Thin, twisted, 3¼ × 2¼ × ¼ in.	10	60	5	235	6	3
Stick, 2¼ in. long	10	3	5	10	Trace	Trace
Rice, white, enriched:						
Instant, ready-to-serve, hot	1 c	165	73	180	4	Trace
Long grain:						
Raw	1 c	185	12	670	12	1
Cooked, served hot	1 c	205	73	225	4	Trace
Parboiled:						
Raw	1 c	185	10	685	14	1
Cooked, served hot	1 c	175	73	185	4	Trace
Roll, enriched:[38]						
Commercial:						
Brown-and-serve (1 oz), browned	1	26	27	85	2	2
Cloverleaf or pan, 2½-in. diam., 2 in. high	1	28	31	85	2	2
Frankfurter and hamburger (8 per 11½-oz package)	1	40	31	120	3	2
Hard, 3¾-in. diam., 2 in. high	1	50	25	155	5	2
Hoagie or submarine, 11½ × 3 × 2½ in.	1	135	31	390	12	4
Homemade:						
Cloverleaf, 2½-in. diam., 2 in. high	1	35	26	120	3	3
Spaghetti, enriched, cooked:						
Firm stage, al dente, served hot	1 c	130	64	190	7	1
Tender stage, served hot	1 c	140	73	155	5	1
Spaghetti (enriched) in tomato sauce with cheese:						
Canned	1 c	250	80	190	6	2
Homemade	1 c	250	77	260	9	9
Spaghetti (enriched) with meat balls and tomato sauce:						
Canned	1 c	250	78	260	12	10
Homemade	1 c	248	70	330	19	12
Toaster pastry	1	50	12	200	3	6
Waffles, made with enriched flour, 7-in. diam.:[38]						
Homemade	1	75	41	210	7	7
From mix, egg and milk added	1	75	42	205	7	8
Wheat flour:						
All-purpose or family flour, enriched:						
Sifted, spooned	1 c	115	12	420	12	1
Unsifted, spooned	1 c	125	12	455	13	1
Cake or pastry flour, enriched, sifted, spooned	1 c	96	12	350	7	1
Self-rising, enriched, unsifted, spooned	1 c	125	12	440	12	1
Whole wheat, from hard wheats, stirred	1 c	120	12	400	16	2

| | Fatty Acids | | | | | | | | | | | |
| Saturated (total) (g) | Unsaturated | | Carbo-hydrate (g) | Calcium (mg) | Phos-phorus (mg) | Iron (mg) | Potassium (mg) | Vitamin A Value (IU) | Thiamin (mg) | Riboflavin (mg) | Niacin (mg) | Ascorbic Acid (mg) |
	Oleic (g)	Linoleic (g)										
1.5	0.2	0.2	5	1	19	0.2	—	—	—	0.01	0.2	0
0.5	0.2	0.4	30	2	47	0.5	—	—	—	0.02	0.4	0
—	—	—	12	4	21	0.2	21	0	0.05	0.04	0.7	0
—	—	—	46	13	79	0.9	78	0	0.20	0.15	2.5	0
—	—	—	2	1	4	Trace	4	0	0.01	0.01	0.1	0
Trace	Trace	Trace	40	5	31	1.3	—	0	0.21	[59]	1.7	0
0.2	0.2	0.2	149	44	174	5.4	170	0	0.81	0.06	6.5	0
0.1	0.1	0.1	50	21	57	1.8	57	0	0.23	0.02	2.1	0
0.2	0.1	0.2	150	111	370	5.4	278	0	0.81	0.07	6.5	0
0.1	0.1	0.1	41	33	100	1.4	75	0	0.19	0.02	2.1	0
0.4	0.7	0.5	14	20	23	0.5	25	Trace	0.10	0.06	0.9	Trace
0.4	0.6	0.4	15	21	24	0.5	27	Trace	0.11	0.07	0.9	Trace
0.5	0.8	0.6	21	30	34	0.8	38	Trace	0.16	0.10	1.3	Trace
0.4	0.6	0.5	30	24	46	1.2	49	Trace	0.20	0.12	1.7	Trace
0.9	1.4	1.4	75	58	115	3.0	122	Trace	0.54	0.32	4.5	Trace
0.8	1.1	0.7	20	16	36	0.7	41	30	0.12	0.12	1.2	Trace
—	—	—	39	14	85	1.4	103	0	0.23	0.13	1.8	0
—	—	—	32	11	70	1.3	85	0	0.20	0.11	1.5	0
0.5	0.3	0.4	39	40	88	2.8	303	930	0.35	0.28	4.5	10
2.0	5.4	0.7	37	80	135	2.3	408	1,080	0.25	0.18	2.3	13
2.2	3.3	3.9	29	53	.113	3.3	245	1,000	0.15	0.18	2.3	5
3.3	6.3	0.9	39	124	236	3.7	665	1,590	0.25	0.30	4.0	22
—	—	—	36	54[60]	67[60]	1.9	74[60]	500	0.16	0.17	2.1	[60]
2.3	2.8	1.4	28	85	130	1.3	109	250	0.17	0.23	1.4	Trace
2.8	2.9	1.2	27	179	257	1.0	146	170	0.14	0.22	0.9	Trace
0.2	0.1	0.5	88	18	100	3.3	109	0	0.74	0.46	6.1	0
0.2	0.1	0.5	95	20	109	3.6	119	0	0.80	0.50	6.6	0
0.1	0.1	0.3	76	16	70	2.8	91	0	0.61	0.38	5.1	0
0.2	0.1	0.5	93	331	583	3.6	—	0	0.80	0.50	6.6	0
0.4	0.2	1.0	85	49	446	4.0	444	0	0.66	0.14	5.2	0

TABLE 5   (continued)

Food	Approximate Measures, Units, or Weight (edible part unless footnotes indicate otherwise)	Weight (g)	Water (%)	Food Energy (kcal)	Protein (g)	Fat (g)
Legumes (dry), Nuts, Seeds; Related Products						
Almonds, shelled:						
Chopped (about 130 almonds)	1 c	130	5	775	24	70
Slivered, not pressed down (about 115 almonds)	1 c	115	5	690	21	62
Beans, dry:						
Common varieties as Great Northern, navy, and others:						
Canned, solids and liquid:						
White with—						
Frankfurters (sliced)	1 c	255	71	365	19	18
Pork and sweet sauce	1 c	255	66	385	16	12
Pork and tomato sauce	1 c	255	71	310	16	7
Red kidney	1 c	255	76	230	15	1
Cooked, drained:						
Great Northern	1 c	180	69	210	14	1
Pea (navy)	1 c	190	69	225	15	1
Lima, cooked, drained	1 c	190	64	260	16	1
Black-eyed peas, dry, cooked (with residual cooking liquid)	1 c	250	80	190	13	1
Brazil nuts, shelled (6–8 large kernels)	1 oz	28	5	185	4	19
Cashew nuts, roasted in oil	1 c	140	5	785	24	64
Coconut meat, fresh:						
Piece, about 2 × 2 × ½ in.	1	45	51	155	2	16
Shredded or grated, not pressed down	1 c	80	51	275	3	28
Filberts (hazelnuts), chopped (about 80 kernels)	1 c	115	6	730	14	72
Lentils, whole, cooked	1 c	200	72	210	16	Trace
Peanuts, roasted in oil, salted (whole, halves, chopped)	1 c	144	2	840	37	72
Peanut butter	1 T	16	2	95	4	8
Peas, split, dry, cooked	1 c	200	70	230	16	1
Pecans, chopped or pieces (about 120 large halves)	1 c	118	3	810	11	84
Pumpkin and squash kernels, dry, hulled	1 c	140	4	775	41	65
Sunflower seeds, dry, hulled	1 c	145	5	810	35	69
Walnuts:						
Black:						
Chopped or broken kernels	1 c	125	3	785	26	74
Ground (finely)	1 c	80	3	500	16	47
Persian or English, chopped (about 60 halves)	1 c	120	4	780	18	77
Sugars and Sweets						
Cake icings:						
Boiled, white:						
Plain	1 c	94	18	295	1	0
With coconut	1 c	166	15	605	3	13
Uncooked:						
Chocolate made with milk and butter	1 c	275	14	1,035	9	38
Creamy fudge from mix and water	1 c	245	15	830	7	16
White	1 c	319	11	1,200	2	21

| | Fatty Acids | | | | | | | Vitamin A | | | | | |
| Saturated (total) (g) | Unsaturated | | Carbo-hydrate (g) | Calcium (mg) | Phos-phorus (mg) | Iron (mg) | Potassium (mg) | Value (IU) | Thiamin (mg) | Riboflavin (mg) | Niacin (mg) | Ascorbic Acid (mg) |
	Oleic (g)	Linoleic (g)										
5.6	47.7	12.8	25	304	655	6.1	1,005	0	0.31	1.20	4.6	Trace
5.0	42.2	11.3	22	269	580	5.4	889	0	0.28	1.06	4.0	Trace
—	—	—	32	94	303	4.8	668	330	0.18	0.15	3.3	Trace
4.3	5.0	1.1	54	161	291	5.9	—	—	0.15	0.10	1.3	—
2.4	2.8	0.6	48	138	235	4.6	536	330	0.20	0.08	1.5	5
—	—	—	42	74	278	4.6	673	10	0.13	0.10	1.5	—
—	—	—	38	90	266	4.9	749	0	0.25	0.13	1.3	0
—	—	—	40	95	281	5.1	790	0	0.27	0.13	1.3	0
—	—	—	49	55	293	5.9	1,163	—	0.25	0.11	1.3	—
—	—	—	35	43	238	3.3	573	30	0.40	0.10	1.0	—
4.8	6.2	7.1	3	53	196	1.0	203	Trace	0.27	0.03	0.5	—
12.9	36.8	10.2	41	53	522	5.3	650	140	0.60	0.35	2.5	—
14.0	0.9	0.3	4	6	43	0.8	115	0	0.02	0.01	0.2	1
24.8	1.6	0.5	8	10	76	1.4	205	0	0.04	0.02	0.4	2
5.1	55.2	7.3	19	240	388	3.9	810	—	0.53	—	1.0	Trace
—	—	—	39	50	238	4.2	498	40	0.14	0.12	1.2	0
13.7	33.0	20.7	27	107	577	3.0	971	—	0.46	0.19	24.8	0
1.5	3.7	2.3	3	9	61	0.3	100	—	0.02	0.02	2.4	0
—	—	—	42	22	178	3.4	592	80	0.30	0.18	1.8	—
7.2	50.5	20.0	17	86	341	2.8	712	150	1.01	0.15	1.1	2
11.8	23.5	27.5	21	71	1,602	15.7	1,386	100	0.34	0.27	3.4	—
8.2	13.7	43.2	29	174	1,214	10.3	1,334	70	2.84	0.33	7.8	—
6.3	13.3	45.7	19	Trace	713	7.5	575	380	0.28	0.14	0.9	—
4.0	8.5	29.2	12	Trace	456	4.8	368	240	0.18	0.09	0.6	—
8.4	11.8	42.2	19	119	456	3.7	540	40	0.40	0.16	1.1	2
0	0	0	75	2	2	Trace	17	0	Trace	0.03	Trace	0
11.0	0.9	Trace	124	10	50	0.8	277	0	0.02	0.07	0.3	0
23.4	11.7	1.0	185	165	305	3.3	536	580	0.06	0.28	0.6	1
5.1	6.7	3.1	183	96	218	2.7	238	Trace	0.05	0.20	0.7	Trace
12.7	5.1	0.5	260	48	38	Trace	57	860	Trace	0.06	Trace	Trace

TABLE 5   (continued)

Food	Approximate Measures, Units, or Weight (edible part unless footnotes indicate otherwise)	Weight (g)	Water (%)	Food Energy (kcal)	Protein (g)	Fat (g)
Candy:						
Caramels, plain or chocolate	1 oz	28	8	115	1	3
Chocolate:						
Milk, plain	1 oz	28	1	145	2	9
Semisweet, small pieces (60 per ounce)	1 c or 6 oz	170	1	860	7	61
Chocolate-covered peanuts	1 oz	28	1	160	5	12
Fondant, uncoated (mints, candy corn, other)	1 oz	28	8	105	Trace	1
Fudge, chocolate, plain	1 oz	28	8	115	1	3
Gumdrops	1 oz	28	12	100	Trace	Trace
Hard	1 oz	28	1	110	0	Trace
Marshmallows	1 oz	28	17	90	1	Trace
Chocolate-flavored beverage powders (about 4 heaping teaspoons per ounce):						
With nonfat dry milk	1 oz	28	2	100	5	1
Without milk	1 oz	28	1	100	1	1
Honey, strained or extracted	1 T	21	17	65	Trace	0
Jams and preserves	1 T	20	29	55	Trace	Trace
	1 packet	14	29	40	Trace	Trace
Jellies	1 T	18	29	50	Trace	Trace
	1 packet	14	29	40	Trace	Trace
Syrups:						
Chocolate-flavored syrup or topping:						
Fudge type	1 fl oz or 2 T	38	25	125	2	5
Thin type	1 fl oz or 2 T	38	32	90	1	1
Molasses, cane:						
Light (first extraction)	1 T	20	24	50	—	—
Blackstrap (third extraction)	1 T	20	24	45	—	—
Sorghum	1 T	21	23	55	—	—
Table blends, chiefly corn, light and dark	1 T	21	24	60	0	0
Sugar:						
Brown, pressed down	1 c	220	2	820	0	0
White:						
Granulated	1 c	200	1	770	0	0
	1 T	12	1	45	0	0
	1 packet	6	1	23	0	0
Powdered, sifted, spooned into cup	1 c	100	1	385	0	0
Vegetables and Vegetable Products						
Asparagus, green:						
Cooked, drained:						
Cuts and tips, 1½- to 2-in. lengths:						
From raw	1 c	145	94	30	3	Trace
From frozen	1 c	180	93	40	6	Trace
Spears, ½-in. diam. at base:						
From raw	4	60	94	10	1	Trace
From frozen	4	60	92	15	2	Trace
Canned, spears, ½-in. diam. at base	4	80	93	15	2	Trace

| | Fatty Acids | | | | | | | | Vitamin A | | | | |
| Saturated (total) (g) | Unsaturated | | Carbo-hydrate (g) | Calcium (mg) | Phos-phorus (mg) | Iron (mg) | Potassium (mg) | Value (IU) | Thiamin (mg) | Riboflavin (mg) | Niacin (mg) | Ascorbic Acid (mg) |
	Oleic (g)	Linoleic (g)										
1.6	1.1	0.1	22	42	35	0.4	54	Trace	0.01	0.05	0.1	Trace
5.5	3.0	0.3	16	65	65	0.3	109	80	0.02	0.10	0.1	Trace
36.2	19.8	1.7	97	51	255	4.4	553	30	0.02	0.14	0.9	0
4.0	4.7	2.1	11	33	84	0.4	143	Trace	0.10	0.05	2.1	Trace
0.1	0.3	0.1	25	4	2	0.3	1	0	Trace	Trace	Trace	0
1.3	1.4	0.6	21	22	24	0.3	42	Trace	0.01	0.03	0.1	Trace
—	—	—	25	2	Trace	0.1	1	0	0	Trace	Trace	0
—	—	—	28	6	2	0.5	1	0	0	0	0	0
—	—	—	23	5	2	0.5	2	0	0	Trace	Trace	0
0.5	0.3	Trace	20	167	155	0.5	227	10	0.04	0.21	0.2	1
0.4	0.2	Trace	25	9	48	0.6	142	—	0.01	0.03	0.1	0
0	0	0	17	1	1	0.1	11	0	Trace	0.01	0.1	Trace
—	—	—	14	4	2	0.2	18	Trace	Trace	0.01	Trace	Trace
—	—	—	10	3	1	0.1	12	Trace	Trace	Trace	Trace	Trace
—	—	—	13	4	1	0.3	14	Trace	Trace	0.01	Trace	1
—	—	—	10	3	1	0.2	11	Trace	Trace	Trace	Trace	1
3.1	1.6	0.1	20	48	60	0.5	107	60	0.02	0.08	0.2	Trace
0.5	0.3	Trace	24	6	35	0.6	106	Trace	0.01	0.03	0.2	0
—	—	—	13	33	9	0.9	183	—	0.01	0.01	Trace	—
—	—	—	11	137	17	3.2	585	—	0.02	0.04	0.4	—
—	—	—	14	35	5	2.6	—	—	—	0.02	Trace	—
0	0	0	15	9	3	0.8	1	0	0	0	0	0
0	0	0	212	187	42	7.5	757	0	0.02	0.07	0.4	0
0	0	0	199	0	0	0.2	6	0	0	0	0	0
0	0	0	12	0	0	Trace	Trace	0	0	0	0	0
0	0	0	6	0	0	Trace	Trace	0	0	0	0	0
0	0	0	100	0	0	0.1	3	0	0	0	0	0
—	—	—	5	30	73	0.9	265	1,310	0.23	0.26	2.0	38
—	—	—	6	40	115	2.2	396	1,530	0.25	0.23	1.8	41
—	—	—	2	13	30	0.4	110	540	0.10	0.11	0.8	16
—	—	—	2	13	40	0.7	143	470	0.10	0.08	0.7	16
—	—	—	3	15	42	1.5	133	640	0.05	0.08	0.6	12

TABLE 5 (continued)

Food	Approximate Measures, Units, or Weight (edible part unless footnotes indicate otherwise)	Weight (g)	Water (%)	Food Energy (kcal)	Protein (g)	Fat (g)
Beans:						
Lima, immature seeds, frozen, cooked, drained:						
Thick-seeded types (Fordhooks)	1 c	170	74	170	10	Trace
Thin-seeded types (baby limas)	1 c	180	69	210	13	Trace
Snap:						
Green:						
Canned, drained solids (cuts)	1 c	135	92	30	2	Trace
Cooked, drained:						
From raw (cuts and French style)	1 c	125	92	30	2	Trace
From frozen:						
Cuts	1 c	135	92	35	2	Trace
French style	1 c	130	92	35	2	Trace
Yellow or wax:						
Cooked, drained:						
From raw (cuts and French style)	1 c	125	93	30	2	Trace
From frozen (cuts)	1 c	135	92	35	2	Trace
Canned, drained solids (cuts)	1 c	135	92	30	2	Trace
Beans, mature. See Beans, dry, and Black-eyed peas, dry.						
Bean sprouts (mung):						
Raw	1 c	105	89	35	4	Trace
Cooked, drained	1 c	125	91	35	4	Trace
Beets:						
Canned, drained, solids:						
Whole, small	1 c	160	89	60	2	Trace
Diced or sliced	1 c	170	89	65	2	Trace
Cooked, drained, peeled:						
Whole, 2-in. diam.	2	100	91	30	1	Trace
Diced or sliced	1 c	170	91	55	1	Trace
Beet greens, leaves and stems, cooked, drained	1 c	145	94	25	2	Trace
Black-eyed peas, immature seeds, cooked and drained:						
From raw	1 c	165	72	180	13	1
From frozen	1 c	170	66	220	15	1
Broccoli, cooked, drained:						
From raw:						
Stalk, medium size	1	180	91	45	6	1
Stalks cut into ½-in. pieces	1 c	155	91	40	5	Trace
From frozen:						
Chopped	1 c	185	92	50	5	1
Stalk, 4½ to 5 in. long	1	30	91	10	1	Trace
Brussels sprouts, cooked, drained:						
From raw, 7–8 sprouts (1¼- to 1½-in. diam.)	1 c	155	88	55	7	1
From frozen	1 c	155	89	50	5	Trace
Cabbage:						
Common varieties:						
Raw:						
Coarsely shredded or sliced	1 c	70	92	15	1	Trace

Nutrients in Indicated Quantity												
Fatty Acids												
Saturated (total) (g)	**Unsaturated**		Carbo-hydrate (g)	Calcium (mg)	Phos-phorus (mg)	Iron (mg)	Potassium (mg)	Vitamin A Value (IU)	Thiamin (mg)	Riboflavin (mg)	Niacin (mg)	Ascorbic Acid (mg)
	Oleic (g)	Linoleic (g)										
—	—	—	32	34	153	2.9	724	390	0.12	0.09	1.7	29
—	—	—	40	63	227	4.7	709	400	0.16	0.09	2.2	22
—	—	—	7	61	34	2.0	128	630	0.04	0.07	0.4	5
—	—	—	7	63	46	0.8	189	680	0.09	0.11	0.4	15
—	—	—	8	54	43	0.9	205	780	0.09	0.12	0.5	7
—	—	—	8	49	39	1.2	177	690	0.08	0.10	0.4	9
—	—	—	6	63	46	0.8	189	290	0.09	0.11	0.6	16
—	—	—	8	47	42	0.9	221	140	0.09	0.11	0.5	8
—	—	—	7	61	34	2.0	128	140	0.04	0.07	0.4	7
—	—	—	7	20	67	1.4	234	20	0.14	0.14	0.8	20
—	—	—	7	21	60	1.1	195	30	0.11	0.13	0.9	8
—	—	—	14	30	29	1.1	267	30	0.02	0.05	0.2	5
—	—	—	15	32	31	1.2	284	30	0.02	0.05	0.2	5
—	—	—	7	14	23	0.5	208	20	0.03	0.04	0.3	6
—	—	—	12	24	39	0.9	354	30	0.05	0.07	0.5	10
—	—	—	5	144	36	2.8	481	7,400	0.10	0.22	0.4	22
—	—	—	30	40	241	3.5	625	580	0.50	0.18	2.3	28
—	—	—	40	43	286	4.8	573	290	0.68	0.19	2.4	15
—	—	—	8	158	112	1.4	481	4,500	0.16	0.36	1.4	162
—	—	—	7	136	96	1.2	414	3,880	0.14	0.31	1.2	140
—	—	—	9	100	104	1.3	392	4,810	0.11	0.22	0.9	105
—	—	—	1	12	17	0.2	66	570	0.02	0.03	0.2	22
—	—	—	10	50	112	1.7	423	810	0.12	0.22	1.2	135
—	—	—	10	33	95	1.2	457	880	0.12	0.16	0.9	126
—	—	—	4	34	20	0.3	163	90	0.04	0.04	0.2	33

TABLE 5 (continued)

Food	Approximate Measures, Units, or Weight (edible part unless footnotes indicate otherwise)	Weight (g)	Water (%)	Food Energy (kcal)	Protein (g)	Fat (g)
Finely shredded or chopped	1 c	90	92	20	1	Trace
Cooked, drained	1 c	145	94	30	2	Trace
Red, raw, coarsely shredded or sliced	1 c	70	90	20	1	Trace
Savoy, raw, coarsely shredded or sliced	1 c	70	92	15	2	Trace
Cabbage, celery (also called pe-tsai or wongbok), raw, 1-in. pieces	1 c	75	95	10	1	Trace
Cabbage, white mustard (also called bokchoy or pakchoy), cooked, drained	1 c	170	95	25	2	Trace
Carrots:						
Raw, without crowns and tips, scraped:						
Grated	1 c	110	88	45	1	Trace
Whole, 7½ by 1⅛ in. or strips, 2½ to 3 in. long	1 carrot or 18 strips	72	88	30	1	Trace
Canned:						
Sliced, drained solids	1 c	155	91	45	1	Trace
Strained or junior (baby food)	1 oz (1¾ to 2 T)	28	92	10	Trace	Trace
Cooked (crosswise cuts), drained	1 c	155	91	50	1	Trace
Cauliflower:						
Raw, chopped	1 c	115	91	31	3	Trace
Cooked, drained:						
From raw (flower buds)	1 c	125	93	30	3	Trace
From frozen (flowerets)	1 c	180	94	30	3	Trace
Celery, Pascal type, raw:						
Pieces, diced	1 c	120	94	20	1	Trace
Stalk, large outer, 8 by 1½ in. at root end	1	40	94	5	Trace	Trace
Collards, cooked, drained:						
From raw (leaves without stems)	1 c	190	90	65	7	1
From frozen (chopped)	1 c	170	90	50	5	1
Corn, sweet:						
Cooked, drained:						
From raw, ear, 5 by 1¾ in.	1	140[61]	74	70	2	1
From frozen:						
Ear, 5 in. long	1	229[61]	73	120	4	1
Kernels	1 c	165	77	130	5	1
Canned:						
Cream style	1 c	256	76	210	5	2
Whole kernel:						
Vacuum pack	1 c	210	76	175	5	1
Wet pack, drained solids	1 c	165	76	140	4	1
Cowpeas. See Black-eyed peas.						
Cucumber slices, ⅛ in. thick (large, 2⅛-in. diam.; small, 1¾-in. diam.):						
With peel	6 large or 8 small	28	95	5	Trace	Trace
Without peel	6½ large or 9 small pieces	28	96	5	Trace	Trace
Dandelion greens, cooked, drained	1 c	105	90	35	2	1
Endive, curly (including escarole), raw, small pieces	1 c	50	93	10	1	Trace

Saturated (total) (g)	Unsaturated Oleic (g)	Unsaturated Linoleic (g)	Carbo-hydrate (g)	Calcium (mg)	Phos-phorus (mg)	Iron (mg)	Potassium (mg)	Vitamin A Value (IU)	Thiamin (mg)	Riboflavin (mg)	Niacin (mg)	Ascorbic Acid (mg)
—	—	—	5	44	26	0.4	210	120	0.05	0.05	0.3	42
—	—	—	6	64	29	0.4	236	190	0.06	0.06	0.4	48
—	—	—	5	29	25	0.6	188	30	0.06	0.04	0.3	43
—	—	—	3	47	38	0.6	188	140	0.04	0.06	0.2	39
—	—	—	2	32	30	0.5	190	110	0.04	0.03	0.5	19
—	—	—	4	252	56	1.0	364	5,270	0.07	0.14	1.2	26
—	—	—	11	41	40	0.8	375	12,100	0.07	0.06	0.7	9
—	—	—	7	27	26	0.5	246	7,930	0.04	0.04	0.4	6
—	—	—	10	47	34	1.1	186	23,250	0.03	0.05	0.6	3
—	—	—	2	7	6	0.1	51	3,690	0.01	0.01	0.1	1
—	—	—	11	51	48	0.9	344	16,280	0.08	0.08	0.8	9
—	—	—	6	29	64	1.3	339	70	0.13	0.12	0.8	90
—	—	—	5	26	53	0.9	258	80	0.11	0.10	0.8	69
—	—	—	6	31	68	0.9	373	50	0.07	0.09	0.7	74
—	—	—	5	47	34	0.4	409	320	0.04	0.04	0.4	11
—	—	—	2	16	11	0.1	136	110	0.01	0.01	0.1	4
—	—	—	10	357	99	1.5	498	14,820	0.21	0.38	2.3	144
—	—	—	10	299	87	1.7	401	11,560	0.10	0.24	1.0	56
—	—	—	16	2	69	0.5	151	310[62]	0.09	0.08	1.1	7
—	—	—	27	4	121	1.0	291	440[62]	0.18	0.10	2.1	9
—	—	—	31	5	120	1.3	304	580[62]	0.15	0.10	2.5	8
—	—	—	51	8	143	1.5	248	840[62]	0.08	0.13	2.6	13
—	—	—	43	6	153	1.1	204	740[62]	0.06	0.13	2.3	11
—	—	—	33	8	81	0.8	160	580[62]	0.05	0.08	1.5	7
—	—	—	1	7	8	0.3	45	70	0.01	0.01	0.1	3
—	—	—	1	5	5	0.1	45	Trace	0.01	0.01	0.1	3
—	—	—	7	147	44	1.9	244	12,290	0.14	0.17	—	19
—	—	—	2	41	27	0.9	147	1,650	0.04	0.07	0.3	5

TABLE 5 (continued)

Food	Approximate Measures, Units, or Weight (edible part unless footnotes indicate otherwise)	Weight (g)	Water (%)	Food Energy (kcal)	Protein (g)	Fat (g)
Kale, cooked, drained:						
From raw (leaves without stems and midribs)	1 c	110	88	45	5	1
From frozen (leaf style)	1 c	130	91	40	4	1
Lettuce, raw:						
Butter head, as Boston types:						
Head, 5-in. diam.	1	220[63]	95	25	2	Trace
Leaves	1 outer, 2 inner, or 3 heart leaves	15	95	Trace	Trace	Trace
Crisp head, as iceberg:						
Head, 6-in. diam.	1	567[64]	96	70	5	1
Wedge, ¼ of head	1	135	96	20	1	Trace
Pieces, chopped or shredded	1 c	55	96	5	Trace	Trace
Loose leaf (bunching varieties including romaine), chopped or shredded pieces	1 c	55	94	10	1	Trace
Mushrooms, raw, sliced, or chopped	1 c	70	90	20	2	Trace
Mustard greens, without stems and midribs, cooked, drained	1 c	140	93	30	3	1
Okra pods, 3 by ⅝ in., cooked	10	106	91	30	2	Trace
Onions:						
Mature:						
Raw:						
Chopped	1 c	170	89	65	3	Trace
Sliced	1 c	115	89	45	2	Trace
Cooked (whole or sliced) drained	1 c	210	92	60	3	Trace
Young green, bulb (⅜-in. diam.) and white portion of top	6 onions	30	88	15	Trace	Trace
Parsley, raw, chopped	1 T	4	85	Trace	Trace	Trace
Parsnips, cooked (diced or 2-in. lengths)	1 c	155	82	100	2	1
Peas, green:						
Canned:						
Whole, drained solids	1 c	170	77	150	8	1
Strained (baby food)	1 oz (1¾–2 T)	28	86	15	1	Trace
Frozen, cooked, drained	1 c	160	82	110	8	Trace
Peppers, hot, red, without seeds, dried (ground chili powder, added seasonings)	1 t	2	9	5	Trace	Trace
Peppers, sweet (about 5 per pound, whole), stem and seeds removed:						
Raw	1 pod	74	93	15	1	Trace
Cooked, boiled, drained	1 pod	73	95	15	1	Trace
Potatoes, cooked:						
Baked, peeled after baking (about 2 per pound, raw)	1	156	75	145	4	Trace
Boiled (about 3 per pound, raw):						
Peeled after boiling	1	137	80	105	3	Trace
Peeled before boiling	1	135	83	90	3	Trace
French-fries, 2 to 3½ in. long:						
Prepared from raw	10	50	45	135	2	7
Frozen, oven heated	10	50	53	110	2	4
Hashed brown, prepared from frozen	1 c	155	56	345	3	18

| | Fatty Acids | | | | | | | | | | | |
| Saturated (total) (g) | Unsaturated | | Carbo-hydrate (g) | Calcium (mg) | Phos-phorus (mg) | Iron (mg) | Potassium (mg) | Vitamin A Value (IU) | Thiamin (mg) | Riboflavin (mg) | Niacin (mg) | Ascorbic Acid (mg) |
	Oleic (g)	Linoleic (g)										
—	—	—	7	206	64	1.8	243	9,130	0.11	0.20	1.8	102
—	—	—	7	157	62	1.3	251	10,660	0.08	0.20	0.9	49
—	—	—	4	57	42	3.3	430	1,580	0.10	0.10	0.5	13
—	—	—	Trace	5	4	0.3	40	150	0.01	0.01	Trace	1
—	—	—	16	108	118	2.7	943	1,780	0.32	0.32	1.6	32
—	—	—	4	27	30	0.7	236	450	0.08	0.08	0.4	8
—	—	—	2	11	12	0.3	96	180	0.03	0.03	0.2	3
—	—	—	2	37	14	0.8	145	1,050	0.03	0.04	0.2	10
—	—	—	3	4	81	0.6	290	Trace	0.07	0.32	2.9	2
—	—	—	6	193	45	2.5	308	8,120	0.11	0.20	0.8	67
—	—	—	6	98	43	0.5	184	520	0.14	0.19	1.0	21
—	—	—	15	46	61	0.9	267	Trace[65]	0.05	0.07	0.3	17
—	—	—	10	31	41	0.6	181	Trace[65]	0.03	0.05	0.2	12
—	—	—	14	50	61	0.8	231	Trace[65]	0.06	0.06	0.4	15
—	—	—	3	12	12	0.2	69	Trace	0.02	0.01	0.1	8
—	—	—	Trace	7	2	0.2	25	300	Trace	0.01	Trace	6
—	—	—	23	70	96	0.9	587	50	0.11	0.12	0.2	16
—	—	—	29	44	129	3.2	163	1,170	0.15	0.10	1.4	14
—	—	—	3	3	18	0.3	28	140	0.02	0.03	0.3	3
—	—	—	19	30	138	3.0	216	960	0.43	0.14	2.7	21
—	—	—	1	5	4	0.3	20	1,300	Trace	0.02	0.2	Trace
—	—	—	4	7	16	0.5	157	310	0.06	0.06	0.4	94
—	—	—	3	7	12	0.4	109	310	0.05	0.05	0.4	70
—	—	—	33	14	101	1.1	782	Trace	0.15	0.07	2.7	31
—	—	—	23	10	72	0.8	556	Trace	0.12	0.05	2.0	22
—	—	—	20	8	57	0.7	385	Trace	0.12	0.05	1.6	22
1.7	1.2	3.3	18	8	56	0.7	427	Trace	0.07	0.04	1.6	11
1.1	.8	2.1	17	5	43	0.9	326	Trace	0.07	0.01	1.3	11
4.6	3.2	9.0	45	28	78	1.9	439	Trace	0.11	0.03	1.6	12

TABLE 5 (continued)

Food	Approximate Measures, Units, or Weight (edible part unless footnotes indicate otherwise)	Weight (g)	Water (%)	Food Energy (kcal)	Protein (g)	Fat (g)
Mashed, prepared from—						
Raw:						
Milk added	1 c	210	83	135	4	2
Milk and butter added	1 c	210	80	195	4	9
Dehydrated flakes (without milk), water, milk,						
butter, and salt added	1 c	210	79	195	4	7
Potato chips, 1¾ by 2½ in. oval cross section	10	20	2	115	1	8
Potato salad, made with cooked salad dressing	1 c	250	76	250	7	7
Pumpkin, canned	1 c	245	90	80	2	1
Radishes, raw (prepackaged) stem ends,						
rootlets cut off	4	18	95	5	Trace	Trace
Sauerkraut, canned, solids, and liquid	1 c	235	93	40	2	Trace
Southern peas. See Black-eyed peas.						
Spinach:						
Raw, chopped	1 c	55	91	15	2	Trace
Canned, drained solids	1 c	205	91	50	6	1
Cooked, drained:						
From raw	1 c	180	92	40	5	1
From frozen:						
Chopped	1 c	205	92	45	6	1
Leaf	1 c	190	92	45	6	1
Squash, cooked:						
Summer (all varieties), diced, drained	1 c	210	96	30	2	Trace
Winter (all varieties), baked, mashed	1 c	205	81	130	4	1
Sweet potatoes:						
Candied, 2½ × 2 in. piece	1 piece	105	60	175	1	3
Canned:						
Solid pack (mashed)	1 c	255	72	275	5	1
Vacuum pack, 2¾ × 1 in. piece	1 piece	40	72	45	1	Trace
Cooked (raw, 5 × 2 in.; about 2½ per pound):						
Baked in skin, peeled	1	114	64	160	2	1
Boiled in skin, peeled	1	151	71	170	3	1
Tomatoes:						
Raw, 2⅗-in. diam. (3 per 12-oz package)	1	135[66]	94	25	1	Trace
Canned, solids and liquid	1 c	241	94	50	2	Trace
Tomato catsup	1 c	273	69	290	5	1
	1 T	15	69	15	Trace	Trace
Tomato juice, canned:						
Cup	1 c	243	94	45	2	Trace
Glass	6 fl oz	182	94	35	2	Trace
Turnips, cooked, diced	1 c	155	94	35	1	Trace
Turnip greens, cooked, drained:						
From raw (leaves and stems)	1 c	145	94	30	3	Trace
From frozen (chopped)	1 c	165	93	40	4	Trace
Vegetables, mixed, frozen, cooked	1 c	182	83	115	6	1

								Nutrients in Indicated Quantity					
Fatty Acids													
Saturated (total) (g)	**Unsaturated**		Carbo-hydrate (g)	Calcium (mg)	Phos-phorus (mg)	Iron (mg)	Potassium (mg)	Vitamin A Value (IU)	Thiamin (mg)	Riboflavin (mg)	Niacin (mg)	Ascorbic Acid (mg)
	Oleic (g)	Linoleic (g)										
0.7	0.4	Trace	27	50	103	0.8	548	40	0.17	0.11	2.1	21
5.6	2.3	0.2	26	50	101	0.8	525	360	0.17	0.11	2.1	19
3.6	2.1	0.2	30	65	99	0.6	601	270	0.08	0.08	1.9	11
2.1	1.4	4.0	10	8	28	0.4	226	Trace	0.04	0.01	1.0	3
2.0	2.7	1.3	41	80	160	1.5	798	350	0.20	0.18	2.8	28
—	—	—	19	61	64	1.0	588	15,680	0.07	0.12	1.5	12
—	—	—	1	5	6	0.2	58	Trace	0.01	0.01	0.1	5
—	—	—	9	85	42	1.2	329	120	0.07	0.09	0.5	33
—	—	—	2	51	28	1.7	259	4,460	0.06	0.11	0.3	28
—	—	—	7	242	53	5.3	513	16,400	0.04	0.25	0.6	29
—	—	—	6	167	68	4.0	583	14,580	0.13	0.25	0.9	50
—	—	—	8	232	90	4.3	683	16,200	0.14	0.31	0.8	39
—	—	—	7	200	84	4.8	688	15,390	0.15	0.27	1.0	53
—	—	—	7	53	53	0.8	296	820	0.11	0.17	1.7	21
—	—	—	32	57	98	1.6	945	8,610	0.10	0.27	1.4	27
2.0	0.8	0.1	36	39	45	0.9	200	6,620	0.06	0.04	0.4	11
—	—	—	63	64	105	2.0	510	19,890	0.13	0.10	1.5	36
—	—	—	10	10	16	0.3	80	3,120	0.02	0.02	0.2	6
—	—	—	37	46	66	1.0	342	9,230	0.10	0.08	0.8	25
—	—	—	40	48	71	1.1	367	11,940	0.14	0.09	0.9	26
—	—	—	6	16	33	0.6	300	1,110	0.07	0.05	0.9	28[67]
—	—	—	10	14[68]	46	1.2	523	2,170	0.12	0.07	1.7	41
—	—	—	69	60	137	2.2	991	3,820	0.25	0.19	4.4	41
—	—	—	4	3	8	0.1	54	210	0.01	0.01	0.2	2
—	—	—	10	17	44	2.2	552	1,940	0.12	0.07	1.9	39
—	—	—	8	13	33	1.6	413	1,460	0.09	0.05	1.5	29
—	—	—	8	54	37	0.6	291	Trace	0.06	0.08	0.5	34
—	—	—	5	252	49	1.5	—	8,270	0.15	0.33	0.7	68
—	—	—	6	195	64	2.6	246	11,390	0.08	0.15	0.7	31
—	—	—	24	46	115	2.4	348	9,010	0.22	0.13	2.0	15

TABLE 5 (continued)

Food	Approximate Measures, Units, or Weight (edible part unless footnotes indicate otherwise)	Weight (g)	Water (%)	Food Energy (kcal)	Protein (g)	Fat (g)
Miscellaneous Items						
Baking powders for home use:						
Sodium aluminum sulfate:						
With monocalcium phosphate monohydrate	1 t	3.0	2	5	Trace	Trace
With monocalcium phosphate monohydrate, calcium sulfate	1 t	2.9	1	5	Trace	Trace
Straight phosphate	1 t	3.8	2	5	Trace	Trace
Low sodium	1 t	4.3	2	5	Trace	Trace
Barbecue sauce	1 c	250	81	230	4	17
Beverages, alcoholic:						
Beer	12 fl oz	360	92	150	1	0
Gin, rum, vodka, whisky:						
80 proof	1½-fl oz (jigger)	42	67	95	—	—
86 proof	1½-fl oz (jigger)	42	64	105	—	—
90 proof	1½-fl oz (jigger)	42	62	110	—	—
Wines:						
Dessert	3½ fl oz	103	77	140	Trace	0
Table	3½ fl oz	102	86	85	Trace	0
Beverages, carbonated, sweetened, nonalcoholic:						
Carbonated water	12 fl oz	366	92	115	0	0
Cola type	12 fl oz	369	90	145	0	0
Fruit-flavored sodas and Tom Collins mixer	12 fl oz	372	88	170	0	0
Ginger ale	12 fl oz	366	92	115	0	0
Root beer	12 fl oz	370	90	150	0	0
Chili powder. See Peppers, hot, red.						
Chocolate:						
Bitter or baking	1 oz	28	2	145	3	15
Semisweet, see Candy: Chocolate.						
Gelatin, dry	7 g	7	13	25	6	Trace
Gelatin dessert prepared with gelatin dessert powder and water	1 c	240	84	140	4	0
Mustard, prepared, yellow	1 t or individual serving pouch or cup	5	80	5	Trace	Trace
Olives, pickled, canned:						
Green	4 medium, 3 extra large, or 2 giant	16[69]	78	15	Trace	2
Ripe, Mission	3 small or 2 large	10[69]	73	15	Trace	2
Pickles, cucumber:						
Dill, medium, whole, 3¾ in. long, 1¼-in. diam.	1 pickle	65	93	5	Trace	Trace
Fresh pack, slices 1½-in. diam., ¼ in. thick	2 slices	15	79	10	Trace	Trace
Sweet, gherkin, small, whole, about 2½ in. long, ¾-in. diam.	1 pickle	15	61	20	Trace	Trace
Relish, finely chopped, sweet	1 T	15	63	20	Trace	Trace
Popcorn. See page A40.						
Popsicle	3 fl oz	95	80	70	0	0

Saturated (total) (g)	Unsaturated Oleic (g)	Linoleic (g)	Carbo-hydrate (g)	Calcium (mg)	Phos-phorus (mg)	Iron (mg)	Potassium (mg)	Vitamin A Value (IU)	Thiamin (mg)	Riboflavin (mg)	Niacin (mg)	Ascorbic Acid (mg)
0	0	0	1	58	87	—	5	0	0	0	0	0
0	0	0	1	183	45	—	—	0	0	0	0	0
0	0	0	1	239	359	—	6	0	0	0	0	0
0	0	0	2	207	314	—	471	0	0	0	0	0
2.2	4.3	10.0	20	53	50	2.0	435	900	0.03	0.03	0.8	13
0	0	0	14	18	108	Trace	90	—	0.01	0.11	2.2	—
0	0	0	Trace	—	—	—	1	—	—	—	—	—
0	0	0	Trace	—	—	—	1	—	—	—	—	—
0	0	0	Trace	—	—	—	1	—	—	—	—	—
0	0	0	8	8	—	—	77	—	0.01	0.02	0.2	—
0	0	0	4	9	10	0.4	94	—	Trace	0.01	0.1	—
0	0	0	29	—	—	—	—	0	0	0	0	0
0	0	0	37	—	—	—	—	0	0	0	0	0
0	0	0	45	—	—	—	—	0	0	0	0	0
0	0	0	29	—	—	—	0	0	0	0	0	0
0	0	0	39	—	—	—	0	0	0	0	0	0
8.9	4.9	0.4	8	22	109	1.9	235	20	0.01	0.07	0.4	0
0	0	0	0	—	—	—	—	—	—	—	—	—
0	0	0	34	—	—	—	—	—	—	—	—	—
—	—	—	Trace	4	4	0.1	7	—	—	—	—	—
0.2	1.2	0.1	Trace	8	2	0.2	7	40	—	—	—	—
0.2	1.2	0.1	Trace	9	1	0.1	2	10	Trace	Trace	—	—
—	—	—	1	17	14	0.7	130	70	Trace	0.01	Trace	4
—	—	—	3	5	4	0.3	—	20	Trace	Trace	Trace	1
—	—	—	5	2	2	0.2	—	10	Trace	Trace	Trace	1
—	—	—	5	3	2	0.1	—	—	—	—	—	—
0	0	0	18	0	—	Trace	—	0	0	0	0	0

TABLE 5   (continued)

Food	Approximate Measures, Units, or Weight (edible part unless footnotes indicate otherwise)	Weight (g)	Water (%)	Food Energy (kcal)	Protein (g)	Fat (g)
Soups:						
Canned, condensed:						
Prepared with equal volume of milk:						
Cream of chicken	1 c	245	85	180	7	10
Cream of mushroom	1 c	245	83	215	7	14
Tomato	1 c	250	84	175	7	7
Prepared with equal volume of water:						
Bean with pork	1 c	250	84	170	8	6
Beef broth, bouillon, consommé	1 c	240	96	30	5	0
Beef noodle	1 c	240	93	65	4	3
Clam chowder, Manhattan type (with tomatoes, without milk)	1 c	245	92	80	2	3
Cream of chicken	1 c	240	92	95	3	6
Cream of mushroom	1 c	240	90	135	2	10
Minestrone	1 c	245	90	105	5	3
Split pea	1 c	245	85	145	9	3
Tomato	1 c	245	91	90	2	3
Vegetable beef	1 c	245	92	80	5	2
Vegetarian	1 c	245	92	80	2	2
Dehydrated:						
Bouillon cube, ½ in.	1 cube	4	4	5	1	Trace
Mixes:						
Unprepared:						
Onion	1½ oz	43	3	150	6	5
Prepared with water:						
Chicken noodle	1 c	240	95	55	2	1
Onion	1 c	240	96	35	1	1
Tomato vegetable with noodles	1 c	240	93	65	1	1
Vinegar, cider	1 T	15	94	Trace	Trace	0
White sauce, medium, with enriched flour	1 c	250	73	405	10	31
Yeast:						
Baker's, dry, active	1 package	7	5	20	3	Trace
Brewer's, dry	1 T	8	5	25	3	Trace

	Fatty Acids											
Saturated (total) (g)	Unsaturated		Carbo-hydrate (g)	Calcium (mg)	Phos-phorus (mg)	Iron (mg)	Potassium (mg)	Vitamin A Value (IU)	Thiamin (mg)	Riboflavin (mg)	Niacin (mg)	Ascorbic Acid (mg)
	Oleic (g)	Linoleic (g)										
4.2	3.6	1.3	15	172	152	0.5	260	610	0.05	0.27	0.7	2
5.4	2.9	4.6	16	191	169	0.5	279	250	0.05	0.34	0.7	1
3.4	1.7	1.0	23	168	155	0.8	418	1,200	0.10	0.25	1.3	15
1.2	1.8	2.4	22	63	128	2.3	395	650	0.13	0.08	1.0	3
0	0	0	3	Trace	31	0.5	130	Trace	Trace	0.02	1.2	—
0.6	0.7	0.8	7	7	48	1.0	77	50	0.05	0.07	1.0	Trace
0.5	0.4	1.3	12	34	47	1.0	184	880	0.02	0.02	1.0	—
1.6	2.3	1.1	8	24	34	0.5	79	410	0.02	0.05	0.5	Trace
2.6	1.7	4.5	10	41	50	0.5	98	70	0.02	0.12	0.7	Trace
0.7	0.9	1.3	14	37	59	1.0	314	2,350	0.07	0.05	1.0	—
1.1	1.2	0.4	21	29	149	1.5	270	440	0.25	0.15	1.5	1
0.5	0.5	1.0	16	15	34	0.7	230	1,000	0.05	0.05	1.2	12
—	—	—	10	12	49	0.7	162	2,700	0.05	0.05	1.0	—
—	—	—	13	20	39	1.0	172	2,940	0.05	0.05	1.0	—
—	—	—	Trace	—	—	—	4	—	—	—	—	—
1.1	2.3	1.0	23	42	49	0.6	238	30	0.05	0.03	0.3	6
—	—	—	8	7	19	0.2	19	50	0.07	0.05	0.5	Trace
—	—	—	6	10	12	0.2	58	Trace	Trace	Trace	Trace	2
—	—	—	12	7	19	0.2	29	480	0.05	0.02	0.5	5
0	0	0	1	1	1	0.1	15	—	—	—	—	—
19.3	7.8	0.8	22	288	233	0.5	348	1,150	0.12	0.43	0.7	2
—	—	—	3	3	90	1.1	140	Trace	0.16	0.38	2.6	Trace
—	—	—	3	17[70]	140	1.4	152	Trace	1.25	0.34	3.0	Trace

[1] Vitamin A value is largely from β-carotene used for coloring. Riboflavin value for powdered creamers apply to products with added riboflavin.

[2] Applies to product without added vitamin A. With added vitamin A, value is 500 IU.

[3] Applies to product without vitamin A added.

[4] Applies to product with added vitamin A. Without added vitamin A, value is 20 IU.

[5] Yields 1 qt of fluid milk when reconstituted according to package directions.

[6] Applies to product with added vitamin A.

[7] Weight applies to product with label claim of 1⅓ cups equal 3.2 oz.

[8] Applies to products made from thick shake mixes with no added ice cream. Products made from milk shake mixes are higher in fat and usually contain added ice cream.

[9] Content of fat, vitamin A, and carbohydrate varies. Consult the label when precise values are needed for special diets.

[10] Applies to product made with milk containing no added vitamin A.

[11] Based on year-round average.

[12] Based on average vitamin A content of fortified margarine. Federal specifications for fortified margarine require a minimum of 15,000 IU of vitamin A per pound.

[13] Fatty acid values apply to product made with regular margarine.

[14] Dipped in egg, milk or water, and bread crumbs; fried in vegetable shortening.

[15] If bones are discarded, value for calcium will be greatly reduced.

[16] Dipped in egg, bread crumbs, and flour or batter.

[17] Prepared with tuna, celery, salad dressing (mayonnaise type), pickle, onion, and egg.

[18] Outer layer of fat on the cut removed to within approximately ½ in. of the lean. Deposits of fat within the cut not removed.

[19] Crust made with vegetable shortening and enriched flour.

[20] Regular margarine used.

[21] Value varies widely.

[22] About one-fourth of the outer layer of fat on the cut removed. Deposits of fat within the cut not removed.

[23] Vegetable shortening used.

[24] Also applies to pasteurized apple cider.

[25] Applies to product without added ascorbic acid. For value of product with added ascorbic acid, refer to label.

[26] Based on product with label claim of 45% of U.S. RDA in 6 fl oz.

[27] Based on product with label claim of 100% of U.S. RDA in 6 fl oz.

[28] Weight includes peel and membranes between sections. Without these parts, the weight of the edible portion is 123 g for pink or red grapefruit and 118 g for white.

[29] For white-fleshed varieties, value is about 20 IU per cup; for red-fleshed varieties, 1,080 IU.

[30] Weight includes seeds. Without seeds, weight of the edible portion is 57 g.

[31] Applies to product without added ascorbic acid. With added ascorbic acid, based on claim that 6 fl oz of reconstituted juice contain 45% or 50% of the U.S. RDA, value is 108 or 120 mg for a 6-fl-oz can and 36 or 40 mg for 1 c of diluted juice.

[32] For products with added thiamin and riboflavin but without added ascorbic acid, values in milligrams would be 0.60 for thiamin, 0.80 for riboflavin, and a trace for ascorbic acid. For products with only ascorbic acid added, value varies with the brand. Consult the label.

[33] Weight includes rind. Without rind, the weight of the edible portion is 272 g for cantaloupe and 149 g for honeydew.

[34] Represents yellow-fleshed varieties. For white-fleshed varieties, value is 50 IU for 1 peach and 90 IU for 1 c of slices.

[35] Value represents products with added ascorbic acid. For products without added ascorbic acid, the values are highly variable; e.g., 10−25 mg for a 10-oz container, and 15−35 mg for 1 c.

[36] Weight includes pits. After removal of the pits, the weight of the edible portion is 258 g for a cup and 133 g for a portion, 43 g for uncooked prunes, and 213 g for cooked prunes.

[37] Weight includes rind and seeds. Without rind and seeds, weight of the edible portion is 426 g.

[38] Made with vegetable shortening.

[39] Applies to product made with white cornmeal. With yellow cornmeal, value is 30 IU.

[40] Applies to white varieties. For yellow varieties, value is 150 IU.

[41] Applies to products that do not contain disodium phosphate. If disodium phosphate is an ingredient, value is 162 mg.

[42] Value may range from less than 1 mg to about 8 mg, depending on the brand. Consult the label.

[43] Applies to product with added nutrient. Without added nutrient, value is trace.

[44] Value varies with the brand. Consult the label.

[45] Applies to product with added nutrient. Without added nutrient, value is trace.

[46] Except for angel food cake, cakes were made from mixes containing vegetable shortening; icings made from butter.

[47] Except for sponge cake, vegetable shortening used for cake portion; butter, for icing. If butter or margarine used for cake portion, vitamin A values are higher.

[48] Applies to product made with a sodium-aluminum-sulfate-type baking powder. With a low-sodium baking powder containing potassium, value would be about twice the amount shown.

[49] Equal weights of flour, sugar, eggs, and vegetable shortening.

[50] Products are commercial unless otherwise specified.

[51] Made with enriched flour and vegetable shortening except for macaroons, which do not contain flour or shortening.

[52] Icing made with butter.

[53] Applies to yellow varieties; white varieties contain only a trace.

[54] Contains vegetable shortening and butter.

[55] Made with corn oil.

[56] Made with regular margarine.

[57] Applies to product made with yellow cornmeal.

[58] Made with enriched degermed cornmeal and enriched flour.

[59] Product may or may not be enriched with riboflavin. Consult the label.

[60] Value varies with the brand. Consult the label.

[61] Weight includes cob. Without cob, weight is 77 g for a raw ear and 126 g for a frozen ear.

[62] Based on yellow varieties. For white varieties, value is trace.

[63] Weight includes refuse of outer leaves and core. Without these parts, weight is 163 g.

[64] Weight includes core. Without core, weight is 539 g.

[65] Value based on white-fleshed varieties. For yellow-fleshed varieties, value is 70 IU for chopped raw onions, 50 IU for sliced raw onions, and 80 IU for cooked onions.

[66] Weight includes cores and stem ends. Without these parts, weight is 123 g.

[67] Based on year-round average. For tomatoes marketed from November through May, value is about 12 mg; from June through October, 32 mg.

[68] Applies to product without calcium salts added. Value for products with calcium salts added may be as much as 63 mg for whole tomatoes, 241 mg for cut forms.

[69] Weight includes pits. Without pits, weight is 13 g for green olives and 9 g for Mission ripe olives.

[70] Value may vary from 6 to 60 mg.

TABLE 6 Common Weights and Measures

Measure	Equivalent	Measure	Equivalent
3 t	1 T	1 fl oz	30 g
2 T	1 oz	½ c	120 g
4 T	¼ c	1 c	240 g
8 T	½ c	1 lb	454 g
16 T	1 c		
		1 g	1 mL
2 c	1 pt	1 t	5 mL
4 c	1 qt	1 T	15 mL
4 qt	1 gal	1 fl oz	30 mL
		1 c	240 mL
1 t	5 g	1 pt	480 mL
1 T	15 g	1 qt	960 mL
1 oz	28.35 g	1 L	1,000 mL

TABLE 7 Weights and Measures Conversions

U.S. System to Metric		Metric to U.S. System	
U.S. Measure	Metric Measure	Metric Measure	U.S. Measure
Length		**Length**	
1 in.	25.0 mm	1 mm	0.04 in.
1 ft	0.3 m	1 m	3.3 ft
Mass		**Mass**	
1 gr	64.8 mg	1 mg	0.015 gr
1 oz	28.0 g	1 g	0.035 oz
1 lb	0.45 kg	1 kg	2.2 lb
1 short ton	907.1 kg	1 metric ton	1.102 short tons
Volume		**Volume**	
1 cu. in.	16.0 cm^3	1 cm^3	0.06 in.^{3}
1 t	5.0 mL	1 mL	0.2 t
1 T	15.0 mL	1 mL	0.07 T
1 fl oz	30.0 mL	1 mL	0.03 oz
1 c	0.24 L	1 L	4.2 c
1 pt	0.47 L	1 L	2.1 pt
1 qt (liq)	0.95 L	1 L	1.1 qt
1 gal	0.004 m^3	1 m^3	264.0 gal
1 pk	0.009 m^3	1 m^3	113.0 pk
1 bu	0.04 m^3	1 m^3	28.0 bu
Energy		**Energy**	
1 cal	4.18 J	1 J	0.24 cal

TABLE 7 (continued)

Temperature

To convert Celsius degrees into Fahrenheit, multiply by $\frac{9}{5}$ and add 32.

To convert Fahrenheit degrees into Celsius, subtract 32 and multiply by $\frac{5}{9}$. For example:

$$30 \text{ °C} = \left(30 \times \frac{9}{5} + 32 \right) \text{ °F}$$

$$= (54 + 32) \text{ °F} = 86 \text{ °F}$$

$$90 \text{ °F} = (90 - 32) \times \frac{5}{9} \text{ °C}$$

$$= 58 \times \frac{5}{9} \text{ °C} = 32.2 \text{ °C}$$

Pounds to Kilograms (for Weight Reference)

Pounds	Kilo-grams	Pounds	Kilo-grams	Pounds	Kilo-grams	Pounds	Kilo-grams	Pounds	Kilo-grams
5	2.3	50	22.7	95	43.1	140	63.5	185	83.9
10	4.5	55	25.0	100	45.4	145	65.8	190	86.2
15	6.8	60	27.2	105	47.6	150	68.0	195	88.5
20	9.1	65	29.5	110	49.9	155	70.3	200	90.7
25	11.3	70	31.7	115	52.2	160	72.6	205	93.0
30	13.6	75	34.0	120	54.4	165	74.8	210	95.3
35	15.9	80	36.3	125	56.7	170	77.1	215	97.5
40	18.1	85	38.6	130	58.9	175	79.4	220	99.8
45	20.4	90	40.8	135	61.2	180	81.6		

Feet and Inches to Centimeters (for Height Reference)

Feet and Inches		Centi-meters	Feet and Inches		Centi-meters	Feet and Inches		Centi-meters	Feet and Inches		Centi-meters	Feet and Inches		Centi-meters
0	6	15.2	2	4	71.1	3	4	101.6	4	4	132.0	5	4	162.6
1	0	30.5	2	5	73.6	3	5	104.1	4	5	134.6	5	5	165.1
1	6	45.7	2	6	76.1	3	6	106.6	4	6	137.1	5	6	167.6
1	7	48.3	2	7	78.7	3	7	109.2	4	7	139.6	5	7	170.2
1	8	50.8	2	8	81.2	3	8	111.7	4	8	142.2	5	8	172.7
1	9	53.3	2	9	83.8	3	9	114.2	4	9	144.7	5	9	175.3
1	10	55.9	2	10	86.3	3	10	116.8	4	10	147.3	5	10	177.8
1	11	58.4	2	11	88.8	3	11	119.3	4	11	149.8	5	11	180.3
2	0	61.0	3	0	91.4	4	0	121.9	5	0	152.4	6	0	182.9
2	1	63.5	3	1	93.9	4	1	124.4	5	1	154.9	6	1	185.4
2	2	66.0	3	2	96.4	4	2	127.0	5	2	157.5	6	2	188.0
2	3	68.6	3	3	99.0	4	3	129.5	5	3	160.0	6	3	190.5

TABLE 8 Milligrams and Milliequivalents Conversion

Sodium (Equivalent Weight 23)		Potassium (Equivalent Weight 39)		
Milligrams	Grams	Milligrams	Grams	Milliequivalents
230	0.23	390	0.39	10
460	0.46	780	0.78	20
—	—	1,000	1.00	25.6
690	0.69	1,170	1.17	30
920	0.92	1,560	1.56	40
1,000	1.00	—	—	43.5
1,150	1.15	1,950	1.95	50
1,380	1.38	2,340	2.34	60
1,610	1.61	2,730	2.73	70
1,840	1.84	3,170	3.17	80
2,170	2.17	3,510	3.51	90
2,300	2.30	3,900	3.9	100
—	—	5,000	5.0	128
5,000	5.00	—	—	217.5
—	—	10,000	10.0	256
10,000	10.00	—	—	435

Note: To convert milligrams to milliequivalents:

$$\text{milliequivalents of sodium or potassium} = \frac{\text{milligrams of sodium or potassium}}{\text{equivalent weight in milligrams}}$$

To convert milliequivalents to milligrams:

milligrams of sodium or potassium = milliequivalents of sodium or potassium × equivalent weight in milligrams

TABLE 9 Weights in Relation to Height and Frame According to the Society of Actuaries and the Metropolitan Life Insurance Company

Weights at Ages 25–29 based on lowest mortality. Weights in pounds according to frame (in indoor clothing weighing 5 pounds for men or 3 pounds for women, shoes with 1–inch heels).

Men					Women				
Height		Small Frame	Medium Frame	Large Frame	Height		Small Frame	Medium Frame	Large Frame
Feet	Inches				Feet	Inches			
5	2	128–134	131–141	138–150	4	10	102–111	109–121	118–131
5	3	130–136	133–143	140–153	4	11	103–113	111–123	120–134
5	4	132–138	135–145	142–156	5	0	104–115	113–126	122–137
5	5	134–140	137–148	144–160	5	1	106–118	115–129	125–140
5	6	136–142	139–151	146–164	5	2	108–121	118–132	128–143
5	7	138–145	142–154	149–168	5	3	111–124	121–135	131–147
5	8	140–148	145–157	152–172	5	4	114–127	124–138	134–151
5	9	142–151	148–160	155–176	5	5	117–130	127–141	137–155
5	10	144–154	151–163	158–180	5	6	120–133	130–144	140–159
5	11	146–157	154–166	161–184	5	7	123–136	133–147	143–163
6	0	149–160	157–170	164–188	5	8	126–139	136–150	146–167
6	1	152–164	160–174	168–192	5	9	129–142	139–153	149–170
6	2	155–168	164–178	172–197	5	10	132–145	142–156	152–173
6	3	158–172	167–182	176–202	5	11	135–148	145–159	155–176
6	4	162–176	171–187	181–207	6	0	138–151	148–162	158–179

Source: Reproduced with permission of Metropolitan Life Insurance Company. Source of basic data: *1979 Build Study*, Society of Actuaries and Association of Life Insurance Medical Directors of America, 1980. Reproduced by permission.

TABLE 10 Guidelines for Body Weight According to the National Institutes of Health

	Metric						Nonmetric					
	Men Weight (kg)*			Women Weight (kg)*				Men Weight (lb)*			Women Weight (lb)*	
Height* (m)	Aver-age	Acceptable weight		Aver-age	Acceptable weight		Height* (ft in)	Aver-age	Acceptable weight		Aver-age	Acceptable weight
1.45				46.0	42	53	4 10				102	92	119
1.48				46.5	42	54	4 11				104	94	122
1.50				47.0	43	55	5 0				107	96	125
1.52				48.5	44	57	5 1				110	99	128
1.54				49.5	44	58	5 2	123	112	141	113	102	131
1.56				50.4	45	58	5 3	127	115	144	116	105	134
1.58	55.8	51	64	51.3	46	59	5 4	130	118	148	120	108	138
1.60	57.6	52	65	52.6	48	61	5 5	133	121	152	123	111	142
1.62	58.6	53	66	54.0	49	62	5 6	136	124	156	128	114	146
1.64	59.6	54	67	55.4	50	64	5 7	140	128	161	132	118	150
1.66	60.6	55	69	56.8	51	65	5 8	145	132	166	136	122	154
1.68	61.7	56	71	58.1	52	66	5 9	149	136	170	140	126	158
1.70	63.5	58	73	60.0	53	67	5 10	153	140	174	144	130	163
1.72	65.0	59	74	61.3	55	69	5 11	158	144	179	148	134	168
1.74	66.5	60	75	62.6	56	70	6 0	162	148	184	152	138	173
1.76	68.0	62	77	64.0	58	72	6 1	166	152	189			
1.78	69.4	64	79	65.3	59	74	6 2	171	156	194			
1.80	71.0	65	80				6 3	176	160	199			
1.82	72.6	66	82				6 4	181	164	204			
1.84	74.2	67	84										
1.86	75.8	69	86										
1.88	77.6	71	88										
1.90	79.3	73	90										
1.92	81.0	75	93										

Source: "Obesity in America," edited by G. A. Bray, U.S. Department of Health, Education, and Welfare, Public Health Service, National Institutes of Health, NIH Publication No. 80-359, 1980, page 7.

*Height without shoes, weight without clothes.

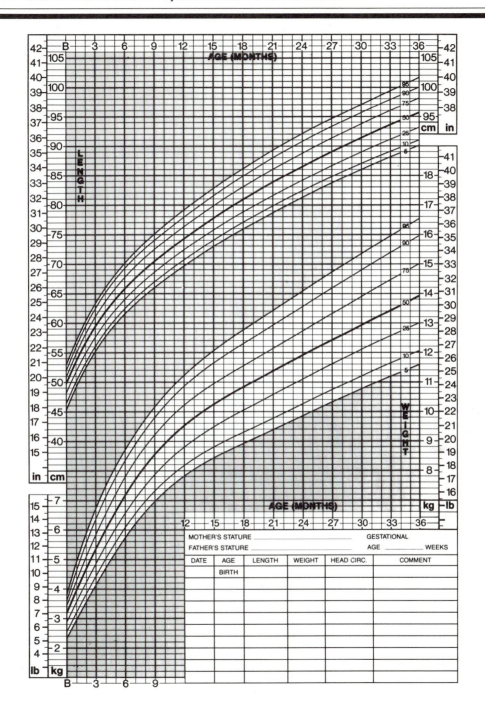

TABLE 11 (continued)

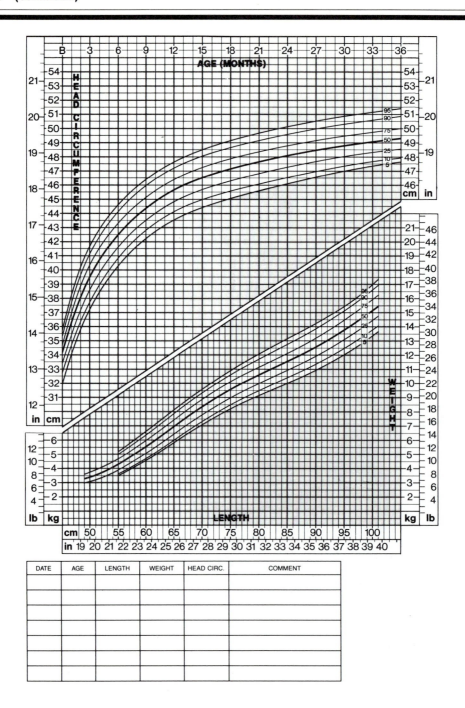

DATE	AGE	LENGTH	WEIGHT	HEAD CIRC.	COMMENT

TABLE 12   Boys: Birth to 36 Months Physical Growth NCHS Percentiles*

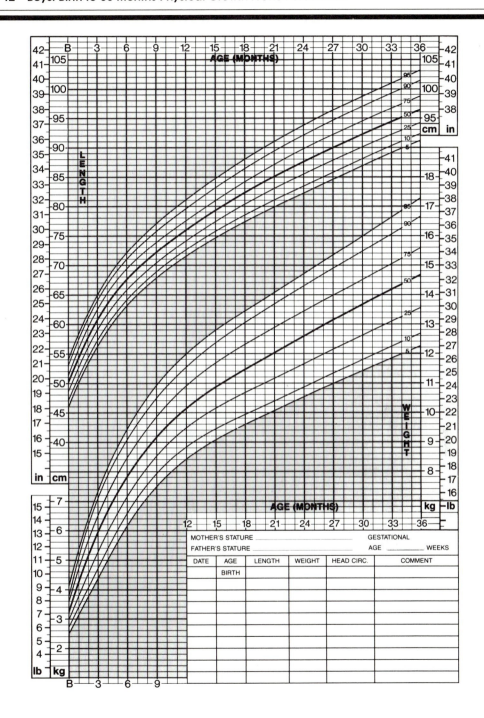

TABLE 12   (continued)

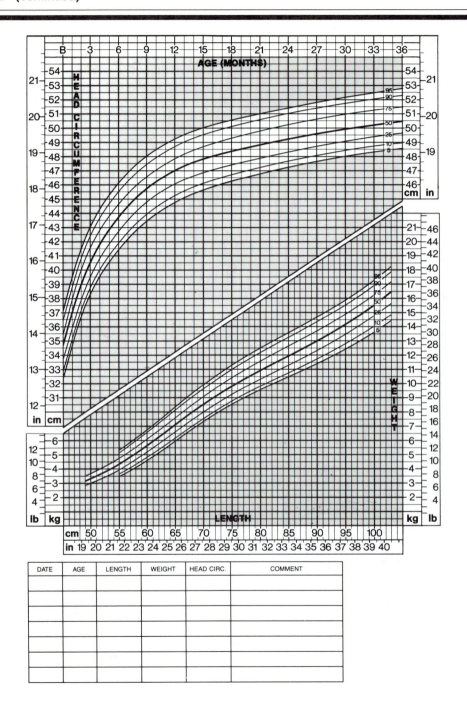

DATE	AGE	LENGTH	WEIGHT	HEAD CIRC.	COMMENT

TABLE 13 Girls: 2 to 18 Years Physical Growth NCHS Percentiles*

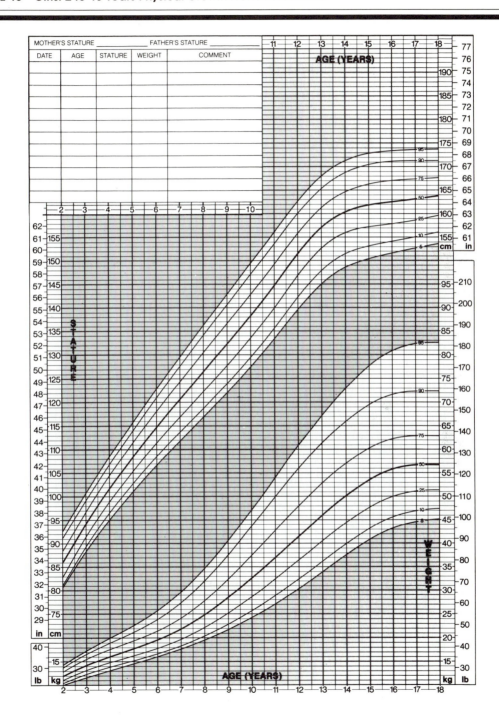

TABLE 13 (continued)

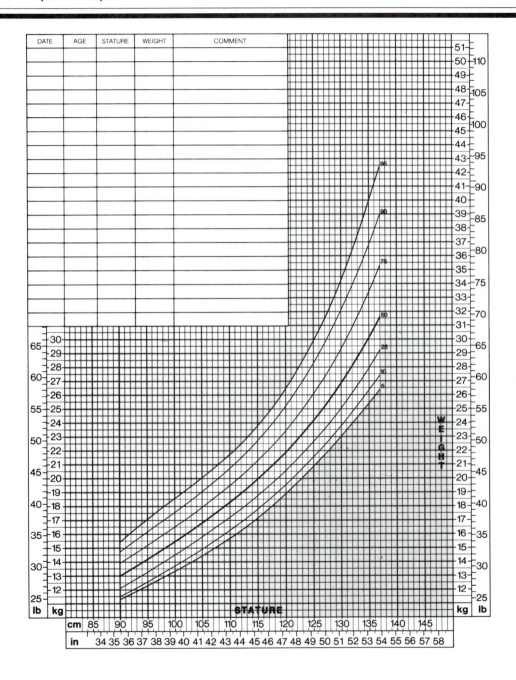

TABLE 14 Boys: 2 to 18 Years Physical Growth NCHS Percentiles*

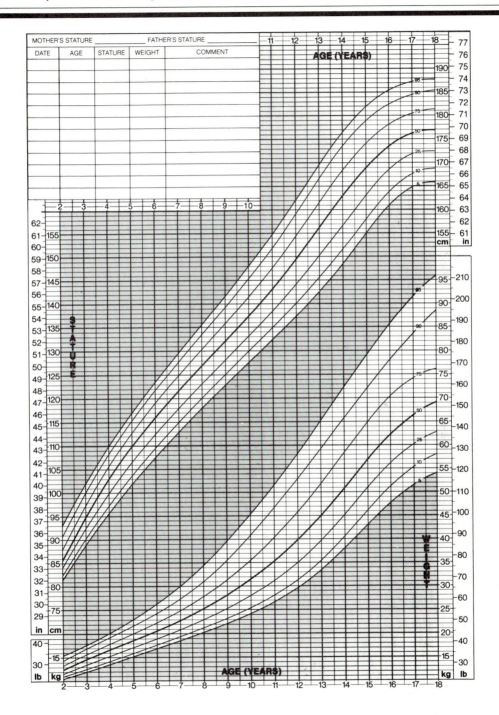

TABLE 14   (continued)

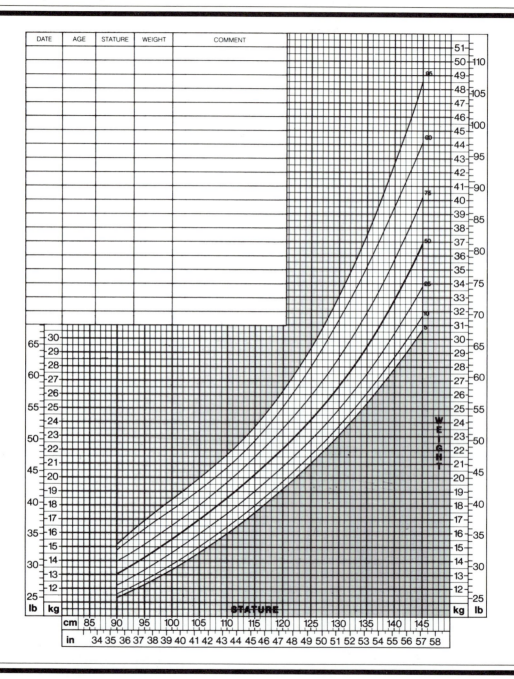

DATE	AGE	STATURE	WEIGHT	COMMENT

*Tables 11–14 adapted from: Hamill PVV, Drizd TA, Johnson CL, Reed RB, Roche AF, Moore WM: Physical growth: National Center for Health Statistics percentiles. AM J CLIN NUTR 32:607–629, 1979. Data from the Fels Research Institute, Wright State University School of Medicine, Yellow Springs, Ohio. © 1982 Ross Laboratories.

TABLE 15 Standard Values for Constituents in the Blood of an Adult

Constituent	Normal Range	Constituent	Normal Range
Physical Measurements		White blood count	
pH	7.37–7.45	(WBC) and differential	
Capillary bleeding time	1–4 min	= 5–10 × 10^3/mm^3	Basophils
Plasma prothrombin time			0%–1.5%
(quick method)	11–19 sec		Eosinophils
Sedimentation rate			0.5%–4%
(Wintrobe method)	Men: 0–9 mm/h		Lymphocytes
	Women: 0–20 mm/h		20%–40%
Specific gravity	1.025–1.030		Monocytes
Viscosity (H$_2$O = 1)	4.5–5.0		4%–10%
Protein			Neutrophils
Albumin, serum	3.5–5.5 g/100 mL		50%–65%
Globulin, serum	1.3–3.0 mg/100 mL	**Nitrogenous Substances**	
Albumin/globulin ratio	1.2–2.5	Amino acid nitrogen, blood	4–8 mg/100 mL
Ceruloplasmin, plasma	15–30 mg/100 mL	Ammonia, blood	40–70 μg/100 mL
Fibrinogen, plasma	0.2–0.4 g/100 mL	Creatine	0.2–0.9 mg/100 mL
Total protein, serum	6–8 g/100 mL	Creatinine	0.7–1.8 mg/100 mL
Hematology		Nonprotein nitrogen, blood	
Cell volume	39%–50%	(NPN)	20–35 mg/100 mL
Coagulation time,		Blood urea nitrogen (BUN)	8–20 mg/100 mL
venous blood (Lee-		Urea, blood	20–35 mg/100 mL
White method)	At 37 °C: 6–12 min	Uric acid, blood	2.5–6 mg/100 mL
	At room temperature:	**Minerals**	
	10–18 min	Base, serum (total)	143–155 mEq/L
Erythrocytes (RBCs)	Men: 4.5–6.2 × 10^6/mm^3	Calcium, serum	9–11 mg/100 mL
	Women: 4.0–5.5 ×		4.5–5.5 mEq/L
	10^6/mm^3	Chlorides, serum	340–372 mg/100 mL
Hematocrit (vol% red			96–105 mEq/L
cells, or PCV)	Men: 40%–52%	Copper	100–240 μg/100 mL
	Women: 37%–47%	Iodine	Total: 7–16 mEq/L
Hemoglobin	Adult:		Protein bound: 3–9 μg/
	Men: 14–18 g/100 mL		100 mL
	Women: 12–16 g/100 mL	Iron, serum	Men: 80–165 μg/100 mL
	Children:		Women: 65–130 μg/
	10–18 g/100 mL		100 mL
	(varies with age)	Magnesium, serum	2–3 mg/100 mL
Leukocytes (WBCs)	5,000–10,000/mm^3		1.65–2.5 mEq/L
Platelets (thrombocytes)	125,000–400,000/mm^3	Phosphate	1.5–2.8 mEq/L
Reticulocytes	0.5%–2% of red cells	Phosphorus, inorganic,	
Whole blood volume	70–100 mL/kg	serum	Child:
			4.0–6.5 mg/100 mL
			Adult:
			2.5–4.5 mg/100 mL
		Potassium, serum	16–22 mg/100 mL
			4.1–5.6 mEq/L

TABLE 15 (continued)

Constituent	Normal Range	Constituent	Normal Range
Sodium, serum	320–335 mg/100 mL	**Liquids**	
	139–146 mEq/L	Fats, neutral	140–300 mg/100 mL
Sulfates, inorganic, serum	2.5–5.0 mg/100 mL	Fatty acids, free	8–31 mg/100 mL
	0.5–1.0 mEq/L	Fatty acids, serum (total)	350–450 mg/100 mL
Zinc(s)	100–140 μg/100 mL	Triglyceride(s)	30–140 mg/100 mL
Amino acids		Cholesterol, serum	Total: 125–240 mg/
Amino acids, total	30–70 mg/100 mL		100 mL
Alanine	3.0–3.7 mg/100 mL		Esters: 90–180 mg/
Arginine	1.2–2.0 mg/100 mL		100 mL
Asparagine	0.4–0.8 mg/100 mL	Cholesterol, free	50–60 mg/100 mL
Aspartic acid	1.01–0.08 mg/100 mL	**Vitamins**	
Cysteine and cystine	1.0–1.4 mg/100 mL	Ascorbic acid	Serum: 0.3–1.4 mg/
Glutamine	5–14 mg/100 mL		100 mL
Glutamic acid	0.5–12 mg/100 mL		White blood cells: 25–
Glycine	1.2–1.6 mg/100 mL		40 mg/100 mL
Histidine	0.9–1.6 mg/100 mL	Folic acid	2–5 μg/100 mL
Isoleucine	0.7–1.3 mg/100 mL	Riboflavin	15–25 μg/100 mL
Leucine	1.4–2.3 mg/100 mL	Thiamin	2–5 μg/100 mL
Lysine	2.5–3.0 mg/100 mL	Vitamin A	50–100 IU/100 mL
Methionine	0.2–0.4 mg/100 mL	Vitamin B_{12}	300–800 μg/100 mL
Ornithine	0.5–0.9 mg/100 mL	Vitamin K, prothrombin time	
Phenylalanine	0.7–1.0 mg/100 mL	(quick method)	10–15 s
Proline	1.8–3.5 mg/100 mL		10–20 s
Serine	1.0–1.2 mg/100 mL		
Threonine	1.2–1.8 mg/100 mL	**Blood Gases**	
Tryptophan	1.0–1.2 mg/100 mL	O_2 capacity, whole blood	16–27 vol%
Tyrosine	0.8–1.5 mg/100 mL	CO_2 content	Serum:
Valine	0.5–3.8 mg/100 mL		45–70 vol%
Carbohydrates			20.3–31.5 mM/L
Fructose	5–9 mg/100 mL		Whole blood:
Glucose	Nelson-Somogyi:		40–60 vol%
	70–100 mg/100 mL		18–27 mM/L
	Folin-Wu: 80–120 mg/	O_2 saturation	Arterial blood: 94%–
	100 mL		96%
Glycogen	5–7 mg/100 mL		Venous blood: 60%–
Hexoses	70–110 mg/100 mL		85%
Pentose, total	2–5 mg/100 mL		

TABLE 16   Standard Values for Constituents in the Urine of an Adult

Constituent	Normal Range	Constituent	Normal Range
Physical Measurements		**Acetone (Ketone) Bodies, continued**	
pH	5.5–8.0		
Specific gravity	1.009–1.030	Glucose	0–0.002 g
Daily volume	900–1,600 mL	Iron	0.001–0.006 g
Total Solid Constituents in Daily		Magnesium (as MgO)	0.14–0.31 g
Volume	50–70 g	Nitrogen	9–18 g
Acetone (Ketone) Bodies		Phosphate (as $PO_4^=$)	2.0–3.5 g
Albumin	0–0.01 g	Potassium	1.5–3.0 g
Ammonia	0.3–1.0 g	Purine bases	0.009–0.05 g
Bile	0	Sodium	3.0–5.5 g
Calcium	0.1–0.4 g	Sulfate (as $SO_4^=$)	1.5–3.0
Chloride (as NaCl)	10–15 g	Urea	20–35 g
Creatine	0–0.1 g	Uric acid	0.5–0.7 g
Creatinine	0.9–1.6 g		

GLOSSARY

acid/base balance The relationship of acidity to alkalinity in the body fluids, normally slightly alkaline

acidosis High acidity in body fluids

adenosine triphosphate The high-energy phosphate molecule which is the major form of stored energy in the human body. Abbreviated "ATP"

alanine A nonessential amino acid

alimentary canal The mucous-membrane lined tube of the digestive system, from mouth to the anus

alkalosis Excess alkalinity of body fluids

allergy An altered immunological state in which pathological reactions are induced by an antigen

amino acids The structural units of protein molecules

amylopectin A constituent of starch, composed of many glucose units joined in branching patterns

amylose A constituent of starch, consisting of many glucose units joined linearly without branching

anabolism The metabolic process within the cells whereby metabolites (e.g., nutrients) are used to synthesize new materials for cellular growth, maintenance, or repair

anemia Pathological deficiency of oxygen-carrying material in the blood

anorexia The loss of appetite

arachidonic acid An essential polyunsaturated fatty acid

arginine An amino acid known to be essential for infants and children

ascorbic acid The chemical name for vitamin C

ash The non-combustible mineral residue left after a substance has been oxidized

asparagine A nonessential amino acid

aspartic acid A nonessential amino acid

atherosclerosis Thickening of the lining of blood vessels as lipid materials are deposited and covered by fibrous connective tissues

atrophy The wasting of tissues

avidin A heat-sensitive glycoprotein found in raw egg white, which can complex with biotin, rendering it unavailable for absorption

basal metabolic rate The least amount of energy required by an individual's body at rest to keep the essential life processes functioning; abbreviated "BMR"

beriberi A syndrome describing vitamin B_1 deficiency

bile The substance stored in the gallbladder and is especially important in fat digestion

biological value The degree to which a protein contains all essential amino acids in the proportions needed by the body

biotin A water-soluble vitamin and part of the B vitamin complex

bomb calorimeter A device in which food samples are oxidized to determine their energy content

butyric acid A saturated fatty acid

cachexia General wasting of the body, especially during chronic disease

calorie The amount of heat energy that will raise the temperature of 1 gm of water from 15 °C to 16 °C

carbohydrate An organic compound containing carbon, hydrogen, and oxygen, with a ratio of carbon to hydrogen to oxygen atoms of $1:2:1$

carcinogenic Cancer-causing

cardiovascular Involving the heart and blood vessels

carotene The precursor of vitamin A, found in plant products

casein Major protein in milk, cheese, and eggs

catabolism Conversion of larger (organized) substances in body into smaller (simpler) ones. The destructive part of metabolism (= catabolism + anabolism)

celiac disease A syndrome resulting from intestinal (small) sensitivity to gluten, a protein in flour

cellulose A polysaccharide made of many glucose molecules and not digestible by man

cheilosis Cracks at the corners of the mouth with yellow crusts, a symptom of deficiency of vitamin B_2, folic acid, vitamin B_{12}, or niacin

chemically defined diet See defined-formula diet

cholecalciferol One chemical form of vitamin D

cholesterol One chemical form of fat, found only in animal products and suspected to play a role in heart disease

choline A substance normally synthesized in the body, important in the biochemistry of metabolism and closely associated with the physiology of vitamins

chylomicron A large, low-density molecule consisting mostly of triglycerides. Its main func-

tion is to transport fat in the body, primarily in the form of triglycerides

citric acid cycle The series of chemical reactions whereby carbohydrate, fat, and/or protein are completely oxidized to carbon dioxide, water, and energy. Also called the "Krebs cycle"

clear liquid diet A diet consisting of fluids that are liquid at body temperature, with mono- and disaccharides as the major sources of calories

cobalamin Vitamin B_{12}, important in all cell metabolism, tissue growth, and maintenance of the central nervous system

coenzyme An accessory substance that facilitates the working of an enzyme, largely by acting as a carrier for products of the chemical reaction

coenzyme A A critical substance in the metabolism of fat, protein, and carbohydrate (it participates in the citric acid cycle and permits the release of energy) which also has other essential functions in the body. Abbreviated CoA. Also see CoQ or Coenzyme Q

coenzyme Q A fat-soluble vitamin-like substance found in most living cells. A perfect biological catalyst, it is an important component of the respiratory chain. Abbreviated CoQ

collagen An insoluble protein that holds together the cells and tissues of skin, cartilage, tendons, ligaments, bones, teeth, and blood vessels

colostomy Surgical creation of an opening between the colon and the surface of the body, usually by establishing a stoma in the abdominal wall

colostrum The thick yellowish fluid that precedes white breast milk, suspected to provide infant with passive immunity

complementary proteins Protein foods which are individually incomplete but which when combined correct each other's deficiencies in essential amino acids

core eating plan On a weight loss diet, specification of the approximate number of servings of each category of food to be consumed daily

cretinism Retardation of infants and children in physical and mental development, associated with a lack of iodine

cysteine A nonessential amino acid

cystic fibrosis An inherited disease of the mucous glands which usually develops during childhood, creating pancreatic insufficiency and lung problems

cystine Though classified as a nonessential amino acid, a substance derived from the essential amino acid methionine

daily food guide A translation of Recommended Daily Allowances into simple-to-follow recommendations of the kinds and amounts of food needed for good nutrition

defined formula diet A commercially-prepared formula for artificial feeding which is considered nutritionally complete. Also called chemically defined diet or elemental diet

dehydration Excessive loss of water from the body; also called "underhydration"

dextran A polysaccharide made of many glucose molecules, with potential clinical usages. Does not occur naturally in food

dextrin A small polysaccharide of five to six glucose units, found in the leaves of starch-forming plants and in the human alimentary canal as a product of starch digestion

diabetes mellitus A disease characterized by excess blood sugar and urine sugar. Caused mostly by a malfunctioning pancreas

dialysis Diffusion of dissolved particles from one side of a semipermeable membrane to the other

dietetics The science and art of human nutrition care

diffusion Movement of a substance from a location of higher concentration to one of lower concentration

digestion The breaking down of ingested foods into particles of a size and chemical composition that the body can readily absorb

digestive system The long tube including the mouth, esophagus, stomach, small intestine, colon, rectum, and associated organs such as pancreas. These structural units and their secretions break food down into units absorbable by the body

diglyceride A glyceride with two molecules of fatty acids

dipeptide Two amino acids chemically joined

disaccharide A carbohydrate composed of two monosaccharides

disaccharidase An enzyme responsible for hydrolysis of disaccharides to monosaccharides in the duodenum, jejunum, and ileum

diuretic A substance that increases urine excretion

diverticulum A blind pouch in the colon, usually developed from some clinical disorders

dumping syndrome A set of symptoms occurring when food passes into the jejunum without first undergoing normal digestion and mixing by the stomach because of partial or complete surgical removal of stomach

edema The presence of an abnormally high amount of fluid in the intercellular spaces; also called "overhydration"

edentulous Lacking teeth previously present

electrolyte A substance that is a charged particle or is separated into charged particles when dissolved in fluid

-emia A suffix indicating the blood

energy The capacity to do work

enter- A prefix indicating intestine

enteral feeding Feeding in which nutrients are delivered to the body via the gastrointestinal tract. May be accomplished by various means including tube-feeding

enterohepatic circulation The cycling of bile salts through the liver, gallbladder, intestinal lumen, portal vein, and liver again

enzyme A protein that catalyzes a specific chemical reaction or a few specific reactions in the body

epidemiology The study of the incidence, distribution, and control of a certain disease or pathogen in a population

ergosterol The form of vitamin D found in plant products

essential Referring to a nutrient that the body needs but is unable to synthesize from ordinary foods

essential amino acid One of the 8 to 10 amino acids that the human body cannot manufacture and that must therefore be consumed in foods

essential fatty acids The polyunsaturated fatty acids lineoleic acid and linolenic acid, which cannot be synthesized by the body and must therefore be consumed in the diet

extracellular Located outside a cell or cells

fat An organic compound whose molecules contain glycerol and fatty acids. Also used in referring to adipose tissue

fatty acid A constituent of fat, a simple lipid containing only carbon, hydrogen, and oxygen

favism A clinical disorder associated with the eating of fava or broad beans by people with an inherited deficiency of glucose-6-phosphate dehydrogenase

fiber Indigestible carbohydrate found in plant foods and connective tissues of meats. Also known as "roughage" or "bulk"

folic acid Part of the B vitamin complex, a substance which participates in many essential biological reactions in its coenzyme form; also called "folacin"

Food Exchange Lists Groups of food in which each group or list contains selected foods, each of which contributes approximately equal amounts of certain nutrients and calories. The American Diabetes Association and the American Dietetic Association originated the Food Exchange Lists for diabetic patients

fortification The addition of nutrients to foods to improve their nutritional value

foundation diet A diet consisting only of the recommended numbers of servings from the Four Food Groups

the Four Food Groups Milk and milk products, meats or meat equivalents, fruits and vegetables, and breads and cereals—the main groups of food now recommended for daily consumption

free amino acid An amino acid existing singly or in free form

fructose A simple carbohydrate found in many fruits, honey, and plant saps. One of the two monosaccharides forming sucrose (table sugar); also called "fruit sugar" or "levulose"

full liquid diet A liquid diet including certain foods and beverages that are liquid at body temperature

galactose A six-carbon monosaccharide usually occurring as one of the two components of lactose, or milk sugar

gastritis Inflammation of the stomach, either chronic or acute

gastrointestinal bypass Surgical stapling of a portion of the stomach or removal of part of the intestine to reduce the amount of food eaten and/or absorbed and thus reduce caloric intake

gastrointestinal system See digestive system

glossitis A smooth red tongue with flat, swollen or pebbled papillae, associated with deficiencies of vitamin B_2, folic acid, vitamin B_{12}, or niacin

glucagon A hormone that can stimulate insulin secretion

glucose A six-carbon monosaccharide found mostly in the blood in the human body, where it provides fuel for immediate energy when oxidized; also called "D-glucose," "fruit sugar," "corn sugar," and "dextrose"

glucose tolerance test A test used to ascertain how well a person tolerates an influx of glucose into the bloodstream, used to determine the presence of hyperglycemia or hypoglycemia. Abbreviated "GTT"

glutamic acid A nonessential amino acid

glutamine A nonessential amino acid

glyceride A simple lipid, an ester of fatty acids and glycerol

glycine A nonessential amino acid

glycogen The polysaccharide form in which energy is stored in an animal; sometimes called "animal starch"

glycolysis The degradation of glucose to pyruvate and/or lactate

goiter A lack of iodine, resulting in enlargement of the thyroid gland

goitrogen A substance capable of inducing goiter

hemocellulose A form of indigestible carbohydrate found in plant foods

hemoglobin The iron-containing protein in red blood cells which carries oxygen to the tissues

heparin A polysaccharide used as a blood anticoagulant

hepatic Pertaining to the liver

hepatic encephalopathy A disorder caused by failure of the liver to remove toxic waste. Also called "portal system encephalopathy"

hexoses Six-carbon sugars, such as glucose, fructose, galactose, and mannose

high density lipoprotein One type of cholesterol carrier in the blood: that which removes deposited cholesterol and carries it away for excretion

high nutrient diet A diet made of nutritionally potent liquids and semi-solid foods of a consistency that can be taken as a beverage or through a straw. Also called "modified full liquid diet"

histidine An amino acid known to be essential for infants and children, and perhaps essential for adults as well

hydrogenation The commercial process by which oils with a high level of unsaturated fatty acids are turned into fats with soft to hard texture

hydrolyze To break down a chemical compound by adding water

hyper- A prefix indicating an abnormal excess

hypercalcemia An excess of calcium in the blood

hypercalciuria Excretion of a large amount of calcium in the urine

hyperglycemia A high blood "sugar" (glucose) level

hyperkalemia An elevated serum level of potassium

hyperlipidemia An elevated level of lipids in the blood serum

hyperlipoproteinemia An elevated level of certain lipoproteins in the blood

hypertension Sustained elevation of systolic and/or diastolic arterial blood pressure

hypo- A prefix indicating an abnormal insufficiency

hypocalcemia A low level of calcium in the blood

hypoglycemia A low blood "sugar" (glucose) level

hypokalemia A decreased serum potassium level

hypoproteinemia An abnormal decrease of protein in the blood

ileostomy Surgical creation of an opening into the ileum, usually by establishing an ileal stoma on the abdominal wall

incomplete protein A protein in which one or more of the essential amino acids is missing or occurs in limited quantity

inorganic Composed of material other than plant or animal in origin

inositol An alcohol form of glucose sometimes called "muscle sugar" because of its high concentration in hair and muscle tissues. Its exact function in the human body is unknown

insensible loss The constant but invisible evaporation of moisture from the skin surface

insulin A pancreatic hormone which controls the body's use of glucose

intra- A prefix meaning within or inside of

intracellular Located inside a cell or cells

intravenous Within a blood vein or veins

intrinsic factor A mucoprotein in the gastric juice which combines with vitamin B_{12} and makes its absorption possible; lack of this substance results in pernicious anemia

isoleucine An essential amino acid

isotonic Referring to a solution with the same osmolarity as human body fluid

Joule One thousand joules: the amount of mechanical energy required when a force of 1 Newton moves 1 kilogram by a distance of 1 meter; preferred by some professionals over the heat energy measurements of the calorie system for calculating food energy. Sometimes referred to as "kilojoule," "Kilojoule," "kJ," or "KJ"

keratinization Degeneration of the epithelial cells (which cover most internal surfaces and organs and the outer surface of the body), a condition associated with vitamin A deficiency

ketone body Describes the three chemicals, acetone, acetoacetic acid, and β-hydroxybutyric acid

ketonuria The presence of ketone bodies in the urine

ketosis A condition in which fatty acids are incompletely oxidized, with resulting accumulation of ketone bodies

kilocalorie The preferred unit of measurement for food energy, equivalent to one thousand calories. Referred to as "Kilocalorie," "Calorie," "Kcal," or "Cal."

Kilojoule See *Joule*

koilonchia A condition in which fingernails and perhaps toenails become thin, flattened, lusterless, and spoon-shaped; associated with long-term iron deficiency

kwashiorkor The syndrome resulting from a severe deficiency in dietary protein, mild to moderate lack of other essential nutrients, but an adequate or even excessive intake of calories

lact-, lacto- A prefix indicating milk

lactase The enzyme that digests lactose in the intestine

lactation Milk secretion; child suckling; period of milk secretion

lacteal system Tiny lymph-carrying vessels that convey finely emulsified fat from the intestine to the thoracic duct

lacto-ovo-vegetarian An individual whose diet contains no meat, poultry, or fish, but does include milk and eggs

lactose The disaccharide made of glucose and galactose; often called "milk sugar"

L-ascorbic acid The chemically active form of vitamin C, a monosaccharide-like six-carbon substance

lathyrism Food poisoning from eating certain peas of the lathyrus family

lauric acid A saturated fatty acid

leucine An essential amino acid

lignins Certain forms of indigestible carbohydrate found in plant foods

limiting amino acids The amino acids that are deficient or missing in vegetable proteins, determining the extent to which the other amino acids present can be used by the body

linoleic acid An essential polyunsaturated fatty acid

lipids A term for fats

lipoprotein A fat combined with a protein, forming a compound which transports both in the blood circulation

liver cirrhosis A serious disease characterized by reduction and death of liver cells, derangement of blood circulation in the liver, and scarring of remaining tissues in the liver

low density lipoprotein One type of cholesterol carrier in the blood: that which carries cholesterol and deposits it in the blood vessels

lumen The open inner space of a tubular organ, such as an intestine or blood vessel

lymphatic system The system of vessels and spaces between organs and tissues through which lymph is circulated in the body

lysine An essential amino acid

macrocytic anemia A form of anemia involving immature red bood cells, resulting from lack of folic acid and/or vitamin B_{12}

macroelements Minerals needed by the body in relatively large quantity: sodium, potassium, calcium, phosphorus, magnesium, chlorine, and sulfur

malabsorption syndrome Failure of the small intestine to absorb nutrients properly

malnutrition Refers to bad (= mal) nutrition. For example: lack of food or eating too much

maltose The disaccharide whose units are each composed of two molecules of glucose; also called "malt sugar"

mannose A six-carbon monosaccharide which sometimes occurs as a free sugar

marasmus The syndrome resulting from a deficiency of calories and nearly all other essential nutrients

mechanical soft diet A diet consisting of foods and beverages that require little chewing

medium chain triglyceride A lipid fractionated from coconut oil, containing only fatty acids with 6 to 12 carbon atoms. Important in diet therapy because these compounds are liquid at room temperature, more water soluble than natural fats, and easily digested and absorbed by the body. Abbreviated "MCT"

megaloblastosis Failure of red blood cells to mature, resulting in a form of anemia which may be associated with deficiency of folic acid and/or vitamin B_{12}

metabolism The complex of processes which food nutrients undergo after absorption, including both their breaking down for energy or excretion or their use in synthesizing new materials for cellular growth, maintenance, or repair

methionine An essential amino acid

microcytic anemia Anemia resulting from a lack of iron and/or other nutrients

microelements Minerals needed by the body in very small amounts; iron, iodine, zinc, fluorine, copper, and other trace elements

monoglyceride A glyceride with only one molecule of fatty acid

monosaccharide One of the simplest carbohydrate molecules, for it cannot be split into simpler forms

monounsaturated fatty acid An unsaturated fatty acid with one double bond

mucin A component of saliva that lubricates food

mucosa The mucous membrane that lines the tubes and body cavities which open to the outside of the body

negative nitrogen balance The condition in which nitrogen losses from the body exceed nitrogen intake

niacin (nicotinic acid) A water-soluble B vitamin that can be synthesized in limited amounts in the body if the amino acid tryptophan is present in an adequate amount

niacinamide The amide of nicotinic acid (niacin)

nitrogen equilibrium The normal condition in which nitrogen intake is equal to nitrogen loss from the body

nonessential amino acid One of the amino acids that can be manufactured in the human body if the proper building blocks are available. These compounds are nonetheless necessary in the diet, in a certain relationship to the "essential" amino acids

normoglycemia A normal level of blood "sugar" (glucose)

nutrient A nourishing organic or inorganic substance in food that can be digested, absorbed, and metabolized by the body

nutrition (1) The sum of the processes by which an animal or plant takes in and utilizes food substances: ingestion, digestion, absorption, and assimilation
(2) The scientific study of these processes

obesity The condition of weighing 15% to 25% more than one's ideal body weight, with the excess consisting of fat rather than water, muscle, or bones

oleic acid A monounsaturated fatty acid

oligosaccharide A carbohydrate containing many units, each made of two to ten chemically joined monosaccharides

oliguria Abnormally low excretion of urine

organic Derived from living organisms

osmolality The concentration of a solute in a solution per unit of solvent

osmolarity The concentration of a solute in a solution per unit volume of the solution

osmosis Passage of dissolved molecules through a semipermeable membrane from an area of higher concentration to an area of lower concentration until the concentration is equal on both sides of the membrane

osteomalacia Bone softening because of impaired mineralization

osteoporosis A clinical disorder characterized by a reduction in the total quantity of bone in the body

overweight The body weighs more than an accepted norm. The excess can be fat, bone, muscle, water, etc.

ovo-vegetarian An individual whose diet contains no meat, poultry, fish, milk, or milk products, but does include eggs

oxalic acid A substance occurring naturally in vegetables such as chard, rhubarb, and spinach which can chelate calcium in the intestinal tract, rendering it unavailable for absorption

oxidation The process in which a substrate takes up oxygen or loses hydrogen

palmitic acid A saturated fatty acid, usually solid at room temperature

pantothenic acid A B vitamin

parenteral feeding Artificial feeding in which nutrients are injected directly into blood veins

parietal cell A cell of a gastric gland which secretes hydrochloric acid and intrinsic factor

pellagra The niacin (a vitamin) deficiency syndrome, characterized by dermatitis, diarrhea, and dementia

pentoses Five-carbon sugars that play an important role in energy release and formation but are not themselves sources of energy

pepsin A protein-digesting enzyme in the gastric juice of the stomach

peptic ulcer An inflammatory lesion found in

the lower end of the esophagus, or in any part of the stomach or duodenum

peptide A compound composed of two or more amino acids joined to each other

peritoneum The membrane that lines the walls of the abdominal cavity and encloses the internal organs

pernicious anemia One form of anemia caused by vitamin B_{12} deficiency, due to a lack of intrinsic factor to facilitate its absorption

phenylalanine An essential amino acid

phospholipid A fat containing glycerol, two fatty acids, phosphate, and a variable chemical, which serves as a structural component of cell membranes

phytic acid A substance found in the outer husks of cereals that can complex with certain minerals including calcium and zinc, making them unavailable for absorption

plaque (1) A deposit of fat and/or fibrous matter in the wall of a blood vessel
(2) a mucus film providing a home for bacteria on a tooth

poly- A prefix meaning "many"

polypeptide 50 to 100 amino acids chemically joined

polysaccharide A carbohydrate containing many units, each made of hundreds to thousands of chemically joined monosaccharides

polyunsaturated fatty acid An unsaturated fatty acid in which two or more carbon atoms have formed double bonds, with each holding only one hydrogen atom; abbreviated "PUFA"

polyuria Excessive urination

positive nitrogen balance The condition in which nitrogen intake exceeds nitrogen losses from the body

precursor A substance from which another substance is derived. Niacin (a vitamin), for instance, can be made from the precursor tryptophan (an amino acid)

preformed vitamins One form of a group of vitamins that the body can synthesize partially. This term applies to niacin and vitamins A and D. Preformed refers to the presence of these vitamins in readily utilizable forms, e.g., in food

proline A nonessential amino acid

protein Any of the large nitrogen-containing organic compounds built of amino acids and found in the cells of all living organisms

protein efficiency ratio In determining protein quality, the gram of body weight gained by experimental animals per gram of a particular protein food eaten; abbreviated "PER"

proteinuria The abnormal presence of protein in the urine

prothrombin A protein important to blood clotting; synthesized in the liver, requiring the presence of vitamin K

provitamins One form of a group of vitamins that the body can synthesize partially. The vitamins include niacin and vitamins A and D. For example, the body can make vitamin A from carotene (found in carrot). Carotene is the provitamin A

ptyalin A digestive enzyme in saliva

pulses The edible seeds of certain pod-bearing plants, such as beans and peas

pureed diet A diet consisting of foods that are easy to digest, with a consistency between liquid and soft

purine A nitrogen-containing structural component of all cells

pyridoxine A term used for vitamin B_6, most important for serving as a coenzyme in many metabolic processes

RDA Recommended Dietary Allowances—the amounts of specific nutrients established by the National Research Council of the National Academy of Sciences as appropriate for daily consumption by people of specific age and sex groups

reduction The process by which a substrate loses oxygen or accepts hydrogen

relactation Stimulation of milk production in women who have not been breastfeeding

renal Referring to the kidney

rhodopsin The red light sensitive pigment in the retinal rods of the eyes, whose formation requires vitamin A. Also called "visual purple," it is responsible for the ability to see at night

riboflavin Vitamin B_2, important in facilitating many biological reactions

rickets The syndrome caused by vitamin D

and/or calcium deficiency, characterized by bone deformities

routine progressive diet The progression from clear liquid, to full liquid, to soft, to solid regular foods traditionally used for certain hospitalized patients

saccharin A controversial artificial sweetener

satiety The satisfying feeling of being full

saturated fatty acid A fatty acid in which each carbon is joined with four other atoms, thus tying up all potential carbon/hydrogen linkages except the carbons at the "carboxyl" end of the chain

scurvy The vitamin C deficiency syndrome characterized by bleeding gums, pain in joints, bone malformation in childhood, and other problems

serine A nonessential amino acid

serum The clear, yellowish fluid within blood, obtained when whole blood is separated into its solid and liquid constituents

soft diet A diet consisting of foods that are easy to chew

sorbitol A six-carbon sugar alcohol, often used to sweeten "diabetic" products because it has little immediate effect on blood glucose level

starch A polysaccharide of many units, each containing hundreds or thousands of glucose molecules; the major form in which energy is stored in plants

steatorrhea The condition in which the fecal waste is bulky, clay-colored, and fatty because fat has not been properly digested and absorbed

sterol Solid alcohol of the steroid group, found in animals and plants

stoma A small opening or pore. In gastroenterology it refers to a surgical opening in the abdominal wall, leading to a part of the small or large intestine

stomatitis Inflammation of the oral mucous tissue

subcutaneous Beneath the skin

sucrose The disaccharide composed of glucose and fructose, often called "table sugar"

systemic blood circulation The vessels carrying blood between the heart and the body tissues with the exception of the lungs

tetany A syndrome resulting from a decreased serum ionizable calcium level, characterized by symptoms such as uncontrolled muscular contractions, seizures, confusion, and increased nervous excitability

thiamin(e) The original chemical name for vitamin B_1, especially important in carbohydrate metabolism

threonine An essential amino acid

tocopherol One chemical form of vitamin E. The term implies "antisterile"

total parenteral nutrition Intravenous feeding which provides a large amount of calories, protein, fat, carbohydrate, vitamins, and minerals. The quality and quantity of nutrients delivered are safe and optimal. Abbreviated "TPN"

toxemia A pathological condition that develops in some pregnant women, characterized by raised blood pressure, edema, nausea, vomiting, liver enlargement and tenderness, headache, the presence of protein in the urine, reduced urine excretion, dizziness, irritability, and sometimes convulsions and coma

triglyceride A fat made of glycerol and three fatty acids; sometimes called a "neutral fat"

tryptophan An essential amino acid and a precursor of niacin

tyrosine Although classified as a nonessential amino acid, it must be derived from the essential amino acid phenylalanine

undernutrition The lack of essential nutrients in the human body as a result of insufficient food

unsaturated fatty acid A fatty acid in which two or more carbon atoms are not joined with all the hydrogen atoms they can hold. If so, the bond between any two such carbons is called a double bond

urea A nonprotein nitrogen-containing substance produced when protein is metabolized in the liver; the main nitrogenous component of urine

uremia The presence of urinary constituents in the blood

-uria A suffix indicating the abnormal presence of a specified substance in the urine

uric acid A nitrogenous substance formed when purines are metabolized, excreted in urine

USRDA The highest level of recommended intakes for population groups excluding pregnant and nursing mothers, described in the 1968 Recommended Dietary Allowances. Used by the Food & Drug Administration in food labeling

valine An essential amino acid

vegan An individual whose diet contains no meat, poultry, fish, milk, milk products, or eggs: a "strict vegetarian"

viral hepatitis A liver disease involving pathologic death of liver cells and caused by a virus

vitamin An organic compound the body requires in very small amounts to perform its essential functions

vitamin B complex All known water-soluble vitamins except vitamin C: B_1, B_2, B_6, niacin, folic acid, B_{12}, pantothenic acid, and biotin

Wernicke-Korsakoff syndrome The neurological problems from vitamin B_1 deficiency that develop in alcoholics, pregnant women experiencing excessive vomiting, and patients deficient in thiamin who are given glucose intravenously

xylitol A five-carbon sugar with potential clinical applications such as use as a sweetener for diabetic patients

INDEX